C0-CDJ-585

OBESITY

PATHOPHYSIOLOGY PSYCHOLOGY AND TREATMENT

CHAPMAN & HALL SERIES IN CLINICAL NUTRITION

Ronni Chernoff, Ph.D., R.D.
Series Editor

Enteral Nutrition

Bradley C. Borlase, M.D.
Stacey J. Bell, M.S., R.D., CNSD
George L. Blackburn, M.D., Ph.D.
R. Armour Forse, M.D., Ph.D.

Pediatric Enteral Nutrition

Susan S. Baker, M.D., Ph.D.
Robert Baker, M.D., Ph.D.
Anne Davis, M.S., R.D., CNSD

Obesity: Pathophysiology, Psychology, and Treatment

George L. Blackburn, M.D., Ph.D.
Beatrice S. Kanders, Ed.D., M.P.H., R.D.

OBESITY
PATHOPHYSIOLOGY PSYCHOLOGY AND TREATMENT

Chapman & Hall Series in Clinical Nutrition
Series Editor: Ronni Chernoff, Ph.D., R.D.

Edited by
George L. Blackburn, M.D., Ph.D.
Harvard Medical School, New England Deaconess Hospital
Beatrice S. Kanders, Ed.D., M.P.H., R.D.
Center for the Study of Nutrition and Medicine Harvard Medical School

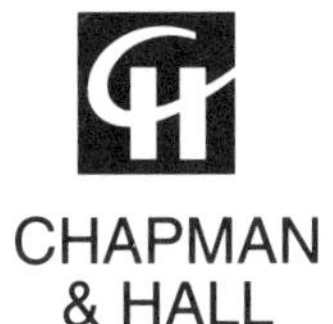

CHAPMAN
& HALL

First published in 1994 by
Chapman & Hall
One Penn Plaza
New York, NY 10119

Published in Great Britain by
Chapman & Hall
2–6 Boundary Row
London SE1 8HN

Printed in the United States of America

Library of Congress Cataloging-in-Publication Data

Obsesity : pathophysiology, psychology, and treatment / [edited by]
George L. Blackburn, Beatrice S. Kanders.
p. cm. — (Chapman & Hall series in clinical nutrition)
Includes bibliographical references and index.
ISBN 0-412-98461-X
1. Obesity. 2. Obesity—Psychological aspects. 3. Obesity—Pathophysiology. I. Blackburn, George L., 1936– . II. Kanders, Beatrice Stefannie. III. Series.
[DNLM: 1. Obesity—therapy. 2. Obesity—physiopathology. 3. Obesity—psychology. WD 210 01256 1994]
RC628.0292 1994
616.3′98—dc20
DNLM/DLC
for Library of Congress 94-5742
CIP

British Library Cataloguing in Publication Data available

Please send your order for this or any other Chapman & Hall book to **Chapman & Hall, 29 West 35th Street, New York, NY 10001, Attn: Customer Service Department.** You may also call our Order Department at 1-212-244-3336 or fax your purchase order to 1-800-248-4724.

For a complete listing of Chapman & Hall's titles, send your request to **Chapman & Hall, Dept. BC, One Penn Plaza, New York, NY 10119.**

To my patients who cared enough to volunteer for essential metabolic and clinical trials in the study of obesity
GLB

To my father and mother with love and appreciation
BSK

Contents

PART II TREATMENT OF OBESITY

Foreword

I am proud that the first Surgeon General's Report on Nutrition and Health was published in 1988, during my tenure as Surgeon General. Its main conclusion came as no surprise: the overconsumption of fat and calories is a major problem for Americans. When this overconsumption is accompanied by a sedentary lifestyle, the result is obesity. Unfortunately, the incidence of obesity has been increasing steadily, and that increase is likely to accelerate. Why? Probably because of a combination of several things.

First, the lag between overeating and its disastrous results is too long for individuals to believe the causal connection. As with smoking, the cause (obesity) and the result (death) are separated by so many years that the fear of natural consequences is diminished. Obesity is a factor in the development of ischemic heart disease, hypertension, stroke, other types of cardiovascular disease, non-insulin-dependent diabetes, sleep apnea, disorders of the gastrointestinal tract, and weight-bearing degenerative arthritis. Yet, the victims of their own obesity see little connection between cause and effect.

Second, as this book is being published, there seems to be growing evidence that the public is tiring of health advice if it involves giving up favorite foods and substituting healthy alternatives.

Early in 1994, the *New York Times* cited several polls to prove the point. A national telephone poll (1,250 adults) showed that the proportion of smokers increased from 25% to 30% from 1991 to 1992. In 1993, the American Dietetic Association found that 39% of 1,000 adults polled said they were doing everything they could to eat a healthy diet compared to 44% the previous year. The annual (23 years) Life Style Survey of 2,500 people in 1993 concluded that "people focus more on how they feel today, rather than looking at the long term benefit of being obedient to the god of good health."

It is hard to be the purveyor of good-health promotion messages without being diagnosed as a bore or a nag.

It has never been easy to understand obesity, and it has been even more difficult to treat it. Therefore, those who attempt to reduce obesity in their patients not only have their work cut out for them, but find that it is getting much more difficult as public resistance increases.

Although much progress has been made in furthering our understanding of obesity, the causes are not well understood, and knowledge of how to prevent and treat the disease remains limited. Controversy exists about every aspect of obesity treatment. Nevertheless, obesity is a major public health problem, and it is clear that more research into its causes, professional training, and patient behavior are needed by the variety of health care professionals who deal with obese patients.

This book can help because it is an authoritative account of the treatment of obesity. Written by leading experts in the field of obesity research and treatment, its 19 chapters describe the scope of the problem and provide in-depth discussion of various treatment modalities: diet, exercise, surgery, pharmacotherapy, and behavior modification. The reader will be exposed not only to the most sophisticated understanding of the diagnosis, risks, causes, and treatment of obesity, but also to the current controversies in each of these areas. Clinicians, nutritionists, scientists, teachers, and students alike should appreciate and benefit from the enormous amount of information presented here.

C. Everett Koop, M.D., Sc.D.
Surgeon General, U.S. Public Health Service, 1981–1989

Series Editor's Foreword

Obesity: Pathophysiology, Psychology, and Treatment, edited by George Blackburn, M.D., Ph.D., and Beatrice S. Kanders, Ed.D., M.P.H., R.D., is a book that addresses both basic and sophisticated approaches to our understanding of and current treatment for obesity, one of the most prevalent medical problems in the United States. The volume is divided into two parts. Part I addresses the problem of obesity and presents an approach to the evaluation of the obese individual. Part II provides an extensive discussion of traditional and innovative treatments for obesity that reflect the expertise and opinions of the most respected investigators and clinicians who work in this field.

Part I of this book includes nine chapters that explore various aspects of understanding and evaluating the obese patient. The authors are all recognized experts in their subject areas and offer a comprehensive discussion of their topics. The problem of obesity is laid out in broad strokes in Chapter 1 by Honig and Blackburn. The medical evaluation and classification of obesity is addressed in Chapter 2 by Dwyer. But classifying obesity is only one step in truly understanding the impact of overweight on individual physiologic function. Chapter 3, by Heshka, Heymsfield, and Buhl, describes the clinical evaluation of body composition and the impact of obesity on energy metabolism.

Plaisted and Istfan describe the relationship between obesity and the manifestation of metabolic abnormalities in Chapter 4. There are other physiologic consequences associated with obesity, some of which may be related to its development and others to its effects. Chapter 5, by Heber, describes the endocrinology of obesity.

Certainly, appetite and its regulation are related to body weight. This topic is discussed in great detail by Drewnowski in Chapter 6. Along with appetite, one area that has received attention and research is exercise and the regulation of body weight. Chapter 7, by Poehlman and Whatley, explores this topic and reviews current knowledge about exercise and obesity.

Wadden and Foster present up-to-date research and clinical findings on the psychology of obesity. They address issues associated with weight loss and weight regain. Anyone who works with patients who have weight problems will recognize this syndrome and will find very useful information in this chapter.

Chapter 9 is a report of research conducted by the book's editors and colleagues on the long-term health benefits of significant weight reduction. It examines the results of positive weight loss outcomes, and risk reduction associated with weight loss in obese subjects.

Part II of this book includes chapters that review the best approaches to the treatment of obesity. Chapter 10, by Coulston and Rock, examines popular dietary interventions and moderate caloric restriction and their success in the treatment of obesity. The book's editors, Kanders and Blackburn, follow this with Chapter 11, a review of the use of very-low-calorie diets in the treatment of obesity.

Often, multifaceted programs are recommended for the treatment of obesity. The following chapters—12 on exercise (Davis and Phinney), 13 on behavior management (Brownell and Kramer), and 14 on stress management (Friedman, Shackleford, Reiff, and Benson)—all discuss state-of-the-art knowledge of the use of these approaches in the treatment of obesity. When these techniques are not appropriate or have not been successful for specific individuals, there are alternative therapies that may be considered. These are surgery (Chapter 15, by Shikora, Benotti, and Forse) or pharmacologic interventions (Chapter 16, by Staten). Any of these therapies, alone or in combination, may prove successful in the correction of obesity. But management does not end with achievement of the weight loss goal; there is a continuing need for support in weight maintenance.

The promotion of long-term weight maintenance is the subject of Chapter 17, by Foreyt and Goodrick. There is an ongoing need to help formerly overweight patients avoid regaining their excess weight. In Chapter 18, Berkowitz presents options for relapse prevention in the treatment of obesity.

Chapter 19, the last chapter of this book, presents some models for interdisciplinary treatment programs that include location options such as the physician's office (Honig), the work site (Quitzau), and a clinic (Norton). It is important that alternative sites, particularly where primary care activities will occur, be considered in this era of health care reform.

The problems associated with obesity, its treatment, and the prevention of relapse should concern all health professionals who are committed to working with patients who have weight problems. This book should be on the shelf of everyone interested in the pathophysiology, psychology, and treatment of obesity.

Ronie Chernoff, Ph.D., R.D.
Series Editor, Chapman & Hall Series in Clinical Nutrition

Preface

Despite progress toward the understanding and treatment of obesity, its prevalence continues to rise in this country. The most recent figures from the National Center on Health Statistics report that one third of adult Americans are obese—an increase from 25% nearly a decade ago. It is also well known that obesity has serious health consequences. It is associated with elevated blood pressure, high serum cholesterol levels and non-insulin dependent diabetes. It also increases the risk for gallbladder disease and certain types of cancer and has been implicated in the development of osteoarthritis. Finally, the negative social and psychological effects of obesity are well documented.

It wasn't until 1985, however, that obesity was first officially designated a disease by the National Institutes of Health. While the benefits of weight loss are well known, long-term reduction of body weight remains elusive. The challenge to develop effective strategies for promoting long-term maintenance of weight loss has become a priority. Over the past two decades much has been learned about the complex nature of the disease of obesity. However, many questions remain unanswered. In addition, the field remains fraught with debate and controversy even on such basic questions as to whether obese individuals should be treated and, if so, by whom and under what circumstances. This book provides a contemporary look at the problem of obesity as well as current treatment options written by leading experts in the field.

Over 37 million Americans are obese, and many will seek treatment from physicians, dietitians, psychologists, and other allied health professionals. This book provides a comprehensive look at both the problem of and current treatment options for obesity. The book is divided into two main sections. The first section of the book reviews the disease of obesity and its metabolic and psychologic complications. The second section of the book provides detailed guidelines for the multidisciplinary treatment of obesity. In addition to traditional approaches (*i.e.* low- and very-low calorie diets, behavior therapy, and weight loss), surgical and drug therapy will be addressed. Specific recommendations for identifying patients who would be appropriate candidates for treatment are presented and the important issues of weight maintenance and relapse prevention discussed. Because obesity treatment is provided in a variety of settings, including worksites, physician offices, and medical clinics, protocols designed for use in these specific situations are included.

Clinicians (whether a physician, dietitian, exercise physiologist, behaviorist, or nurse) will find essential information and guidance for treating the obese patient. However, researchers in the overlapping disciplines that study obesity will also find this book useful. The chapters provide an overview of the broad field of obesity and review of both laboratory and clinical studies. Reference lists are extensive and current.

We hope that this book will assist clinicians and scientists with their continued effort to understand and treat this serious and complex disease.

Acknowledgments

We wish to thank many people for their assistance in preparing this book. First and foremost, we wish to thank the many contributors to this book who took the time and effort to write the scholarly and insightful chapters.

We wish to acknowledge Michelle Kienholz for her editorial assistance and Joan Long, Barbara Ainsley, and Tracey Doyle for their assistance in handling many of the often overwhelming details involved in producing this book.

We thank Ronie Chernoff, Ph.D. the series editor, for her editorial assistance. We also wish to acknowledge with gratitude the help and support of the staff at Chapman and Hall, in particular, Eleanor Riemer, the Food Science Editor, for supporting this effort.

Finally we thank our spouses, Sue and Jeff, for their love, support, and encouragement.

George L. Blackburn, M.D., Ph.D.
Beatrice S. Kanders, Ed.D., M.P.H., R.D.

Contributors

Peter N. Benotti, M.D.
Chief
Professor of Surgery
Tufts University School of Medicine
Boston, Massachusetts

Herbert Benson, M.D.
Director
Mind Body Medical Institute
Department of Behavioral Medicine
New England Deaconess Hospital
Boston, Massachusetts
Associate Professor of Medicine
Harvard Medical School
Boston, Massachusetts

Robert I. Berkowitz, M.D.
Assistant Professor of Psychiatry and Pediatrics
University of Pennsylvania School of Medicine
Philadelphia, Pennsylvania

George L. Blackburn, M.D., Ph.D.
Director
Center of Study of Nutrition and Medicine
New England Deaconess Hospital
Boston, Massachusetts
Associate Professor
Department of Surgery
Harvard Medical School
Boston, Massachusetts

Kelly D. Brownell, Ph.D.
Professor of Epidemiology and Public Health and Co-Director

Yale Center for Eating and Weight Disorders
Yale University
New Haven, Connecticut

Kathleen Buhl, M.A.
Obesity Research Center
St. Luke's-Roosevelt Hospital
New York, New York

Ann M. Coulston, M.S., R.D.
Research Dietitian
General Clinical Research Center
Stanford University Medical Center
Stanford, CA

Peter Davis, Ph.D.
Sports Physiologist
Australian Institute of Sport
Australia

Adam Drewnowski, Ph.D.
Professor and Director Human Nutrition Program
School of Public Health
University of Michigan
Ann Arbor, Michigan

Johanna T. Dwyer, D.Sc., R.D.
Professor of Medicine and Community Health
Tufts University Medical School
Boston, Massachusetts
Director, Francis Stern Nutrition Center
New England Medical Center Hospitals
Boston, Massachusetts

John P. Foreyt, Ph.D.
Professor of Medicine
Director, Nutrition Research Center
Baylor College of Medicine
Houston, Texas

R. Armour Forse, M.D., Ph.D.
Associate Professor of Surgery
Department of Surgery
New England Deaconess Hospital
Boston, Massachusetts

Gary D. Foster, M.S.
Obesity Research Group
Department of Psychiatry
University of Pennsylvania School of Medicine
Philadelphia, Pennsylvania

Richard Friedman, Ph.D.
Associate Professor of Psychiatry and Psychology
State University of New York at Stony Brook
Stony Brook, New York

G. Ken Goodrick, Ph.D.
Assistant Professor of Medicine
Baylor College of Medicine
Houston, Texas

David Heber, M.D., Ph.D.
Chief
Division of Clinical Nutrition
Professor of Medicine
University of California, Los Angeles School of Medicine
Los Angeles, California

Stanley Heshka, Ph.D.
Research Scientist
Obesity Research Center
St. Luke's-Roosevelt Hospital
New York, New York

Steven B. Heymsfield, M.D.
Associate Professor Medicine
Columbia University
College of Physicians and Surgeons
Director, Weight Control Unit
St. Luke's-Roosevelt Hospital Center
New York, New York

Jaimy F. Honig, M.D.
Research Fellow
Center of Study of Nutrition and Medicine
New England Deaconess Hospital
Boston, Massachusetts

Nawfal W. Istfan, M.D., Ph.D.
Assistant Professor of Medicine
Harvard Medical School
Boston, Massachusetts

Beatrice S. Kanders, Ed.D., M.P.H., R.D.
Instructor in Surgery
Harvard Medical School
Boston, Massachusetts
President of Nutrition Consultants of Atlanta
Atlanta, Georgia

C. Everett Koop, M.D., Sc.D.
Surgeon General U.S. Public Health Service 1981–1989
Senior Scholar
C. Everett Koop Institute at Dartmouth
Hanover, New Hampshire

F. Mathew Kramer, Ph.D.
Research Psychologist
US Army
Natick Research Development and Engineering Center
Natick, Massachusetts

Philip T. Lavin, Ph.D.
Clinical Associate Professor of Surgery (Biostatistics)
Harvard Medical School
Boston, Massachusetts
Director, Boston Biostatistics Research Foundation
Newton, Massachusetts

Dawn E. Norton, B.S.
Program Manager
Center for the Study of Nutrition and Medicine
New England Deaconess Hospital
Boston, Massachusetts

Francis J. Peterson, Ph.D.
Director of Technical Development
Sandoz Nutrition, Inc.
Minneapolis, Minnesota

Stephen D. Phinney, M.D., Ph.D.
Associate Professor of Medicine
University of Caliornia at Davis
Davis, California

Claudia S. Plaisted, M.S., R.D.
Clinical Research Analyst
Sarah W. Stedman Center for Nutritional Studies
Duke University Medical Center
Durham, North Carolina

Eric T. Poehlman, Ph.D.
Associate Professor of Medicine
University of Maryland
Baltimore, Maryland

Sarah Reiff, B.A.
Department of Psychiatry & Psychology
State University of New York
Stony Brook, New York

Cheryl Rock, Ph.D., R.D.
Assistant Professor
Program in Human Nutrition
The University of Michigan
Ann Arbor, Michigan

Alan Shackelford, M.D.
Fellow, Behavioral Medicine
Mind Body Medical Institute
Department of Behavioral Medicine
New England Deaconess Hospital
Boston, Massachusetts

Scott A. Shikora, M.D.
Assistant Professor of Surgery
Uniformed Service University of the Health Sciences
Staff Surgeon
Wilford Hall USAF
San Antonio, Texas 78236

Myrlene A. Staten, M.D.
Senior Director
Clinical Research
Cardiovascular and Metabolic Diseases
American Cyanamid Company
Lederle Laboratories
Medical Research Division
Pearl River, New York

Karen Quitzau, B.S.
Worksite Wellness Coordinator
Life Signs
Brookline, Massachusetts

Thomas A. Wadden, Ph.D.
Professor
School of Medicine
Obesity Research Group
University of Pennsylvania
Philadelphia, Pennsylvania

Janet E. Whatley, Sc.D.
Assistant Professor
Human Performance Laboratory
University of Nebraska
Kearney, Nebraska

UNDERSTANDING AND EVALUATING THE OBESE PATIENT

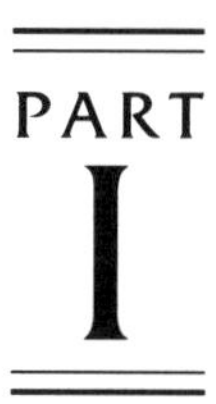

The Problem of Obesity: An Overview

CHAPTER **1**

Jaimy F. Honig, M.D.
and George L. Blackburn, M.D., Ph.D.

Overwhelming evidence now exists to support the fact that obesity is a complex disease of heterogeneous and multifactorial etiology. The treatment of obesity requires extensive assessment and monitoring, which should not be left in the hands of lay therapists if weight loss in excess of 10% of starting weight or rapid weight reduction (>1.5%/week) is entertained.

Tens of thousands of people are involved in weight reduction programs, both medically supervised and unsupervised commercial enterprises. The public health implications of the comorbidities associated with obesity have been highlighted in such recent publications as *Healthy People: 2000* (U.S. Department of Health and Human Services, 1900), *The Diet and Health Report* (National Research Council, 1988), and the *Surgeon General's Report on Nutrition and Health* (U.S. Department of Health and Human Services, 1988). Treatment, with the goal of a long-term successful outcome (i.e., weight maintenance, absence of weight cycling, improvement in clinical status and quality of life), has, however, often been frustrating to physicians and other practitioners due to incomplete understanding of the factors that contribute to the development, perpetuation, and seemingly refractory nature of obesity. The experts who contributed work to this textbook have devoted extensive time and research to the pathophysiology and treatment of obesity, and they provide the readers with as complete and comprehensive a reference as currently exists.

This book is designed to provide an authoritative account of factors contributing to the etiology of obesity and multidisciplinary treatment, including adjuvant therapies such as surgery and pharmacotherapy. Physicians, nutritionists, psychologists, exercise physiologists, and other allied health care professionals who treat obese patients or who are interested in learning more about the state of the art in obesity research and treatment will find this text a valuable and practical resource.

UNDERSTANDING AND EVALUATING THE OBESE PATIENT

Chapter 2 presents the different classifications of obesity in terms of etiology. Genetics, environment, and personal behaviors all contribute to body weight; recent research has clarified the relative contributions of each in different patient populations. In this chapter, Dr. Johanna Dwyer discusses components of a thorough evaluation of the obese patient to ensure that treatment is appropriate for the particular type of obesity, as well as to ensure that medical attention is paid to any accompanying comorbidities. The obese patient must give a history and must have a physical exam and laboratory studies that are specific to the medical problems of that population, with high index of suspicion in regard to hypertension, diabetes, cardiovascular disease, sleep apnea, musculoskeletal problems, and gallstones, as well as other conditions. Distribution of body fat (upper body vs. lower body) affects the degree of medical risk associated with obesity and is also covered.

For many years, the treatment of obesity has stressed the caloric consumption side of the energy balance equation, with caloric expenditure being largely ignored. Research by physicians such as Drs. Steven Heymsfield, Eric Poehlman, and Janet Whatley has brought to light the essential roles that defects in thermogenesis and lack of physical activity play in contributing to the development of obesity and in perpetuating the obese state, as well as how specific types of exercise can help reduce obesity, increase lean body mass, modify resting metabolic rate, and assist in long-term weight maintenance.

Factors affecting body composition, basal metabolic rate, and weight loss, both diet and exercise mediated, are discussed by Drs. Steven Heymsfield, Eric Poehlman, and Janet Whatley. Subtle differences in resting metabolic rate and postprandial and exercise-induced thermogenesis exist among obese, nonobese, and postobese populations that can affect body weight over the long term, as well as contributing to the efficiency with which dietary caloric restriction and exercise can reduce body fat. The research supporting and contesting these findings is presented, underscoring the importance of thorough evaluation of obese patients and individualization of weight loss programs.

How body composition affects energy expenditure, and how different types of exercise affect fat loss and preservation of lean body mass during weight reduction, are at the forefront of obesity research. Initially, aerobic activity was recognized for its ability to help expend calories. Recent research has focused on strength training and its effects on lean body mass, basal metabolic rate, and overall weight loss. In addition, the type of diet used, its caloric level, and its protein content, interact with aerobic and strengthening exercise regimens to induce changes in metabolic rate and composition of weight loss. These complex interrelationships are covered in Chapters 3 and 7 by Drs. Heymsfield, Poehlman, and Whatley. Studies are analyzed for their design, methodology, and results. Many existing inconsistencies are discussed. It is clear from these chapters that much research is needed to develop the optimal combination of diet and exercise for most effective weight reduction, with preservation of basal metabolic rate and lean body mass.

There exists an interesting, evolving story demonstrating a connection between the obese state and specific metabolic abnormalities. While it has long been recognized that obese patients suffer from cardiovascular abnormalities, hypertension, type 2 diabetes, dyslipidemias, and gout, the mechanism that underlies each condition has only recently been identified as hyperinsulinemia. Indeed, as Claudia Plaisted and Dr. Nawfal Istfan discuss in Chapter 4, physiologic testing, such as the use of the euglylcemic insulin clamp technique during an intravenous glucose tolerance test can detect the existence of hyperinsulinemia and glucose intolerance prior to the overt manifestation of disease. Weight reduction has been demonstrated as the treatment of choice for obese patients with hyperinsulinemia, as it reverses completely the metabolic dysfunction. Use of medications to treat the diseases that have collectively come to been known as *syndrome X* do nothing to reverse the hyperinsulinemic state and therefore must be considered palliative rather than curative.

Hyperinsulinsmia, glucose intolerance, and overactivity of the sympathetic nervous system are all endocrinologic sequelae of obesity. Other endocrine abnormalities can both cause and result from the obese state. Dr. David Heber conducts endocrinologic research related to obesity at UCLA and contributes his expertise in the area to this text.

Dr. Heber begins Chapter 5 with a discussion of the endocrine syndromes that promote obesity, stressing their rarity. Endocrine changes secondary to obesity are then covered in detail, including effects on growth hormone, insulin, prolactin, parathyroid hormone, and testosterone. Finally, Dr. Heber cautions against the use of hormones in the treatment of obesity, since none have been found to be successful.

For the majority of adults, body weight remains remarkably stable from month to month and from year to year. Such observations and research in both humans and animals have led to the theory of the existence of a genetically determined body weight set point. In the obese, the body weight set point appears to be aberrant or is "set" higher than is compatible with good health.

Determinants of body weight and appetite regulation are discussed in Chapter 6 by Dr. Adam Drewnowski. He has conducted research in the area of taste preferences among obese patients, and he covers the role of food cravings and preferences in the development and perpetuation of the obese state. Some obese patients have been shown to prefer foods that combine higher fat and carbohydrate contents than their lean counterparts in taste experiments, consuming greater amounts of test foods and/or beverages.

The proportion of fat in relation to the total caloric content of the diet is the most recent area of interest in the search for the causes of obesity. Dr. Drewnoski emphasizes that human obesities must be categorized on the basis of genetic, metabolic, and behavioral variables, including additional criteria such as familial risk of obesity, age at onset, and history of weight loss and weight cycling. Much research remains to be conducted on the etiology of taste preference among the obese and whether it can be modified or merely controlled over the long term.

Is there a unique psychological profile that predicts the development of obesity or failure to respond to weight loss efforts? Does an "obese" personality exist? What are the psychological ramifications of being obese in a world that is preoccupied with thinness? In Chapter 8, Gary Foster and Dr. Thomas Wadden review these questions. They also discuss the effects of weight loss and regain on the psychological functioning of the obese.

A historical perspective on cultural ideals of beauty brings to light the fact that, over the centuries, perspectives have changed dramatically. The authors point out that our ideal of beauty has become so lean that it has become almost impossible to attain the physical proportions desired. Most of the pressure to comply with standards of beauty falls on women, and so do the psychological stresses involved in the pursuit of an impossible goal.

It is difficult to determine whether a psychological predisposition results in overeating or whether the prejudice experienced by obese persons creates a vicious cycle resulting in the persistence of emotionally stimulated overconsumption. Certainly obese persons are as subject to psychiatric disease as their lean counterparts. Reviewing the clinical research, Mr. Foster and Dr. Wadden conclude that some obese individuals display mild or moderate psychological distress compared to controls but that in general, no specific profile exists in the obese population.

Some of the timely topics of discussion include issues of self-regulation, perception of internal versus internal locus of control, responsiveness to food cues and the *externality* hypothesis, and how repeated cycles of weight loss and gain affect the psychological profile of the dieter. The complexity of human eating behavior, as well as the multiplicity of causes leading to obesity, makes difficult the search for psychological factors unique to obese persons. The authors detail the complex nature of research in the area of the psychogenesis of obesity.

It is well known that weight loss confers significant health benefits. However, few studies have investigated the amount of weight loss needed to achieve these benefits or the long-term effects of sustained weight loss on health outcomes. In Chapter 9, Drs. George Blackburn, Beatrice S. Kanders, and colleagues address these important issues though the analyses of 18 months of medical outcome data for 783 obese individuals who participated in a medically supervised, multidisciplinary very-low-calorie diet program. Particular attention was paid to diabetes and hypertension as these chronic diseases are most frequently associated with obesity.

The results presented in Chapter 9 suggest that a dose response relationship exists between percent weight loss and health outcome. Greater weight loss in this significantly obese population resulted in better control of diabetes and hypertension. Improvement in health status remained evident in many patients one year after treatment, even among those who had regained weight. These results underscore the importance of weight loss in ameliorating obesity-related diseases. The results of this and other studies will be useful in helping health professionals set appropriate weight loss goals for obese patients.

TREATMENT OF OBESITY

The most common method of weight reduction is the use of moderate caloric and fat restriction. These diets vary widely but generally provide 1000–1200 kcal/daily, with no more than 30% of calories derived from fat. In Chapter 10, Ann Coulston and Dr. Cheryl Rock review the more popular diets with respect to nutrient composition, nutritional adequacy, safety, and efficacy.

Various "novelty" diets are discussed, as well as nutritionally balanced regimens. A summary of criteria to help clinicians and consumers select a weight management program with the greatest likelihood for long-term weight loss maintenance is provided.

Over 15 million people worldwide have been on very-low-calorie diets. There is no universally accepted definition of these diets; however, there is general agreement that they provide 800 kcal or less per day. Because of the severity of the caloric restriction, these diets require greater medical supervision.

Chapter 11, by Drs. Kanders and Blackburn, reviews the historical development and current use of very low-calorie-diets. It then focuses on the clinical application of such diets, including the indications for use, safety, and efficacy.

The research behind the practical application of a structured exercise program is presented in Chapter 7. Chapter 12, written by Drs. Peter Davis and Steven Phinney, translates theory into practice for use by clinicians involved in weight control. The authors briefly discuss the use of exercise alone in the treatment of obesity, a modality that is not effective by itself. They also address problems with patient resistance to initiating an activity program, outline the basic approach needed for exercise instruction, and discuss the optimization of diet composition to enhance the exercise process.

It is established that all responsible weight reduction and maintenance programs require a behavioral component. In Chapter 13, Drs. Kelly Brownell and F. Matthew Kramer review the history of behavior modification in weight reduction, both when used by itself and when combined with either low or very low caloric diets and exercise. The authors provide a detailed discussion of the components of a behavioral treatment program for weight control and concrete suggestions for implementation. They address new directions for maximizing weight loss, such as improved screening techniques, matching treatment modalities to specific patient needs, and increasing the length of treatment duration and the rate of weight loss.

Strategies for long-term weight maintenance are covered as well. Above all, Drs. Brownell and Kramer stress the need for tailoring programs to specific patient requirements, as well as ensuring that patients who embark on weight loss programs are emotionally ready for that long-term commitment.

Adjuncts to dietary intervention in the treatment of obesity include exercise, behavior modification, pharmacotherapy, surgery, and stress management. Dr. Herbert Benson and the coauthors of Chapter 14 have developed and use the relaxation response as part of their stress management program. They explain why behavior modification techniques alone do not work for most restrained eaters (whether obese or of normal weight) during times of stress. They review the research on the ways that stressors disinhibit restraint on eating behavior and describe how eliciting the relaxation response after a patient has been trained appropriately can prevent emotional arousal and reduce the probability of inappropriate eating.

Use of the relaxation response induces physiologic alteration similar to those that occur during meditation, yoga, biofeedback, and related secular and religious techniques. Dr. Benson's group explains the mechanics of instruction and how training sessions are conducted. More obesity treatment and weight maintenance programs will incorporate training in and use of the relaxation response to complement their other components and increase the likelihood of patient success.

Surgical treatment of obesity began in the late 1950s, and the procedures have been continuously refined to reduce morbidity and mortality and lessen long-term side effects. The Department of Surgery at the New England Deaconess Hospital has a well-established surgical obesity program. In Chapter 15, Drs.

Scott A. Shikora, Peter N. Benotti and R. Armour Forse describe surgical indications, complications, treatment of surgical failures, and the various operative procedures performed.

Careful patient selection is essential for long-term success. Patients must understand that the operation is only an adjunct to permanent dietary change and regular exercise. Surgery is an appropriate treatment option in patients who have 100% excess body weight (body mass index >40 kg/m^2) and who have failed conservative therapy. The authors describe in detail the screening process for surgery as well as preoperative assessment and postoperative management.

Pharmacologic approaches to treating obesity remain poorly accepted by most medical professionals. Negative attitudes toward pharmacologic therapy of obesity result from a number of factors, including the high abuse potential of formerly used amphetamines. Dr. Myrlene Staten is a researcher in the use of pharmacologic agents as adjuncts to obesity treatment. In Chapter 16, she cites reasons for the poor acceptance of pharmacologic treatment of obesity and defines the characteristics of an ideal antiobesity agent. Currently available and investigational agents for weight loss therapy are reviewed. These fall into two categories: those that decrease energy availability and those that increase energy outflow.

The goal of weight reduction in a medical context is to reverse the adverse health outcomes that result from obesity. This goal can be achieved only if weight loss is maintained. The norm, unfortunately, is that patients regain all the weight they worked so hard to lose; many regain even more and experience the further frustration of weight cycling. Scientific data now document the health consequences of weight cycling. This new information, when added to the negative impact that weight regain has on self-esteem, makes it essential that we develop more effective programs for ensuring weight maintenance.

Drs. John P. Foreyt and G. Ken Goodrick are conducting research on tactics to help patients maintain weight loss. They begin Chapter 17 with the premise that many obese patients suffer from food dependence and that a lifetime commitment to weight maintenance must be made; patients should view themselves as perpetually "in recovery" rather than as cured of obesity. Emphasis is placed on motivating patients to accept the continued need for social support, exercise, a low-fat diet, and overcoming inappropriate eating urges.

Periods of dietary indiscretion and lack of regular physical activity can be described as slips, lapses, or relapses, depending on their severity, duration, and the psychological upheaval they induce. In Chapter 18, Dr. Robert I. Berkowitz reviews the literature on the weight loss relapse, incorporating discussions of how the set point theory and the environment may both contribute to the problem. He describes the psychological, behavioral, and demographic characteristics of successful maintainers and outlines a model for relapse prevention.

Having thoroughly covered the understanding and evaluation of the obese patient and state-of-the-art therapeutic modalities, this textbook concludes with a description of three different venues in which comprehensive multidisciplinary obesity treatment programs can be conducted: the physician's office, the worksite, and a clinic setting. Each section of Chapter 19 has been written by a professional with extensive experience in clinical obesity treatment. Dr. Jaimy Honig trained with Dr. Blackburn at the New England Deaconess Hospital and treated patients at the Center for the Study of Nutrition and Medicine as well as at the Deaconess Health Management Clinics. Karen Quitzau organizes and implements worksite obesity treatment programs for Life Signs, a Boston-based firm. She describes the worksite approach and its components. Dawn Norton manages the Center for Nutrition Research, an obesity treatment clinic in Boston. She describes the organization, marketing, staffing, physical plant, management, finances, and other key elements required to conduct a successful multidisciplinary obesity treatment program in a clinic setting.

Medical Evaluation and Classification of Obesity

CHAPTER 2

Johanna T. Dwyer, D.Sc., R.D.

REASONS FOR CONCERN

The reason for concern about obesity is that there is good evidence that obesity is prevalent in the United States and that it contributes to premature mortality, morbidity, and social disadvantage.[1]

Prevalence of Obesity

Obesity is prevalent in the United States today. A body mass index (BMI) of 27, or 120% of desirable height for weight, is a commonly used standard to define obesity. A recent national population-based survey found that about 24%

Partial support for preparation of this chapter was provided by Grant MCJ9120 to Dr. Dwyer and by training grant 8421 from the MCH Service, U.S. Department of Health and Human Services, and by Training Grant 8421. Partial salary support was also provided with federal funds from the U.S. Department of Agriculture, Agricultural Research Service, under Contract 53–3K06–5–10. The contents of this chapter do not necessarily reflect the views and policies of the U.S. Department of Agriculture.

of American men and 27% of women were overweight, using a BMI of 27.3 for women and 27.8 for men to define obesity. In that same study, about 8% of men and 11% of women were severely overweight, with a BMI exceeding 31.1 for men and 32.3 for women (about 140% of insurance company tables). One percent of both sexes were morbidly obese, twice their normal weights or 100 kg overweight, with a BMI of over 45.4 in men or 44.8 in women.[2]

In addition to sex, obesity differs by ethnic group, with a prevalence of 44% in black women versus 25% in white women. More black women are also severely and morbidly obese. Hispanic women have obesity rates intermediate between those of whites and blacks.[3] In contrast to women, black and white men do not differ in the prevalence of obesity, although both exhibit a substantially increased prevalence in middle age. Hispanic men also closely resemble black and white men in their obesity levels.

Obesity increases with age in both sexes, but to an older age in women than in men. White women tend to continue to gain weight until old age; black women stop gaining after peaking at ages 45–54.

Rates of obesity among native Americans vary. Some tribes, such as the Pimas, have extremely high rates of obesity, whereas rates are relatively low in other groups.

Other Western countries, such as Canada, Australia, and New Zealand, also have large numbers of obese individuals. For example, obesity in Canada ranges from 20% to 29% among adults males and from 14% to 19% among adult women 20–69 years of age.[4]

ASSESSMENT OF OBESITY

Age of Obesity Onset

The age at which obesity began and its duration are significant both prognostically and for setting treatment goals. Obesity of early onset is relatively uncommon. But when it is already established by childhood or adolescence, the possibility of a strong genetic influence is increased, and it is more likely to be severe and to continue into adulthood. Duration of obesity is also of prognostic significance in adults.[5]

At least two-thirds to three-quarters of all obese adults become so in adulthood. When obesity does develop in individuals below 35 or 40 years of age, it seems to be fraught with greater health risks than when it begins later in life. Both the increased severity of the obesity and the metabolic and structural risks it imposes may contribute to these increases risks.

Obesity is also often associated with age and with certain life or physiologic events. Many women gain excessive fat during pregnancy. The effects of lactation on obesity are more variable. An extended period of lactation does not necessarily confer protection in the small number of studies that exist.[6] Menopause may also be associated with an increase in body fatness. Many men become fatter in the early adult years, perhaps because they become more sedentary after marriage and settling down in careers. Cessation of smoking is often associated with an increase in fatness, perhaps because of the anorectic or metabolic effects of smoking. Needless to say, the adverse health effects of smoking greatly exceed the small weight gains that some patients experience when they stop smoking. The hypothesis that childbearing accounts for the greater age-associated changes in women compared with men is borne out by many recent studies.[7–10] Although weight gains between pregnancies do exceed age-related increases,[11,12] parity exerts fewer effects than age. It may be that changes in lifestyle associated with marriage are just as important as, if not more important than, parity. This is borne out by a recent study that showed excess weight gain in men after marriage.[13] Changes in physical activity, income, stress, menopause, and other factors may be involved as well.[14]

Use of certain drugs, such as the tricyclic antidepressants, cyproheptadine, medroxyprogesterone, phenothiazines, glucocorticoids, and lithium, as well as surgery, are associated with increased body weight and fatness.

Periods of physical inactivity and excessive food intake in comparison to energy needs owing to changes in occupation, lifestyle, or psychological state also appear to be linked to rapid gains in fatness[15].

Differential Diagnosis

The medical evaluation of the obese patient is well described in several recent publications.[16–19] Both the cause of the obesity and various comorbidities need to be assessed. A complete physical examination, including routine biochemical and metabolic tests, diet and nutritional history, psychological assessment, and fitness assessment are in order. The pathophysiology of the obesity must be fully evaluated. Endocrine and other disease processes that might be involved in its causation need to be assessed and treatment initiated if they are present. These sources provide guidance in the differential diagnosis. In the vast majority of obese individuals, however, there is no clear pathologic process that accounts for the development of the obesity.

Risks, Signs, and Symptoms Associated with Obesity

Metabolic disease. Obesity is strongly associated with gallbladder disease; the dyslipidemias, including hypercholesterolemia, high very low density lipoprotein (VLDL) and low density lipoprotein (LDL) cholesterol levels, low high density lipoprotein (HDL) cholesterol levels, and hypertriglyceridemia; disorders in carbohydrate metabolism such as insulin resistance and hyperglycemia; and other metabolic disorders, including hyperuricemia and hypertension.[20] These are all either caused or worsened by the obesity, and its treatment reduces their severity.

The risk of gallstones is increased with age, parity, and at least twofold by obesity, owing to increased production and output of cholesterol in bile. Among individuals who have deficient hepatic secretion of bile acids or a tendency to form cholesterol crystals in bile, obesity increases the likelihood of gallstone development.[21] Other dietary and metabolic factors may also predispose some individuals to develop gallstones.[22,23] For example, in a recent population-based study, dietary risk factors for hospitalization with gallbladder disease among women included obesity, as well as long overnight fasting periods, dieting, and low fiber intake.[24] There is some evidence that the lithogenicity of bile rises during weight loss, particularly when reducing involves very low calorie diets.[25] Such dieting decreases gallbladder emptying, and thus increases the risk, in a manner similar to other conditions also known to increase the incidence of gallstones, such as pregnancy or diabetes.[26,27] In addition, the saturation of bile with cholesterol is increased in weight loss[28] and in fasting.[29,30] For example, with fasting, saturation of bile with cholesterol rises very quickly, from about 5% after 9 hr to 55% after 16 hr. Thus obese individuals known to be at risk of gallbladder disease should approach weight reduction very carefully, and should especially avoid very low calorie diets and extended fasts.

The risk of cardiovascular disease is positively associated with obesity even after other associated factors, such as hypertension, hypercholesterolemia, smoking, glucose intolerance, and left ventricular hypertrophy, are taken into account.[31] The heightened risks result from elevated production of VLDL. When a genetic defect in the clearance of VLDL or of LDL is present, this overproduction of VLDL leads to increased VLDL, triglycerides, and LDL cholesterol. The mechanism by which HDL cholesterol is decreased in obesity is less clear; it may be that excess adipose tissue removes the HDL.

The risk of adult-onset diabetes becoming manifest among those who are genetically susceptible also rises in obesity. One estimate suggests that for every 20% excess of body weight, the risk rises 150%.[32] If the underlying genetic defect in insulin secretion by the beta cells of the pancreas is present, obesity heightens resistance to the peripheral action of insulin, possibly reducing both cell surface insulin receptors and postreceptor insulin action. This increases hepatic secretion of glucose. The result is that in genetically predisposed people, hyperglycemia develops more rapidly and glucose tolerance worsens in obesity; blood glucose levels increase by about 2 mg/dL for each 10% rise in body weight. Weight loss improves blood glucose levels and brings insulin secretin down to more normal values, thus improving glucose tolerance and insulin sensitivity. Since hyperinsulinemia and insulin resistance have an important role, not only in diabetes but also in hypertension, dyslipidemia, and cardiovascular disease, obesity treatment may be especially important in those with adult-onset diabetes.

Obesity also worsens high blood pressure by poorly understood, probably genetic, mechanisms. Increased plasma volume and cardiac output due to the obesity may interact with a genetic defect in peripheral vascular resistance. In addition, the hyperinsulinemia caused by the obesity may raise peripheral resistance by impairing sodium excretion.

The cancers for which obesity causes a sharply increased risk include endometrial and ovarian cancer in women and prostate and colon cancer in men. The means by which obesity increases the risk of cancer are unknown, although hormonal mechanisms are likely. Obesity seems to act as a promoter rather than an initiator of the carcinogenic process. Reduction in fatness is not known to be preventive.

Structural problems. Some obesity-associated pathology is due simply to the structural burdens created by a vastly increased fat mass. This is especially apparent in massive obesity. Obese individuals with osteoarthritis of weight-bearing joints may experience particular orthopedic difficulties. Ventilatory demand may rise by two to four times in massive obesity, causing pulmonary impairment. Surgical mortality risk also rises owing to the increased anesthesia risk, time in surgery, and skill demanded from the surgeon. The increased risk of complications, including postoperative wound infections, wound dehiscence, hematomas, and atelectasis, increases surgical morbidity.

Social problems. Finally, the adverse effects of obesity on body image, psychosocial functioning, social relationships, and employability must be considered. In a weight-conscious society such as ours, obesity is a handicap. These disadvantages may be more potent than medical risks in motivating many patients to seek obesity treatment. It is thus helpful to find out which problems particularly bother the patient and to develop realistic goals for improving function in these areas.

Other Comorbid Conditions and Behaviors Associated with Obesity

In addition to being subject to increased risks of the various problems listed above, obese patients may suffer from a variety of other disorders that coexist with the obesity, although they are not necessarily directly caused or affected by it.[33]

The medical risks of obesity are heightened by the presence of concurrent illnesses, lifestyle habits such as smoking or physical inactivity, poor control of diabetes or high blood pressure, and coexisting dysfunctions of the organs or limbs due to obesity or other causes.

Correction of obesity is warranted because it can improve many associated medical conditions, endocrine disturbances, and lipid abnormalities, thus reducing morbidity and mortality. Among the benefits associated with weight loss are improved glucose tolerance (although not all of the increased risks associated with type II diabetes are caused by obesity or reversed by weight loss).[34,35] Also, weight loss often results in decreased blood pressure[36] and improved serum lipid profiles (e.g., lessened triglycerides, total cholesterol, LDL, VLDL, and apolipoprotein B, and increased HDL and apolipoprotein A).[37–39]

Associated Symptoms

Relief of symptoms is another benefit of weight reduction. Obesity treatment may lessen symptoms from early arthritis or gout. Reduction in adiposity often decreases symptoms of hypoventilation syndrome, congestive heart failure, chronic obstructive pulmonary disease, sleep apnea, angina pectoris, and cardiomyopathy. Certain gynecologic problems such as menstrual abnormalities and some forms of infertility may be lessened. Weight reduction may also delay progression of nephropathy in obese diabetic patients.[40]

Associated Symptoms

In addition to medical evaluation of the above disorders, it is important to review other symptoms that may be associated with obesity and lessened by its treatment. These include diaphoresis (excessive sweating), fatigue, dyspnea on exertion or at rest, difficulties with walking, and joint pain. Poor sleep, daytime somnolence, anginal pain, and orthopnea (needing to sit up to breathe) are common among the very obese. Digestive distress including reflux esophagitis, heartburn after eating, and biliary colic also occurs. Menstrual abnormalities are also more common. These symptoms are often ameliorated or eliminated by weight loss, and their relief helps to provide patients with objective evidence that they are reaching more healthy weights.

Evaluation of the Fat Mass: BMI

In adults, most of the differences between a body weight in the normal range and overweight is excess adipose tissue. At most, only about 10% of excess weight is due to muscle or bone. Of excess fat weight, about 75% is lipid and the other 25% is lean tissue.[41] The sheer bulk of this mass of fat is associated with both the structural and metabolic complications of obesity. It is measured clinically by the BMI. This is a single number that adjusts for height; thus, it better reflects fatness than weight alone. Since over 90% of the variation in weight for any given height is due to fat, most of the differences from person to person that remain after adjusting for height and sex are due to fat.[42] For research purposes, a variety of more exact techniques are available, such as underwater weighing, but these are impractical in clinical practice. For this reason, BMI is preferred.

BMI is calculated from the following formula: weight (kg)/height (m^2). For metric conversions, pounds are multiplied by 0.45. The result is then divided by height in inches multiplied by .025 to convert to meters, which are then squared.

A simpler method for estimating BMI that can be programmed into hand calculators is: BMI = (pounds divided by inches squared) × 705.[43] Conversion of an individual's known height and weight to BMI is facilitated by the use of nomograms from which one can read the BMI directly from a table. Unfortunately, several incorrectly drawn nomograms have been published lately, but correct versions are available.[44]

For practitioners who are more familiar with tables of "ideal" weight for height for lowest mortality published by insurance companies, a BMI of 25 corresponds roughly to 115% of ideal weight, a BMI of 27 to about 120% of ideal weight (usually defined as obese), a BMI of 30 to 130% of ideal weight, and a BMI of 32 to 140% of ideal weight.

A range of BMI from 19 to 25 is usually regarded as acceptable. Even in the acceptable range, an upward drift in BMI is not advisable and is associated with increasing risk. Above the upper cutoff of about 27, obesity is usually present, but the risks of hypertension, type II diabetes, hyperlipidemia, and other chronic conditions increase with adiposity above BMI 25 or so. Since a gradient of risk rather than a single sharp cutoff point exists, individual factors need to be taken into account in determining at what point actions may be warranted to restore body fatness to more normal levels. That is, for many individuals, weight reduction may be in order below BMI 27.

Men and women differ in the proportion of their bodies that consist of fat. In young men, approximately 15–18% of body weight is fat, whereas in young women it is 20–25%. These differences in body composition between men and women mean that, at a given weight for height, men are likely to be leaner than women. Thus, sometimes slightly higher cutoffs for obesity are used for men than for women (e.g., 27.8 for men and 27.3 for women). However, for most practical purposes, a cutoff of BMI 27 suffices for both sexes. Treatment is definitely called for if BMI exceeds 26.4 for men or 25.8 for women when there is a family history or current indication of diseases that are complicated by obesity.[45] Many experts recommend obesity treatment for anyone with a BMI over 25 and any of these risk factors: high blood pressure, hyperglycemia, type II diabetes, a history of gestational diabetes, sleep apnea, hyperlipidemia, gallbladder disease, a high risk of cardiovascular disease, sedentary lifestyle, and structural problems associated with obesity.

Just as there are sex-related differences in body fatness, but similar BMI standards for treatment, so too the healthiest BMI levels may be constant, at least until old age, even though age-related increases in body fatness are often present. However, there is currently controversy over whether there should be age-specific standards for BMI in adults. The latest edition of the *Dietary Guidelines for Americans* allows for slightly higher weights for individuals aged 35 years and over than for younger adults. Its justification is based on actuarial analysis of insured people's mortality experience done in 1983 and on recent National Health Survey data on average weight of Americans. Only when no other risk factors, including a high waist:hip ratio, are present does the recommendation apply, although these caveats are often forgotten by those who read the guidelines as justifying higher weights. The upper ranges of normal permitted in the *Dietary Guidelines* are thus higher than previous limits, but only for those who have no other risk factors. The standards for those over 35 allow for an increase amounting to approximately 10 to 15 lb between early and later adulthood. The ranges of younger adults are simply increased by this amount at the upper end and a similar amount is subtracted at the lower end, with the ranges given for both sexes together. The lower end of the range is suggested as being appropriate for women, especially those lower in muscle and bone, and the higher end for men.[46]

The Committee on Diet and Health of the National Academy of Sciences also proposed cutoffs for desirable BMI that rise from 21–26 at ages 45–54 in increments by decade up to 24–29 at ages over 65. Reasoning was based on data showing that the BMI associated with the lowest mortality increased with age.[47,48]

Currently there is much dispute about the appropriate BMI standards to use for aging individuals. The rationale behind the recommendations suggesting that small weight gains are not harmful has been questioned. It is argued by opponents that young adults are the individuals most likely to gain excessive weight. Thus standards that imply that such gains are healthy may be misguided, since they may encourage young people to gain weight in early or midadulthood, which will increase their later risks for obesity-associated disease. Additional adiposity with age is associated with an increased risk of morbidity from adult-onset diabetes, high blood pressure, and reduced HDL levels in some studies.[49] There is also a good deal of disagreement about the validity of the analyses on which the recommendations for age-adjusted BMIs are based. The effects of obesity on morbidity and mortality over the very long term[50] are negative in some studies. In any event, the Dietary Guidelines represent upper acceptable limits for BMI.

Because of changes in body composition, which include decreased bone, body water, and lean tissue and increased fatness, different BMI standards may apply for those over age 65. Further research is needed. Special BMI standards for those with certain physiologic conditions are available, such as for persons under age 20 who may still be growing[51,52] or for pregnancy,[53] in which there is growth of the fetus, placenta, and maternal lean as well as fat tissue. Recommendations have also been made for weight loss in lactation.[54] Clinical judgment is needed to assess obesity in advanced renal or cardiovascular disease, in which edema has an important influence on body weight. Other disease states must also be considered on an individual basis.

Assessment of Fat Distribution: Waist:Hip Ratio

The total amount of excess fat on the body is roughly reflected in the BMI. Another useful metric for classifying obesity involves fat distribution: the waist:hip ratio (WHR). This value is particularly associated with the metabolic complications of obesity. Some workers prefer a single circumference at the level of the waist, since they feel that it more directly assess the mesenteric fat which is thought to be associated with these adverse effects. The waist measurement is taken as the circumference at the smallest place below the rib cage and above the level of the umbilicus; the hip is measured at the largest circumference over the posterior extension of the buttocks. These measurements may be taken in a recumbent position if the individual is very fat. The ratio between the two is then calculated. Nomograms for determining the WHR (or abdominal:gluteal circumference ratio) are also available.[55]

Distribution of body fatness carries its own risks even after adjustment for the sheer amount of weight. Concentration of fat in an android, central, or upper body pattern is more strongly associated with metabolic derangements than a more gynoid, femoral, or lower body pattern.[56] Abdominal adiposity appears to be more subject to environmental influences than does gynoid adiposity, and it may also be a marker for differences in lipid metabolism. Abdominal adipose tissues, particularly mesenteric fat cells, that mobilize their free fatty acids into the portal vein, are highly lipolytic. As abdominal adiposity increases, so does lipolytic activity.[57] It is thought that abdominal obesity thus induces a particular endocrine profile, and this is how metabolism is altered. However, the morphologic alterations in android obesity are not found solely in adipose tissue, since muscle from low-WHR individuals has a higher content of highly glycolytic fast-twitch muscle fibers and a lower content of slow-twitch fibers.[58] Thus it is also possible that underlying differences in both fat and muscle tissue may cause the pathologic events associated with upper body obesity. Sorting out these differences is currently an active area of investigation.

Relative risks associated with WHR have been calculated from several large studies. A WHR of 1.0 or greater in men, or of 0.8 or greater in women (since women normally have smaller waists and wider hips than men), corresponds to the upper 10th percentile. Above this level, risks appear to be elevated for various chronic degenerative diseases.[59–62]

When the BMI is over 30, morbidity and mortality risks are evident. But the advantage of assessing both BMI and WHR is that WHR is much more sensitive than BMI alone in identifying obese individuals at high risk of morbidity and mortality when obesity is in the moderate range (e.g., under BMI 30 or a body weight of about 130–140% of ideal body weight). Non-insulin-dependent diabetes mellitus shows a strong association with BMI.[63] The hyperinsulinism and insulin resistance correlate very well with the degree of abdominal obesity. Insulin excess causes alterations in metabolism of the arterial wall and possibly in clotting as well. Android obesity also is associated with high total serum cholesterol and triglycerides, low HDL cholesterol, high blood pressure, gout, and uric acid. Thus, with the android pattern, many risk factors for atherosclerosis are present, and diabetogenic android obesity also tends to be atherogenic.[64] It is thought that the relatively refractory nature of upper body fatness to sex hormones may be part of the reason for the high rates of metabolic and arterial complications of obesity. Abdominal obesity is largely genetically determined; once present, it unmasks other genetic predispositions to metabolic and cardiovascular disorders.[65] This is probably due to the differential response of the various tissues to hormones.[66,67]

Ratios such as the WHR are fatness dependent. With increasing fatness, the abdominal region adds fat more quickly than the gluteal-femoral region. Thus it is likely that some (but not all) of the increased risks associated with high WHR are simply due to the level of fatness itself, especially in women, who do not develop an android pattern unless they are very obese.[68–71] Therefore the adverse metabolic effects of obesity may be due both to the distribution of fat and to the total amount of fat. By reducing the total amount of body fat, WHR may also be affected. There is no specific reducing regimen that can reduce fatness only at that specific depot, however. Fat tends to be lost proportionally from all subcutaneous depots. Loss from the mesentery is now being studied.

Like BMI, WHR rises with age, although this may not be desirable from the health standpoint. At present, age-specific WHR have not been proposed, since data are sparse.[72]

In research studies, skinfold thicknesses on the trunk and extremities or more sophisticated methods such as computer tomography (CT) scans and magnetic resonance imaging (MRI) have also been used to describe body fat distribution. But these require special equipment, are expensive, have poor reliability, are time-consuming, and therefore are usually inappropriate for clinical use. For most purposes, WHR suffices.[73]

Evaluation of Healthy Body Weight, Desirable Weight, and Ideal Weight, and Setting Weight Targets

"Ideal" weight derived from height and weight tables of insurance companies are based on ill-defined frame or build standards. They focus solely on weights associated with the lowest mortality rates collected in past years on insured persons. They do not account for differences in fat distribution or other known risk factors associated with mortality, such as high blood pressure, elevated blood glucose level, and smoking, which worsen the risks of any given level of obesity. In fact, less than desirable or ideal reductions in body weight may also improve health and may decrease morbidity. Desirable or ideal body weights for minimal mortality have outlived their usefulness as weight targets. In the light of newer knowledge about the many factors that influence the association between obesity and health risk, it is apparent that the concept of a single best weight for height, frame, and sex may be simplistic. No one single weight is best for all persons of a given height; other risk factors must also be taken into account. Weights associated with maximal health and well-being, as well as minimal mortality, are determined not only by how much of the weight is fat but also by where the fat is located, the age of the individual, whether weight-related medical problems or a history of such problems exist, and whether other risk factors, such as smoking, are present. Also, under some circumstances, physiologic or psychological factors such as long-standing obesity may militate against achieving a BMI in the normal range. Nevertheless, some progress and health benefits may still be possible if weight control efforts are initiated and some weight is lost, even if "ideal" weights or BMI are not achieved.

The concept of *healthy* body weight has become popular in the past few years. It is more useful than the concept of *ideal* weight popularized by insurance companies, since it emphasizes that a range of healthy weights exists for most people, and that associations of weight with morbidity as well as mortality are important. A healthy weight is one at which the BMI is within the normal range of 19–25 (and stable within it) for individuals between 18 and 35 or within the normal range of 21–25 for those over 35 years of age, *assuming that no other risk factors* are *present*. In the range 25–27, if upper body obesity (e.g., WHR above 1.0 in men or above 0.8 in women) or family history or concurrent evidence of chronic disease risk factors such as heart disease, type II diabetes, hypercholesterolemia or hypertension is present, therapeutic intervention may help to achieve a healthier weight. Weight gains of more than 10 pounds should trigger reassessment and action to blunt further gains. For individuals over 65, intervention is called for if BMI is over 27 and other factors increasing risk, including high WHR, are present. Whether intervention is warranted when other risk factors are absent in older people depends on careful medical evaluation. Recently, a formula for possible weight has been developed that takes into account the individual's age, duration of obesity, and maximum overweight attained. It was tested using a group of formerly obese women who had successfully reduced their weights and kept them at lower levels for 1 year or more, and was found to correspond to their actual weights over the long term.[74] In the end, the validity of such formulas will depend on long term outcomes with respect to morbidity.

The formula is:

Possible weight = ideal weight from 1959 Metropolitan Life Insurance Co. tables + 0.405 Maximum weight ever achieved/ideal weight

Patients often have unrealistically low goals for their body weights; these are based more on cosmetic than medical considerations. Medically and psychologically, it may be better to strive for more modest, healthy weight goals. These bring gains in health, as well as some improvement in body image and appearance, without requiring the individual to be obsessive about weight control, and perhaps they auger better for keeping weight off over the long term.

Healthy body weights are the range of acceptable body weights that are compatible with health in most persons, and with decreased metabolic and other risk factors in individual patients. They minimize preoccupation on the part of both physician and patients with achieving a single ideal or desirable weight.

For most people there is no one perfect weight, but rather a range of healthy weights and BMI values that are appropriate and within which disease risks are likely to be lowered. This healthy weight or BMI level for an individual is one at which some correction of underlying metabolic abnormalities such as hypertension, hyperglycemia, and hyperlipidemia is likely. Healthy weight goals are those toward which patients should be urged to strive. In clinical practice, even smaller amounts of weight loss may be associated with lowered risks for some of the structural or metabolic problems associated with obesity. Thus intermediate weight targets may also be helpful medically and emotionally. They represent healthier weights than present ones. As such, they are worthy *interim* goals. For some individuals, it may never be possible to achieve their personal goal weights based on cosmetic considerations, or even ultimate medically desirable weights, but a lower weight than their current one is reasonable and may be satisfactory in these other respects as well. Other persons may be able to achieve and sustain lower weights. The clinical reality is that some sustained weight reduction is better than none. Therefore, rather than discouraging patients by insisting that the only target is perfection, practitioners should emphasize the importance of lasting weight reduction even of smaller amounts of weight. For example, weight targets for individuals who have always been obese should be realistic; usually it is best to set them at the upper limits of healthy weight ranges. Weight goals for those who are not yet obese are lower; in the range of 19–25 BMI with gains of no more than 5–10 pounds from healthy weights in young adulthood.

Behavioral and Psychological Evaluation

Another critical function of the primary physician in evaluation of obesity is screening the patient's readiness for a long-term weight management program.[75]

Among the factors that need to be probed are the presence of social support for weight loss efforts, relative stability of life situation (e.g., the patient is not in the midst of changing jobs or personal relationships), positive patient attitude toward losing weight, and concern about the excess weight. Having the patient keep and analyze a food and activity diary often helps increase awareness of the need for changes. Attitudes toward eating and exercise, the positive or negative influences of social relationships on weight management, and views about nutrition also need to be explored.

Once the patient has begun the process of weight control, the physician plays a critical role in helping to sustain motivation even when lapses occur, as they inevitably do.[76,77] It may be helpful to provide patients with self-help materials to help assess readiness, motivate, and teach skills to minimize the probability of later lapses.[78,79] Individuals who have always been obese are likely to need special support in weight reduction. Social and psychological support is particularly critical for them. Later in therapy, physician support is also vital.

Improvement in long-term maintenance of lowered weight is best achieved by emphasizing exercise, gradual changes in diet to more healthy overall patterns, and provision of proper support to help sustain these changes.[80] The physician, who sees the patient on a continuing basis, is in an ideal situation to help sustain efforts to keep weight off.

Energy and Nutrient Intake: Dietary Aspects of Assessment

Assessment of the nutritional aspects of current intake is important. While energy intake may need to be reduced during the weight loss phase, intakes of other nutrients must be maintained or increased to promote health. Nutritional evaluation can be performed by a physician who is knowledgeable about food composition or it can be delegated to a registered dietitian.

Dietary assessment starts with a nutritional and weight history, including a review of weight control efforts since childhood. This portion of the interview sheds some light on the individual's past successes and failures and may provide useful clues to the type of therapy that is most likely to succeed in the future. Familial aggregation is also important. Some families have metabolic predispositions, as well as habits of diet and physical activity, that may favor obesity. Special attention needs to be paid to periods during which there was particularly rapid weight gain, as well as to any social, psychological, or physical factors that may have been associated with it. Fluctuations up and down in body weight may have negative consequences, especially for coronary heart disease. They may also be indicative of an eating disorder. Therefore, swings in weight should also be noted.[81,82] Wide swings may indicate that an eating disorder is present. It is unclear if repeated bouts of dieting and regaining alter body composition, although there is some evidence that they may.[83]

Questions about desired weights and weights that the individual has been able to maintain without extreme effort in the past are helpful for setting attainable initial healthy weight targets. The patient should also be questioned specifically and in a nonthreatening manner about binging and the use of self-induced vomiting, diuretics, laxatives, and diet pills, since this information is often not provided voluntarily and indicates eating disorders that must be treated when discovered. Any previous adverse reactions such as depression, fatigue, or illness associated with weight control efforts should also be identified. If the history reveals past eating disorders or depression associated with weight control efforts, consultation with a clinical psychologist or psychiatrist is in order before embarking on new efforts. At the very least, such histories should alert the counselor to the need for especially careful supervision of the patient during therapy.

Finally, any conditions requiring therapeutic diets, including chronic diseases, allergies, and intolerances, need to be identified so that weight reduction and maintenance plans can incorporate appropriate modifications.

Caloric intake and energy deficits. There are many different ways to assess energy intake.[84] A rough estimate sufficient for clinical purposes is based on the method of Owen et al.[85,86] Energy needs for resting metabolism in men are calculated by taking the patient's weight in kilograms multiplied by 10 and then adding 900. For women, the patient's weight in kilograms is multiplied by 7 and 800 is added. To adjust further for physical activity, multiply the result by 1.2 if the patient is sedentary (as many obese patients are), by 1.4 for those who are moderately active, or by 1.6 for those who are very active. The result is the energy intake that is needed to maintain current weight.

By subtracting 500 calories a day from current intakes, loss of about 1 lb of fat tissue will result. Subtracting 1000 calories/day will cause losses of about 2 lb a week. The actual caloric deficit achieved on a reducing diet will depend not only on the individual's typical food intake but also on physical activity level, adherence, and water losses or shifts due to diuresis.

Rate, pattern, and composition of weight loss. The lower the calorie level of the reducing diet, the more rapid the weight loss, and the more quickly the patient is likely to reach a healthier level of body fatness and a healthy weight reflecting it. But the lower the calorie level, the more the therapy is likely to be associated with medical and psychological risks, other side effects, and disruption of daily life.

Gradual losses of 0.5–2 lb/week (0.25–1 kg/week) are the maxima for most individuals who must lose weight. More rapid losses usually involve such dramatic deficits of energy and other nutrients. The risks of excessive losses of lean body mass, other nutrient deficiencies, metabolic abnormalities, fatigue, and other adverse effects they engender are not advisable. Moreover, weight losses exceeding 0.5–2 lb are rarely sustainable in outpatient treatment settings. Losses of less than 0.5 lb/week are not associated with any particular risks, but the patient may lose motivation with slow weight loss since progress may not be apparent.

The usual tissue of gain when excess fat is being accumulated is about 75% lipid and 25% lean tissue, that is, a gain of about 3 pounds (2.9 lb or 1.3 kg) in weight for about every 2 pounds (2.2 lb or 1 kg) gain in fat. A similar proportion of fat to lean should be strived for in healthy weight loss. Some reducing regimens begin with a low-calorie, low-carbohydrate, ketogenic diet to speed weight (although not fat) loss by inducing fluid shifts and diuresis.

Healthy weight loss is best achieved by keeping the carbohydrate level sufficient to maintain the blood sugar level within the normal range and ensuring that protein intake is satisfactory so that lean tissue does not have to be catabolized. Also, the reducing regimen should not be so extreme that most physical activity and exercise are contraindicated or unlikely.

Total fasting involves catabolism of excessive amounts of protein and lean tissue to maintain blood sugar levels, so that the tissue lost is roughly half fat and half lean. Total fasting is contraindicated because of the excessive losses in lean body mass; the risks of nutrient inadequacies, electrolyte imbalances, and counterproductive decreases in resting metabolism as well as voluntary physical activity; and increased adverse side effects of weight loss such as fatigue and postural hypotension. Similarly, use of thyroid hormone for weight loss increases the loss of lean tissue; for this reason, it is not recommended.

Very low calorie diets (VLCD) are regimens involving fewer than 800 (or occasionally 600) calories/day.[87] Diets at such energy levels are below the resting metabolic rates of virtually all adults. Thus caloric levels might be expected to, and do, produce major metabolic adjustments. They cause a rapid initial weight loss, due in part to the initial diuresis that accompanies them. Mild ketosis usually continues for the duration of VLCD. In addition, electrolyte abnormalities, hyperuricemia with precipitation of gout, flareups of gallbladder disease, postural hypotension, and other side effects may occur. For these reasons, VLCD can be used safely only with a good deal of medical support and guidance. Under appropriate medical supervision, VLCD can be safe and effective for some patients, particularly those with immediate and pressing medical reasons for losing weight. However, there is no evidence that the initial rapid weight losses VLCD often engender are any better sustained over the long term than those in any other type of weight loss program. Thus both short-term (1 year) and long-term effectiveness of weight loss programs need to be evaluated.

A wide variety of programs are available to assist the individual in losing weight. They include self-help and commercial weight loss programs with varying amounts of social support and medical surveillance, smaller-scale weight loss programs run by various health professionals such as registered dietitians, spas and live-in programs, and diet books.

In general, if there is a medical reason for the patient to lose weight, a formal program is probably in order because most people, on their own, are unlikely to achieve success in weight loss.

The weight loss methods that involve more modest caloric deficits with nutrition education, a physical activity and exercise program, behavior modification, psychological support, and a sound program for consolidating and maintaining lower, healthier weights after the weight loss phase is over are less risky.

Food records. It is helpful to have the patient keep food records during the period of obesity evaluation and assessment, as well as later during treatment. Such records help to motivate, educate, and provide the patient with a self-monitoring tool and supply data on food intake to the counselor.

Contrary to popular opinion, not all obese individuals have grossly increased energy intakes in comparison to their thinner peers, especially after the increased lean body mass of the obese is taken into account. Nevertheless, if obese people are to lose weight and keep it off, they must decrease their energy intakes. The data from food records are helpful in the weight loss phase for planning therapeutic approaches if these involve modifications of the usual diet. Even if a fixed-menu, hypocaloric diet with food choices unrelated to current intakes is prescribed during the weight loss phase, information on previous food intakes will be helpful to both patient and counselor for developing maintenance eating plans after weight is lost. Food intakes at the new, lower levels that will be required for weight maintenance and to achieve long-term weight management can be tailored to include familiar and preferred items.

It is important for obese patients to become aware of the physiologic as well as psychological implications of their food intake. Food record keeping can also help to do this. Among the common patterns that can be identified, even without recourse to food tables, are excessive intake of alcoholic beverages. These provide 7 calories per gram of absolute alcohol. Also, excessive amounts of foods high in fat (which provides 9 calories/g), and of sweetened fatty foods, which are highly palatable and low in bulk, make it easy to overeat. Finally, chronic intakes of large amounts of high-calorie snacks and desserts or patterns of binging associated with depression, with weekends, or with changes in location may be evident even on preliminary inspection of the records.

Finally, a simple daily food guide can be used to evaluate the soundness of the diet with respect to protective nutrients. If intakes are less than 3–5 servings of vegetables, 2–4 servings of fruits, 6–11 servings of breads, cereals, and pastas, 2–3 servings of milk and milk products such as yogurt and cheese, and 2–3 servings of high-protein products such as meats, poultry, fish, dry beans or peas, eggs, and nuts, protective nutrient needs and prudent dietary guidelines are unlikely to be met, even though energy and dietary fat intakes are likely to be excessive.[88] Often the very process of keeping food records will sensitize the patient sufficiently so that food intake will drop slightly.

We find it helpful to analyze food records using computerized nutrient data bases, but such analyses can also be done by hand using food exchange lists or the USDA food guidance pyramid or tables of food composition. Since the purpose is largely educational, the more the patient can be involved in the process of analyzing the food record, as well as in reviewing and analyzing the implications of intakes of protective nutrients, the better.

Ideally, the patient should be mailed a food record with instructions for measuring food intakes to keep for a week before the first visit, so that patient and counselor can review the food records together. If this is not done prior to the visit, a 24-hr recall or other computerized assessment may be helpful for focusing the discussion, and the records can be given to the patient at the visit itself to be mailed in at a later time.

Keeping food records assists the patient in assessing overall intake of the various food groups providing needed nutrients other than energy. It also sensitizes the individual to the eating component of his or her lifestyle. But keeping food records is unhelpful for establishing the exact level of caloric intake at which the individual is currently in energy balance at his or her excess weight for several reasons. First, there is a tendency to underestimate intakes, particularly among the obese. When records are compared to less subjective techniques, such as estimates of energy intake derived from doubly labeled water or from intakes obtained under metabolic ward conditions, they are usually much (e.g. 10% or more) lower in calories.[89,90] Also, the relative excess of energy intake over energy output can be precisely determined only if energy output as well as energy intake is known. This cannot be done with precision in clinical practice using food records for a few days. Caloric intakes in excess of energy needs may occur even at relatively low levels of energy intake if the individual is extremely sedentary, as many obese people are. Moreover, energy balance is not achieved from day to day, but usually only over longer cycles of several weeks. Therefore, many days' worth of intakes are required to determine true levels of energy intakes even under the best circumstances. Finally, a small but significant number of individuals exhibit eating disorders such as bulimia, which involve periodic overeating in massive proportions. This may not be captured by a few days' food records. However, food record keeping may help such patients to become more aware of these eating aberrations. Thus records are also useful for them to begin the self monitoring process.

Nutrient needs during weight loss. Although energy intakes must decrease if fat loss is to be achieved, intakes of carbohydrate, protein, essential fatty acids, water, vitamins, and minerals must be maintained at safe levels.[91] Recommendations for safe weight reduction programs have recently been summarized.[92,93] In developing specific and individualized plans for weight loss and maintenance, registered dietitians can provide helpful treatments to accompany physicians' efforts and the more standardized approaches provided by commercial weight management programs.

CARBOHYDRATE. Carbohydrate levels must be adequate in weight loss diets to spare protein, minimize ketosis, and prevent large shifts in weight owing to imbalances in body water. At least 100 g is desirable to do this while minimizing ketosis. On very low calorie diets, at least 50 g is mandatory, but when intakes are that low, mild ketosis is likely. As long as carbohydrate intakes stay low, the individual will remain relatively dehydrated.

PROTEIN. Protein deserves particular attention during weight loss because when energy intakes are marginal, protein needs rise to maintain blood glucose levels and to provide energy.[94] This is a particular concern on VLCD under 600 kcal, since nitrogen balance is greatly affected by the level of protein these diets provide.[95] Most recommendations are for at least 1.5 g of high-quality protein per kilogram of ideal body weight (corresponding roughly to the target BMI values stated earlier). Intakes of 65–70 g/day or more are thought to protect the nitrogen balance.[96,97] The importance of adequate amounts of high-quality protein for the health of individuals on VLCD became evident in the late 1970s, when a variety of electrocardiographic abnormalities and even deaths resulted from the use of inadequate regimens in these and other respects.[98] This exposé of the hazards led to more rigorous controls over the sales of VLCD. Presently, two types of VLCD are in use: those based on animal protein foods such as meat, fish, or fowl as the source of high-quality protein and liquid formula diets employing milk- or egg-based protein sources.[99] Both types are supplemented with vitamins and minerals. They appear to produce equal amounts of weight loss. Costs and carbohydrate levels vary.

It becomes increasingly difficult to include both sufficient protein and carbohydrate on VLCD as energy intakes decline. For this reason alone, very careful medical monitoring of patients on VLCD is in order, and patients should never be permitted to embark on regimes of their own devising.

Patients consuming 600–1200 calories/day should eat at least 1 g/kg/ideal body weight per day of protein, and those consuming 1200 calories/day or more should eat no less than 0.8 g/kg/ideal body weight per day.

ESSENTIAL FATTY ACIDS. At least 10 g of linoleic acid from various food sources is needed (the equivalent of slightly more than a tablespoon of corn oil a day) to provide the essential fatty acid needs. Above this minimum, weight loss diets vary greatly in the percentage of calories they provide from fat. In general, fat intakes should not exceed 30% of total calories on weight loss diets.

In fact, lower intakes are desirable, since more food can then be eaten without exceeding energy restrictions. This is because fat is calorically dense and because, as fat intakes rise, so do intakes of saturated fatty acids and cholesterol, which are known to increase atherogenic risks. It is difficult to plan palatable menus with usual foods below about 20% of calories. Specially prepared foods are now available in frozen, canned, and dried forms that are very low in fat, and for some patients these may be helpful as meal replacements.

Dietary cholesterol levels should not exceed 300 mg/day; this is the amount of three egg yolks per week. Alcohol, providing 7 calories/g, is not recommended on reducing diets since it provides high amounts of energy and little else.

WATER. Water and other noncaloric fluids should be provided in amounts of at least 1 to 2 L/day.

FIBER. Dietary fiber helps to prevent constipation, provides no calories, and may have other positive effects by reducing the risk of certain chronic degenerative diseases. For this reason, 20–30 g/day of fiber should be provided on weight loss diets. On VLCD this goal may need to be modified slightly and lesser amounts of fiber provided.

VITAMINS AND MINERALS. It is very difficult to meet the recommended dietary allowances,[100] as well as the need for iron, calcium, and several other nutrients, including copper, zinc, magnesium, and vitamin B_6, at intakes below about 1200 calories/day. Since most weight loss diets are at least that low in calories, a multivitamin, multimineral preparation is advisable in addition to stressing foods high in nutrients and low in calories. Electrolyte levels also deserve careful monitoring. Supplements are mandatory for vitamins and minerals as well when diets for weight loss are below 800 calories/day. Minimal needs for sodium and potassium must be met. These prescriptions may need to be individualized, depending on coexisting health conditions, physical activity levels, and other factors.[101,102]

Weight maintenance. After satisfactory weight loss has been achieved, fewer calories will be needed to maintain energy balance. This is because decreases in lean body mass accompany weight loss. Also, the slimmer individual has less weight to move around and greater efficiency in performing physical activity. For long-term weight management, the recommendations of the National Academy of Sciences' Committee on Diet and Health are a useful basis for a healthful eating pattern.[103] Briefly, they suggest carbohydrate intakes exceeding 55% of kilocalories, with emphasis on complex carbohydrates and dietary fiber–rich foods. This goal can be fulfilled by eating five or more servings of vegetables and fruits a day, with six or more servings of starches or other complex carbohydrates such as whole-grain breads and cereals, pastas, and legumes. Dietary fat intakes should not exceed 30% of total kilocalories, with no more than 10%

from saturated fat sources. This is accomplished by emphasizing lean meats, poultry, and fish prepared with minimal added fat, using low-fat or nonfat dietary products, and limiting egg yolks to about three per week (to keep dietary cholesterol intake low). Spreads and baked or fried foods high in fat should be deemphasized. Alcohol intake should not exceed about one drink a day for women or two for men, and for those who can avoid alcohol altogether, this is preferable. Water and other noncaloric fluids should be consumed in liberal amounts. At the same time, physical activity and exercise levels need to stay high. Both need to be scheduled rather than left to chance.

Energy Output: Evaluation of Physical Activity

Obese adults have higher energy outputs than the nonobese, largely because of their higher lean body masses, which result in elevated resting metabolic rates.[104] Also, the costs of moving their larger bodies increase energy outputs in physical activity.

As people lose weight, they lose some lean body mass, decreasing their resting metabolic rates.[105] The best method for maintaining as much lean body mass as possible while losing weight is to keep energy outputs high by a combination of vigorous aerobic exercise and physical activity. In addition, obese individuals who achieve weight loss by decreasing their energy intakes and increasing physical activity lose more weight than those who only diet.[106] Finally, those who use both strategies are more likely to sustain reduced weights during maintenance.[107] Aerobic exercise also improves cardiovascular function, increasing the ability to use oxygen and decreasing cardiac work.[108] High density lipoprotein (HDL) cholesterol levels may be increased, and blood pressure is decreased.[109] Improved insulin sensitivity and normalization of blood sugar levels are also common. Thus, there is good evidence that increased physical activity in daily life, as well as structured exercise, are useful supplements to low-calorie diets for weight loss.[110]

The primary physician has the responsibility to evaluate the patient's capacity for physical activity. This begins with a comprehensive medical evaluation, which includes a medical history, physical exam, and laboratory tests including blood lipids and glucose.[111] It is also important to review coexisting medical conditions such as hypertension, diabetes, and cardiovascular disease and medications for them, as well as the musculoskeletal system, with particular attention to any orthopedic problems that might affect exercise capacity or tolerance.[112,113] Even those with conditions that are adversely affected by weight-bearing exercise may be candidates for swimming, water walking, water aerobics, and biking, which reduce the impact on joints.

Next, the physician must help motivate obese patients to include structured exercise in their long-term weight management efforts. This is assisted by designing an exercise program that is appropriate for them. The program must be tailored to the individual's physiologic capacities, needs, and preferences. The basic principle is to help patients gradually increase their physical activity to more appropriate levels over time.

The exercise prescription must be appropriate for diet during the weight loss phase.[114] On VLCD with appropriate vitamin and mineral supplementation, exercise should not exceed low-intensity activities such as walking, shopping, and gardening. Low-carbohydrate, low-calorie VLCD decrease endurance and the ability to perform work, especially during high-intensity exercise.[115]

Physical activity of low to moderate intensity, that is, exercise that is within the individual's capacity and is noncompetitive, such as speed walking, can usually be sustained for about 1 hr on a low-calorie diet (LCD). Both everyday activities and more structured activities requiring planning, such as swimming, biking, and speed walking also need to be included.

On reducing diets of 1200 kilocalories/day or more, in addition to physical activity in daily life, exercise of moderate to high intensity, including vigorous exercise that challenges the individual and causes fatigue in about 20 min, can be added, assuming that there are no health-related contraindications.

The maximal heart rate is best determined by monitoring it. Starting exercise intensity at 60% of the maximal heart rate and gradually increasing the duration of the exercise helps to condition the patient gradually. Attention must be paid to warmup periods to increase flexibility and blood flow through muscles, the aerobic phase of exercise itself, and a cooling-down period to prevent venous pooling in exercised muscles and side effects such as dizziness, nausea, and fainting.

After the active weight loss phase, it is important to sustain higher physical activity levels.[116] The physician can help by encouraging patients to stay physically active in daily life and to include structured exercise programs several times a week.

Evaluating the Risks of Obesity Treatment

The treatment of obesity always involves some medical and psychological risks. These vary from trivial to life-threatening, depending on the patient's characteristics and the method chosen. The primary physician, who knows the patient's overall health status, can help the dieter achieve and maintain healthier levels of body fatness while minimizing risks and discomfort. This is accomplished by taking an active role in assessing the risks of various therapies, advising, and guiding the patient in selecting appropriate treatment options.

IMPORTANCE OF THE PRIMARY PHYSICIAN IN OBESITY TREATMENT

The primary physician's role in obesity treatment varies, depending on four factors: the patient's health risks and other characteristics, the physician's interest and expertise in clinical nutrition and metabolism, the type of obesity therapy to be employed, and the time and resources available in the medical practice setting. Nevertheless, there are certain basic aspects of care that the physician must carry out, regardless of how much of the burden he or she is able to shoulder in treating obesity directly.

With low-risk cases of obesity, the primary physician is either the provider of direct care or the coordinator of obesity treatment. When the physician provides obesity treatment directly, integration of this therapy with other treatment and medical surveillance is easy. Follow-up can be built into ongoing health care visits.

The steps to take to incorporate weight management more fully into primary health care have recently been summarized.[117,118] They include deciding what to do and who will do it in the office. Then it is important to assess the knowledge and skills of those who will provide the nutrition services and to develop a plan for building skills if these are not present. Additional details on screening and assessing patients at high risk, informing and motivating patients, triaging by risk, setting dietary change priorities, establishing a treatment plan, determining how best to implement the treatment plan in the particular setting, and both initiating and assisting in maintaining long-term weight management are provided in recent publications[117,118] along with details on monitoring, evaluating, and dealing with long-term maintenance problems.

Obesity therapy takes a good deal of time and requires knowledge of food and diet. Thus, many primary physicians may opt to delegate treatment to a registered dietitian working within or associated with the practice, some other health professional working within the practice, or a reputable commercial weight loss group while continuing to provide medical supervision and surveillance. Totally self-directed weight loss programs in which patients are left completely on their own are unlikely to succeed in most cases. In any event, all obese patients need their primary physicians to assess the causes and health risks of their obesity and of coexisting diseases and conditions, especially those that might be affected by treatment. Thus the physician must assess the type and severity of the obesity, the need for therapy, and possible risks or contraindications to certain weight loss strategies. For example, coexisting diseases and conditions may require therapy in addition to weight loss. The obesity therapy chosen must be optimal for both the patient's health and personal preferences. Patients need frequent physician encouragement to adopt and maintain appropriate weight management methods. They also need advice and guidance to discourage the use of inappropriate methods. The primary physician's motivation, advice, and surveillance of patients who are undergoing obesity treatment are vital, regardless of where the patient receives obesity therapy. It cannot be assumed that complications of obesity therapy will always be recognized in commercial diet treatment settings. Vigilance is therefore warranted, especially if the patient has other health problems.

In order to help the patient make wise treatment choices, the physician must be knowledgeable and informed about obesity and weight control therapies. This is facilitated by access to unbiased, objective, up-to-date sources of information on the topic. Groups such as the local, state, or national offices of the American Dietetic Association, state public health agencies, and cooperative extension groups, provide useful literature and articles on the subject and may be helpful.

The primary physician coordinates care and arranges for referrals if needed while continuing as the manager of the patient's overall health care. Diagnostic medical or psychological consultation is often appropriate for severe or complex and involved cases. These include the very obese, those with complicated medical or emotional problems, and those on VLCD. Such patients are likely to require so much assistance, ongoing surveillance, and psychological and group support to reach healthy body weights that their needs are best met in specialized practice settings. Unless the individual physician is especially knowledgeable about obesity and clinical nutrition, referral of complex and involved cases of obesity (e.g, those exceeding 150% ideal body weight or a BMI of ≥30, especially if coexisting or obesity-related diseases that may be affected by therapy are present) is usually in order. Also, if VLCD are to be used and the physician has not had extensive training and experience (e.g., treatment under supervision of 50 or more such cases) in dealing with them, referral is a better option. Members of the American Dietetic Association, the American Society for Clinical Nutrition, the North American Association for the Study of Obesity, and the American Society for Parenteral and Enteral Nutrition who specialize in obesity are helpful sources of consultation and referral for such individuals.

The options for high-risk patients or those at lower risk whom the physician does not treat directly include registered dietitians, formal (commercial) weight loss programs, and hospital-based programs. Before referring patients, the physician needs to determine if the potential treatment incorporates safe, sensible weight loss techniques and education about healthy eating, behavior modification, and exercise, as well as a weight loss diet. Patient and physician together need to determine if the treatment is a good fit for the patient in terms of the patient's lifestyle, degree of commitment, psychological outlook, and need for group support. Long-term outcomes and costs need to be assessed, since many programs are very expensive. Ways for the physician to obtain feedback and to refer those who have health problems or may develop them need to be clearly stated. Above all, the high-risk patient must continue to be encouraged and supervised to some extent by the primary physician.

In conclusion, there is an appropriate long-term weight management program for every obese patient. But there is no program that is right for every single person.[119] If we want patients to turn out the same, with good, long-lasting outcomes from their obesity control efforts, we must individualize our assessment and therapies. The problem is to find the program that is right for each patient. With the interest of knowledgeable primary physicians, the patient's ability to do this will be dramatically increased.

REFERENCES

1. Pi-Sunyer FX. Health implications of obesity. *Am J Clin Nutr* 53:15955, 1991.
2. Najjar MF, Rowland M. *Anthropometric Reference Data and Prevalence of Overweight, United States*, 1976–80. Vital and Health Statistics Series 11, No. 238, DHHS Publication No (PHS) 87–1688. Washington, D.C., National Center for Health Statistics, Public Health Service, 1987.
3. Centers for Disease Control. Prevalence of Overweight for Hispanics—United States, 1982–84. *MMWR* 38:838, 1989.
4. Health Services and Promotion Branch, Health and Welfare, Canada. Promoting healthy weights: A discussion paper. Catalogue No. H39–131, 1988E. Ottawa, Ontario, Ministry of National Health and Welfare, 1988.
5. Bray GA, Gray DS. Obesity: Part I. Pathogenesis. *West J Med* 149:429, 1988.
6. Subcommittee on Nutrition During Lactation, Committee on Nutritional Status During Pregnancy and Lactation, Food and Nutrition Board, Institute of Medicine, National Academy of Sciences. *Nutrition During Pregnancy and Lactation*. Washington, DC, National Academy Press, 1991, pp. 201–204.
7. Billewicz WZ, Thomason AM. Body weight in parous women. *Br J Prev Soc Med* 24:87, 1970.
8. Pi-Sunyer FX, Obesity. In Shils ME, Olson JA and Shike M, eds. *Modern Nutrition in Health and Disease*, 8th edition, vol. 2, 1994, pp 984–1006.
9. Rockus MA, Rokebrand P, Burema J. et al. The effect of pregnancy on the body mass index 9 months postpartum in 49 women. *Int J Obes* 11:609, 1987.
10. Kritz-Silverstein D, Barrett-Connor E, Wingard DL. The effects of parity on the later development of non-insulin dependent diabetes mellitus or impaired glucose tolerance. *N Engl J Med* 321:1214, 1989.
11. Forsum E, Sadurski A, Wager J. Resting metabolic rate and body composition of healthy Swedish women during pregnancy. *Am J Clin Nutr* 47:942, 1988.
12. Weiss N, Jackson EC, Niswander K, et al. The influence on birthweight of change in maternal weight gain in successive pregnancies in the same women. *Int J Gynecol Obstet* 7:210, 1969.
13. Rona RJ, Morris RW. National study of health and growth: Social and family factors and overweight in English and Scottish parents. *Ann Hum Biol* 9:147, 1982.
14. Willett W, Stampfer MJ, Bain C, et al. Cigarette smoking, relative weight, and menopause. *Am J Epidemiol* 117:651, 1983.

15. Bray GA. Classification and evaluation of the obesities. *Med Clin North Am* 73:161, 1989.
16. Kanders BS, Forse RA, Blackburn GA. Obesity, in Rakel RE (ed), *Conns Current Therapy*. Philadelphia, PA, WB Saunders, 1991, pp. 524–531.
17. Frankel RT, Yang MY. *Obesity and Weight Control: The Health Professional's Guide to Understanding and Treatment*. Rockville, MD, Aspen, 1988.
18. Bray GA. *The Obese Patient*, Philadelphia, WB Saunders, 1976.
19. Pi-Sunyer FX. Obesity, in Shils ME, Young VR (eds), *Modern Nutrition in Health and Disease*, ed 7. Philadelphia, Lea & Febiger, 1988, pp. 795–816.
20. Wood FC, Bierman EL. Is diet the cornerstone in management of diabetes? *N Engl J Med* 315(19):1224–7, 1986.
21. Grundy SM, Barnett JP. Metabolic and health complications of obesity. *Disease-a-Month* 36:643, 1990.
22. Sauerbruch T, Paumgartner G. Gallbladder stones: Management. *Lancet* 338:1121, 1991.
23. Paumgartner G, Sauerbruch T. Gallstones: Pathogenesis. *Lancet* 338:1117, 1991.
24. Sichieri R, Everhart JE, Roth H. A prospective study of hospitalization with gallstone disease among women: Role of dietary factors, fasting period, and dieting. *Am J Pub Health* 81:880, 1991.
25. Jorgensen T. Gallstones in a Danish population. Relation to weight, physical activity, smoking, coffee consumption, and diabetes mellitus. *Gut* 30:528, 1989.
26. Everson GT, McKinley KC, Lawson M, et al. Gallbladder function in the human female: Effect of the ovulatory cycle, pregnancy, and contraceptive steroids. *Gastroenterology* 82:711, 1982.
27. Stone, BG, Gavaler JS, Belle SH, et al. Impairment of gallbladder emptying in diabetes mellitus. *Gastroenterology* 95:170, 1988.
28. Bennion LJ, Grundy SM. Effects of obesity and caloric intake on biliary lipid metabolism in man. *J. Clin Invest* 56:996, 1976.
29. Metzger AL, Adler R, Heymsfield S, et al. Diurnal variation in biliary lipid composition: Possible role in cholesterol gallstone formation. *N Engl J Med* 288:333, 1973.
30. Williams CN, Morse JWI, MacDonald IA, et al. Increased lithogenicity of bile on fasting in normal subjects, *Dig Dis Sci* 22:189, 1977.
31. Hubert HB, Feinleib M, McNamara PM, et al. Obesity as an independent risk factor for cardiovascular disease: A 26-year follow-up of participants in the Framingham Heart Study. *Circulation* 67:968, 1983.
32. Bierman EM. Unpublished manuscript, 1991.
33. Bray G. Complications of obesity. *Ann Intern Med* 103:1052, 1985.
34. Osei K. Predicting type II diabetes in persons at risk. *Ann Intern Med* 113:905, 1990.

35. Caro JF, Dohm LG, Pories WJ, et al. Cellular alterations in liver, skeletal muscle, and adipose tissue responsible for insulin resistance in obesity and type II diabetes. *Diabetes/Metab Rev* 5:665, 1989.
36. Landsberg L. Obesity, metabolism, and hypertension. *Yale J Biol Med* 62:511, 1989.
37. Wolf RN, Grundy SM. Influence of weight reduction on plasma lipoproteins in obese patients. *Arteriosclerosis* 3:160, 1983.
38. Wood PD, Stefanick ML, Dreon DM, et al. Changes in plasma lipids and lipoproteins in overweight men during weight loss through dieting as compared with exercise. *N Engl J Med* 319:1173, 1988.
39. Wood PD, Stefanick ML, Williams, PT, et al. The effects on plasma lipoproteins of a prudent weight reducing diet, with or without exercise, in overweight men and women. *N Engl J Med* 325:461, 1991.
40. Solderte B, Fioravanti M, Shifino N, et al. Effects of diet therapy on urinary protein excretion, albuminuria, and renal haemodynamic function in obese diabetic patients with overt nephropathy. *Int J Obes* 13:203, 1989.
41. Garrow JS, Webster J. Quetelet's index (W/H2) as a measure of fatness. *Int J Obes* 9:147, 1985.
42. Garrow JS. Energy balance in man: An overview. *Am J Clin Nutr* 45:1114, 1987.
43. Stensland, S, Margolis S. Simplifying the calculation of body mass index for quick reference. *J Am Diet Assoc* 90:856, 1990.
44. Kahn HS. A major error in nomograms for estimating body mass index. *Am J Clin Nutr* 54:435, 1991.
45. Rowland ML. A nomogram for computing body mass index. *Ross Diet Curr* 16:1, 1989.
46. *Dietary Guidelines for Americans*, ed 3. Washington, DC, US Dept of Agriculture and US Dept of Health and Human Services, 1990.
47. Committee on Diet and Health. *Implications for Reducing Chronic Disease Risk*, Washington, DC, National Academy Press, 1989, pp. 21–22.
48. Andres R, Elahi D, Tobin JD, et al. Impact of age on weight goals. *Ann Intern Med* 103:1030, 1985.
49. Willett WC, Stampfer M, Manson, JA, et al. New weight guidelines for Americans: justified or injudicious? *Am J Clin Nutr* 53:1102, 1991.
50. Garrison RJ, Castelli WP. Weight and 30-year mortality of men in the Framingham study. *Ann Intern Med* 103:1006, 1985.
51. Rosenbaum M, Leibel RL. Obesity in childhood. *Pediatr Rev* 11:43, 1989.
52. Hammer LD, Kraemer HC, Wilson DM, et al. Standardized percentile curves of body mass index for children and adolescents. *Am J Dis Child* 145:259, 1991.
53. Institute of Medicine. *Nutrition During Pregnancy. Part I: Weight Gain. Part II: Nutrient Supplements*. Washington, DC, National Academy Press, 1990.
54. Institute of Medicine. *Nutrition During Lactation*. Washington, DC, National Academy Press, 1991.

55. Bray GA, Gray DS. Obesity: Part I, Pathogenesis. *West J Med* 149:429, 1988.
56. Bjorntorp P. Regional patterns of fat distribution. *Ann Intern Med* (Part II):994, 1985.
57. Rebuffe-Scrive M. Regional adipose tissue metabolism in men and in women during menstrual cycle, pregnancy, lactation, and menopause, in *Proceedings of the 5th International Congress on Obesity, Jerusalem.* London, John Libbey, September 1986.
58. Krotkiewski M, Bjorntorp P. Muscle tissue in obesity with different distribution of adipose tissue: Effects of physical training. *Int J Obes* 10:331, 1986.
59. Kissebah AH, Freedman DS, Peris AN. Health risks of obesity. *Med Clin North Am* 73:111, 1989.
60. Vague J. Willendorf Lecture: Diabetogenic and atherogenic fat. In: Oomura Y, Tarui S, Inoue S, Shimazu T. Progress in Obesity Research 1990. London: John Libbey, 1991, pp. 343–358.
61. Ostlund RE, Staten M, Kohrt WM, et al. The ratio of waist to hip circumference, plasma insulin level and glucose intolerance as independent predictors of the HDL2 cholesterol level in older adults. *N Engl J Med* 322:229, 1990.
62. Bjorntorp P. Criteria of obesity, in Oomura Y, Tarui S, Shimazu T (eds), *Progress in Obesity Research.* London, John Libbey, 1990, pp 655–658.
63. Bjorntorp P. How should obesity be defined? *J Intern Med* 227:147, 1990.
64. Vague J. Diabetogenic and atherogenic fat, in Oomura Y, Tarui S, Shimazu T (eds), *Progress in Obesity Research.* London, John Libbey, 1990, pp. 343–358.
65. Rebuffe-Scrive M. Regional differences in visceral adipose tissue metabolism in Oomura Y, Tarui S, Inoue S, et al. (eds), *Progress in Obesity Research 1990.* London, John Libbey, 1991, pp. 313–316.
66. Despres JP. Lipoprotein metabolism in abdominal obesity, pp. 285–90.
67. Bouchard C. Genetic and environmental influences on regional fat distribution, in Oomura Y, Tarui S, Inoue S, et al. (eds), *Progress in Obesity Research 1990.* London: John Libbey, 1991, pp. 303–08.
68. Garn SM, Sullivan T, Hawthorne VM. Differential fatness remodelling rates at different body sites. *Int J Obes* 11:519, 1988.
69. Garn SM, Sullivan TV, Hawthorne VM. Evidence against functional differences between centeral and peripheral fat. *Am J Clin Nutr* 47:836, 1989.
70. Garn SM, Sullivan TV, Hawthorne VM. Fatness dependence of skinfold ratios and its implications to fat patterning. *Ecol Food Nutr* 21:151, 1988.
71. Garn SM. Implications and applications of subcutaneous fat measurement to nutritional assessment and health risk evaluation, in Himes J (ed) *Anthropometric Assessment of Nutritional Status.* New York, Wiley Liss, 1991, pp. 123–130.
72. Bray GA. Overweight: Basic considerations and clinical approaches. *Disease-a-Month* 7:451, 1989.
73. Bray GA. Epidemiology of obesity, in Oomura Y, Tarui S, Shimazu T (eds), *Progress in Obesity Research.* London, John Libbey, 1990, pp. 639–643.

74. Carmillot A, Fuch SA. Possible weight, in Oomura Y, Tarui S, Inoue S, Shimazu T (eds), *Progress in Obesity Research*. London, John Libbey, 1990, pp 663–664.
75. Brownell KD. The psychology and physiology of obesity: Implications for screening. *J Am Diet Assoc* 84:406, 1984.
76. Brownell KD, Kramer FM. Behavioral management of obesity. *Med Clin North Am* 73:185, 1989.
77. Brownell KD. *The LEARN Program for Weight Control*. Dallas, American Health Pub Co, 1990.
78. Brownell KD, Rodin J. *The Weight Maintenance Survival Guide*. Dallas, American Health Publ Co, 1990.
79. Brownell KD. *The LEARN Program for Weight Control*. Dallas, American Health Pub Co, 1990.
80. Foreyt JP, Goodrick GK. Factors common to successful therapy for the obese patient. *Med Sci Sports Exerc* 23:292, 1991.
81. Lissner L, Odell PM, D'Agostino RB. Variability of body weight and health outcomes in the Framingham population. *N Engl J Med* 324:1939, 1991.
82. Blackburn GL, Wilson GT, Kanders BS, et al. Weight cycling: The experience of human dieters. *Am J Clin Nutr* 49:1105, 1989.
83. Manore MM, Berry TE, Skinner JS, et al. Energy expenditure at rest and during exercise in nonobese female cyclical dieters and in nondieting control subjects. *Am J Clin Nutr* 54:41, 1991.
84. Dywer JT. Assessment of energy intake and expenditure, in Micozzi M, Moon R (eds), *Diet and Cancer: Role of Macronutrients*. Bethesda, MD, Aspen, 1992, pp. 125–57.
85. Owen OE, Kavle E, Owen RS, et al. A reappraisal of caloric requirements in healthy women. *Am J Clin Nutr* 44:1, 1986.
86. Owen OE, Holup JL, D'Allessio DA, et al. A reappraisal of the caloric requirements of men. *Am J Clin Nutr* 46:875, 1987.
87. Life Sciences Research Office. *Research Needs in Management of Obesity by Severe Caloric Restriction*. FASEB Contract FDA 223–75–0290. Washington, DC, Federation of Societies of Experimental Biology, 1979.
88. US Dept of Agriculture, Human Nutrition Info Service. *Preparing Foods and Planning Menus Using the Dietary Guidelines*. House and Garden Bulletin 232–8. Hyattsville, MD, US Dept of Agriculture, 1989.
89. Schoeller DA, Fjeld CR. Human energy metabolism: What have we learned from the doubly-labeled water method? *Ann Rev Nutr* 11:355, 1991.
90. Livingstone MBE, Prentice AM, Strain JJ, et al. Accuracy of weighed dietary records in studies of diet and health. *Br Med J* 300:708, 1990.
91. VanItallie TB, Yang MU. Diet and weight loss. 297:1158, 1977.
92. *Federal Trade Commission Facts for Consumers: Diet Programs*. Washington, DC, Federal Trade Commission, September 1990.

93. Dwyer JT. *Nutrient Needs in Weight Management*. Piscataway, NJ, Health Learning Systems, 1991.
94. VanItallie TB, Yang MU. Diet and weight loss. *N Engl J Med* 297:1158, 1977.
95. Report on Joint FAO/WHO Expert Consultation on Energy Intake and Protein Requirements. In Rand WM, Uauy R, and Scrimshaw NS. *Protein Energy Requirement Studies in Developing Countries: Results of International Research*. U.N. University Food and Nutrition Bulletin. Supplement 10. Tokyo: U.N. University 1984, pp. 331–369.
96. Gelfand RA, Handler R. Effect of nutrient composition on the metabolic response to very low calorie diets: Learning more and more about less and less. *Diabetes Metab Rev* 5(1):17, 1989.
97. Week M, Fischer S, Hinefeld M, et al. Loss of fat, water, and protein during very low calorie diets and complete starvation. *Klin Wochenschr* 65:1142, 1987.
98. Sours HE, Frattali VP, Brand CD, et al. Sudden death associated with very low calorie weight reduction regimens. *Am J Clin Nutr* 34:453, 1981.
99. Wadden TA, Stunkard AJ, Brownell KD. Very low calorie diets: Their efficacy, safety, and future. *Ann Intern Med* 99:675, 1983.
100. Committee on Dietary Allowances, Food and Nutrition Board, National Academy of Sciences. *Recommended Dietary Allowances* ed. 10. Washington, DC, National Academy Press, 1989.
101. Wadden TA, VanItallie TB, Blackburn GL. Responsible and irresponsible use of very low calorie diets in the treatment of obesity. *JAMA* 263:83, 1990.
102. Atkinson RL. Low and very low calorie diets. *Med Clin North Am* 73:203, 1989.
103. National Academy of Sciences Diet and Health. *Implications for Reducing Chronic Disease Risk*. Washington, DC, National Academy Press, 1989.
104. Prentice AM, Black AE, Coward WA, et al. High levels of energy expenditure in obese women. *Br Med J* 292:983, 1986.
105. Sims EAH. Storage and expenditure of energy in obesity and their implications for management. *Med Clin North Am* 73:97, 1989.
106. Stern JS, Titchenal CA, Johnson PR. Obesity: Does exercise make a difference?, in Berry EM, Blondheim SH, Eliahou HE, et al (eds), *Recent Advances in Obesity Research: V. Proceedings of the 5th International Congress on Obesity*. John Libbey, London, 1987, pp 352–364.
107. Pavlou KN, Krey S, Steffee WP. Exercise as an adjunct to weight loss and maintenance in moderately obese subjects. *Am J Clin Nutr* 49:1115, 1989.
108. McHenry PL, Ellestad MH, Fletcher GF, et al. Statement on exercise: A position statement for health professionals by the Committee on Exercise and Cardiac Rehabilitation of the Council on Clinical Cardiology, American Heart Association *Circulation* 81:936, 1990.
109. Pi-Sunyer FX. Exercise in the treatment of obesity, in Frankel RT, Yang MU (eds), *Obesity and Weight Control: The Health Professional's Guide to Understanding and Treatment*. Rockville, MD, Aspen, 1988, pp. 241–255.

110. Pavlou KN, Whatley JE, Jannace PW, et al. Physical activity as a supplement to a weight loss dietary regimen. *Am J Clin Nutr* 49:1110, 1989.

111. Ward A, Mallowy, P, Rippe J. Exercise prescription guidelines for normal and cardiac populations. *Cardiol Clin* 5:197, 1987.

112. Pate RR, Blair SN, Durstine JL, et al. *American College of Sports Medicine Guidelines for Exercise Testing and Prescription*. ed 4. Philadelphia, Lea & Febiger, 1991.

113. Fletcher GF, Froelicher VF, Hartley LH, et al. American Heart Association Exercise Standards. A statement for health professionals from the American Heart Association. *Circulation* 82:2286, 1990.

114. McArdle WD, Toner MM. Application of exercise for weight control: The exercise prescription, in Frankel RT, Yang MU (eds), *Obesity and Weight Control: The Health Professional's Guide to Understanding and Treatment*. Rockville, MD, Aspen, 1988, pp 257–274.

115. Horton ES. Metabolic aspects of exercise and weight reduction. *Med Sci Sports Exerc* 18:10, 1985.

116. King AC, Frey-Hewitt B, Dreon DM, et al. Diet vs exercise in weight maintenance: The effects of minimal intervention strategies on long term outcomes. *Arch Intern Med* 149:2741, 1989.

117. Dwyer JT. Steps to take in primary care for achieving lasting dietary change. *Topics Clin Nutr* 6:22, 1991.

118. University of Washington School of Medicine. *Contemporary Management of the Obese Patient*. Little Falls, NJ, Health Learning Systems, 1991.

119. Brownell MD, Wadden TA. The heterogeneity of obesity: Fitting treatments to individuals. *Behav Ther* 22:153, 1991.

Obesity: Clinical Evaluation of Body Composition and Energy Expenditure

CHAPTER 3

Stanley Heshka, Ph.D., Kathleen Buhl, M.A., and Steven B. Heymsfield, M.D.

INTRODUCTION

Assessment of body composition and energy expenditure are two important and related components of the obese patient's evaluation. This chapter reviews the clinical approach to estimating body composition and energy expenditure in obese patients and presents research in a historical context. An emphasis is placed on physiologic concepts that provide the groundwork and rationale for patient studies.

BODY COMPOSITION

Body Weight Indices

Obesity in the adult represents the accumulation of excess adipose tissue and a gain in body weight. Since body weight is easily measurable, the diagnosis of obesity is first suggested by an increase in body weight adjusted for stature. At present, two approaches are used to determine if an individual's body weight is suggestive of obesity.

The first is to express body weight as a percentage of *ideal* or *desirable*. The concept of a desirable body weight began in the 1920s, when tables were prepared that indicated that the average weight for height at age 30 was ideal in terms of mortality.[1] The Build and Blood Pressure Study of 1959 combined the experience of 26 life insurance companies for enrollees between the ages of 15 and 69 years.[2] Height and weight data were gathered in subjects wearing shoes and indoor clothing. The results of this study, which excluded individuals with heart disease, cancer, and diabetes, presented the average weight for height in about 5 million people. The 1959 Metropolitan Life Insurance Company's desirable body weights (Table 3–1) were derived from this data base, using weights associated with the lowest mortality. A frame size designation was provided in the table, although no method of estimating skeletal dimensions was included.

The 1979 Build Study[3] indicated that the gap between average population weights and weights associated with the lowest mortality has narrowed from

TABLE 3–1 Desirable Weights for Men and Women Age 25 and Over (in lbs by Height and Frame, in Indoor Clothing and Shoes)

Men					Women				
Height		Frame			Height		Frame		
Feet	Inches	Small	Medium	Large	Feet	Inches	Small	Medium	Large
5	2	112–120	118–129	126–141	4	10	92–98	96–107	104–119
5	3	115–123	121–133	129–144	4	11	94–101	98–110	106–122
5	4	118–126	124–136	132–148	5	0	96–104	101–113	109–125
5	5	121–129	127–139	135–152	5	1	99–107	104–116	112–128
5	6	124–133	130–143	138–156	5	2	102–110	107–119	115–131
5	7	128–137	134–147	142–161	5	3	105–113	110–122	118–134
5	8	132–141	138–152	147–166	5	4	108–116	113–126	121–138
5	9	136–145	142–156	151–170	5	5	111–119	116–130	125–142
5	10	140–150	146–160	155–174	5	6	114–123	120–135	129–146
5	11	144–154	150–165	159–179	5	7	118–127	124–139	133–150
6	0	148–158	154–170	164–184	5	8	122–131	128–143	137–154
6	1	152–162	158–175	168–189	5	9	126–135	132–147	141–158
6	2	156–167	162–180	173–194	5	10	130–140	136–151	145–163
6	3	160–171	167–185	178–199	5	11	134–144	140–155	149–168
6	4	164–175	172–190	182–204	6	0	138–148	144–159	153–173

Source: Data adapted from the *Statistical Bulletin,* Metropolitan Life Insurance Company, New York. Derived primarily from data of the *1959 Build and Blood Pressure Study,* Society of Actuaries.

TABLE 3–2 Metropolitan Height-Weight Tables, 1983 (lb)

Men					Women				
Height		Frame			Height		Frame		
Feet	Inches	Small	Medium	Large	Feet	Inches	Small	Medium	Large
5	2	128–134	131–141	138–150	4	10	102–111	109–121	118–131
5	3	130–136	133–143	140–153	4	11	103–113	111–123	120–134
5	4	132–138	135–145	142–156	5	0	104–115	113–126	122–137
5	5	134–140	137–146	144–160	5	1	106–118	115–129	123–140
5	6	136–142	139–151	140–164	5	2	108–121	118–132	128–143
5	7	138–145	142–154	149–168	5	3	111–124	121–135	131–147
5	8	140–148	145–157	152–172	5	4	114–127	124–138	134–151
5	9	142–151	148–160	155–176	5	5	117–130	127–141	137–155
5	10	144–154	151–163	156–180	5	6	120–133	130–144	140–159
5	11	146–157	154–166	161–184	5	7	123–136	133–147	143–163
6	0	149–160	157–170	164–188	5	8	126–139	136–150	146–167
6	1	152–164	160–174	168–192	5	9	129–142	139–153	149–170
6	2	155–168	164–178	172–197	5	10	132–145	142–156	152–173
6	3	158–172	167–182	176–202	5	11	132–148	145–159	155–176
6	4	102–176	171–187	181–207	6	0	138–151	148–162	158–179

Weight according to frame (ages 25 to 59) for men wearing indoor clothing weighing 5 lb, shoes with heels; for women, indoor clothing weight 3 lb.

Source: Reprinted with permission from the Metropolitan Life Insurance Company, New York.

that observed in 1959. The 1983 height-weight tables of the Metropolitan Life Insurance Company (Table 3–2) take this finding into consideration, and the result is that desirable body weights are higher than those reported in 1959. The 1983 table avoids the use of terms such as *ideal weight* or *desirable weight* due to misinterpretations of their meaning.

An estimate of frame size is included in the 1983 tables, and approaches to evaluating skeletal dimensions are described in the next section. Body weight, expressed as a percentage of desirable, is used to classify subjects as normal or as mildly ($\geqslant 15 < 30\%$), moderately ($\geqslant 30 < 50\%$), severely ($\geqslant 50 < 100\%$), or morbidly obese ($\geqslant 100\%$).

The second approach to adjusting body weight for stature is the calculation of a *height-normalized* index. Although many such indices have been developed, the most widely used at present is the body mass index (BMI) calculated as weight (in kilograms) divided by height (in meters) squared. The main assumptions of the BMI are that it agrees with other measures of adiposity and that it is independent of height.[4–7]

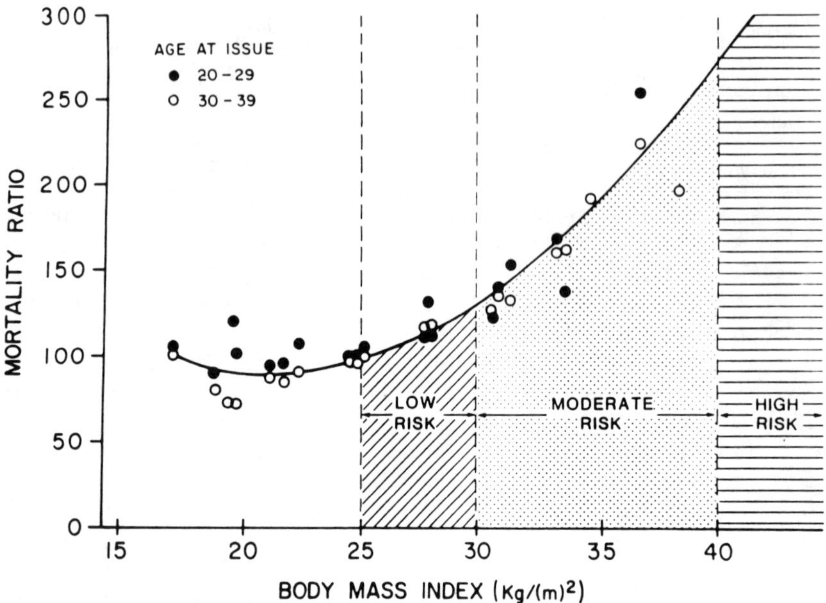

Figure 3–1. Use of BMI and excess mortality to provide an estimate of risk from obesity. Solid circles show persons aged 20 to 29 years, and open circles show persons aged 30 to 39 years.

Population studies demonstrate a U- or J-shaped mortality curve for BMI (Figure 3–1). Cutoff points for BMI vary, but the generally accepted range for good health is 20–23 kg/m^2. The BMI for men and women with a medium frame calculated from the 1959 desirable weight table is 21–22 kg/m^2. A BMI of 25–27 kg/m^2 may lead to health problems in some people, and BMIs in excess of 27 kg/m^2 are associated with an increased health risk.[8] A nomogram for calculating BMI from height and weight, and the corresponding health risk for each level of BMI, are presented in Figure 3–2.

BMI may have a small stature dependence, as people with short legs for their height will have higher BMI values independent of fatness.[9] In addition, BMI is not a very precise measure of total body adiposity, as athletes or muscular individuals may have a BMI considered in the obese range. The relation between BMI and total body fat in mixed groups of subjects is generally between r = 0.5 and r = 0.8.[4,10] The range in total body fat associated with any specific BMI is relatively wide. For example, Smalley et al.[7] found that a man with a BMI of 27 kg/m^2 could have a total body fat ranging from 10% to 31% of body weight.

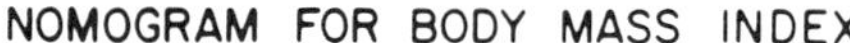

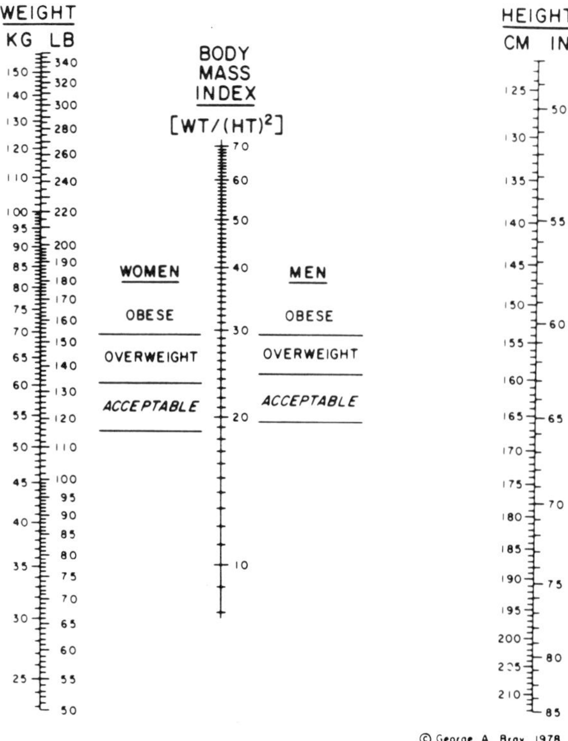

Figure 3–2. A nomogram for determining BMI. To use this nomogram, place a ruler or straight edge between the body weight in kilograms or pounds (without clothes), located on the left-hand line, and the body weight in centimeters or inches (without shoes), located on the right-hand line. The BMI is read from the middle of the scale and is in metric units.

(Reprinted with permission; copyright 1978 George A. Bray)

Body weight should be measured under standardized or at least reproducible conditions. The standard conditions include leaving shoes on, changing into a dressing gown, evacuating the bladder, and then measuring body weight. Body weight should be measured using a calibrated physician's scale to the nearest 0.1 kg. Serial weights should be measured at the same time each day.

Stature is measured without shoes, using the sliding stick that is attached to most physician's scales. A more desirable method is to use a separate standiometer attached to a wall. Stature measurements are usually made to the nearest 0.1 cm.

Although not well studied, frame size is assumed to influence body weight independently of height and percentage of body fat. Frame size is usually estimated from limb circumferences or bone breadths, although no consensus exists on the ideal approach. Small, medium, and large frames are usually classified according to population percentiles for specific anatomic measurements.[11]

The 1983 Metropolitan height-weight table includes an estimate of frame size. Elbow breadth measurements were taken from the 1971–1975 National Health and Nutrition Examination Survey,[12] and the population distribution was divided into small (<25th percentile), medium (25th to 74th percentiles), and large (≥75th percentile) frames. The procedure for estimating frame size from elbow breadth and height for men and women is presented in Table 3–3.

Body weight and BMI are inaccurate guides to the amount of adipose tissue present in an individual patient. It is therefore useful to use additional techniques in evaluating body composition.

Body weight can be divided into adipose tissue, skeletal muscle, skeleton,

TABLE 3–3 Height and Elbow Breadth for Men and Women

Height	Elbow Breadth
MEN	
5′2″–5′3″	2 1/2″–2 1/4″
5′4″–5′7″	2 5/8″–2 7/8″
5′8″–5′11″	2 3/4″–3″
6′0″–6′3″	2 3/4″–3 1/8″
6′4″	2 7/8″–3 1/4″
WOMEN	
4′10″–4′11″	2 1/4″–2 1/2″
5′0″–5′3″	2 1/4″–2 1/2″
5′4″–5′7″	2 3/8″–2 5/8″
5′8″–5′11″	2 3/8″–2 5/8″
6′0″	2 1/2″–2 3/4″

Procedure: Extend your arm and bend the forearm upward at a 90° angle. Keep fingers straight and turn the inside of your wrist toward your body. If you have a caliper, use it to measure the space between the two prominent bones on either side of your elbow. Without a caliper, place the thumb and index finger of your other hand on these two bones. Measure the space between your fingers against a ruler or tape measure. Compare it with these tables that list elbow measurements for medium-frame men and women. Measurements lower than those listed indicate that you have a small frame. Higher measurements indicate a larger frame.

Source: Reprinted with permission from Metropolitan Life Insurance Company, New York.

and remaining tissue that consists mainly of organs and viscera. Although it would be desirable to subdivide body weight into these four major organ tissue compartments, the needed methods are not clinically available or practical. An alternative is to base body composition estimates on the molecular or chemical model. Body weight according to the chemical model is divided into fat and fat-free body mass, the latter including water, protein, and mineral. Adipose tissue and fat differ, although the two compartments are highly correlated with each other.[13] Adipose tissue consists of adipocytes, extracellular fluid, vascular endothelium, and connective tissue. The remainder of body weight after removal of adipose tissue is referred to as *adipose tissue-free mass* (Figure 3–3). Fat is usually defined as the total lipid extract of homogenized tissue, most of which is adipose tissue triglycerides.[14] The remainder of body weight after extraction of fat is defined as fat-free body mass (Figure 3–3).

Figure 3–3. The relation between chemical [fat plus fat-free body mass (FFM)] and organ tissue [adipose tissue (AT) + adipose tissue free mass (ATFM)] models of body composition. Fat-free body mass represents the sum of ATFM and the fat-free portion of adipose tissue (FFAT).

(Adapted from Ref. 14 with permission)

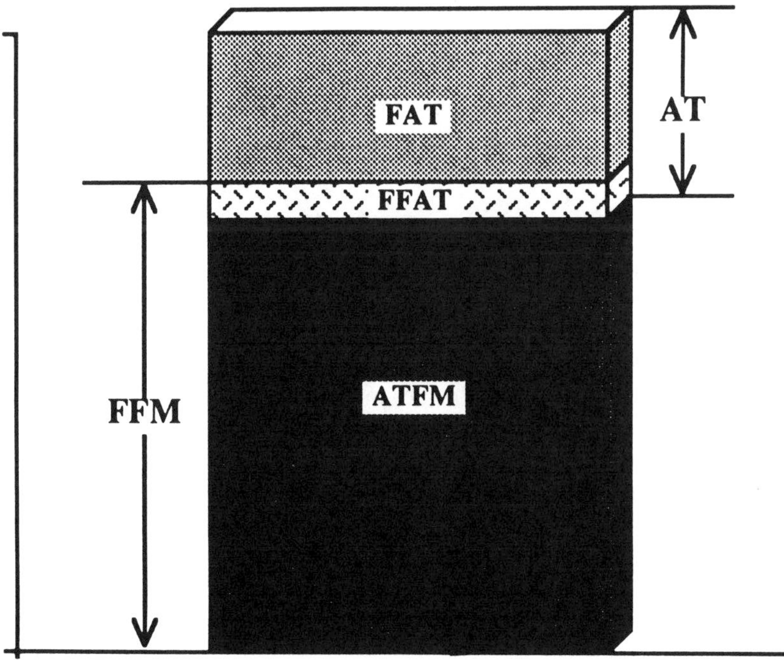

Anthropometry

Anthropometry in the evaluation of obese patients provides both absolute circumferential and skinfold measurements and derived estimates of body composition. Anthropometric measurements are made using simple devices such as a tape measure for circumferences and skinfold calipers for skinfolds. The tape measure should resist stretching, be durable, and have an accuracy of ±0.1 cm. Fiberglass and linen tapes are recommended, and calibration should be confirmed at regular intervals using a reference meter stick. When taking a circumference measurement, it is important not to apply too much pressure in order to avoid compressing the underlying adipose tissue and musculature. Several skinfold calipers are available. The best calipers are light, rugged, and maintain a standard jaw pressure throughout the skinfold range.[15] A calibration block should be provided with the instrument.

Some errors involved in skinfold measurement are related to selection of the skinfold sites, choice and use of the proper caliper, accurate definition of the measurement area, and tester reliability. Both intra- and inter-tester reliability studies indicate that circumference measurements are less variable than skinfold measurements in general, although skinfold thickness correlates better with total body fatness.[16]

The techniques of measurement, reproducibility, and other technical aspects of anthropometry are reviewed in the Airlie Conference proceedings, a highly recommended monograph for all individuals who use anthropometry in their practice.[17]

The locations of commonly used skinfold sites and circumferences are described in Table 3–4. In addition, normative values for triceps and subscapular skinfold thicknesses in both men and women are presented in Tables 3–5 to 3–8.

The use of skinfolds in estimating body fat is based on two assumptions. First, skinfold thickness is assumed to be strongly related to total subcutaneous adipose tissue. Second, the use of skinfolds as a measure of body fat assumes that the relationship between subcutaneous adipose tissue and total body fat is known.[18] Both of these assumptions are valid under selected conditions, including use of a minimum of three skinfold sites to predict total body fat, and selecting a skinfold equation that was developed on a population of subjects similar to ethnicity, gender, and body composition to the patients under study.[19]

Several problems occur when measuring circumferences and skinfolds in the obese. It is difficult to locate the proper site for measurement, and in some patients the skinfold may be too large for the caliper (50–70 mm, depending on the brand) to measure. Moreover, the reliability of skinfold measurements exceeding 45–50 mm is not well known.[19] In morbidly obese patients, circumfer-

TABLE 3–4 Anatomic Location of Skinfold and Circumference Measurement Sites

Skinfold	Anatomic Site
Bicep	A vertical fold taken anteriorly halfway between the acromian and olecranon processes
Tricep	A vertical fold taken posteriorly to the bicep skinfold
Subscapular	A diagonal fold taken just below the inferior angle of the scapula
Suprailiac	A diagonal fold taken just above the iliac crest at the midaxillary line
Chest	A diagonal fold taken halfway between the armpit and the nipple for men and one-third the distance for women
Thigh	A vertical fold taken anteriorly halfway between the hip and the knee
Circumference	**Anatomic Site**
Upper arm	Measured halfway between the acromian and olecranon processes
Chest	Measured at the nipple line in men; at the largest circumference above the breasts in women
Abdomen	The smallest circumference in the abdominal area
Waist	Measured at the umbilicus
Hips	The largest circumference below the umbilicus
Buttocks	The largest circumference in the gluteal area
Thigh	Measured just below the gluteal fold
Calf	The largest circumference below the knee

ences may be the only means of anthropometric evaluation.[16] Hence, a tape measure of sufficient length should always be available.

Several studies have examined the use of anthropometry to predict fatness in obese patients. Gray[20] studied fat estimates provided by skinfolds in obese patients in comparison to fat measured by underwater weighing. A similar relationship was observed between skinfold estimates and underwater weighing in both lean and obese subjects. The investigators also found an overestimation of percentage body fat by skinfolds at lower levels of body fat and an underestimation of percentage fat in more obese patients. They attributed the underestimation of fat by subcutaneous skinfold measurement in obese patients to a relative increase in the deposition of intra-abdominal fat. Roche[18] found that the fat content of adipose tissue was higher in obese subjects than in lean individuals. Thus an absolute skinfold measurement in an obese patient may reflect a higher fat content at that site compared to a lean subject.

Several studies have investigated the use of skinfold measurements in obese subjects after weight loss. These studies illustrate the importance of choosing an appropriate equation for the population under study. Some equations were

TABLE 3–5 Triceps Skinfold Thickness: Adult Men, United States, 1971–1974

Race and Age in Years	Number in Sample	Estimated Population in Thousands	Mean	SD	Percentile								
					5th	10th	15th	25th	50th	75th	85th	90th	95th
ALL RACES*													
	5,261	61,180	12.0	5.9	4.5	6.0	6.5	8.0	11.0	15.0	18.0	20.0	23.0
18–19	260	3,673	11.0	6.1	4.5	5.0	6.0	7.0	8. 5	15.0	18.0	19.5	23.5
20–24	513	8,110	11.2	6.2	4.0	5.0	6.0	7.0	10.0	14.0	17.5	20.0	23.0
25–34	804	13,003	12.6	6.4	4.5	5.5	6.0	8.0	12.0	16.0	18.5	21.5	24.0
35–44	664	10,676	12.4	5.5	5.0	6.0	7.0	8.5	12.0	15.5	17.5	20.0	23.0
45–54	765	11,150	12.4	5.9	5.0	6.0	7.0	8.0	11.0	15.0	18.0	20.0	25.5
55–64	598	9,073	11.6	5.2	5.0	6.0	6.5	8.0	11.0	14.0	16.5	18.0	21.5
65–74	1,657	5,496	11.8	5.5	4.5	5.5	6.5	8.0	11.0	15.0	17.0	19.0	22.0
WHITE													
	4,344	54,694	12.2	5.8	5.0	6.0	6.5	8.0	11.0	15.0	18.0	20.0	23.0
18–19	203	3,206	11.3	5.9	5.0	5.5	6.0	7.0	9.0	15.0	18.0	20.0	23.0

20–24	423	7,094	11.5	6.0	4.0	5.0	6.0	7.0	10.0	15.0	18.0	21.0	23.0
25–34	672	11,594	12.7	6.2	5.0	6.0	6.5	8.0	12.0	16.0	18.5	21.0	24.0
35–44	569	9,516	12.6	5.4	5.0	6.0	7.0	9.0	12.0	15.5	17.5	20.0	23.0
45–54	628	10,039	12.6	5.9	5.5	6.5	7.0	8.5	11.0	15.0	18.0	20.0	26.0
55–64	505	8,275	11.7	5.0	5.0	6.0	7.0	8.0	11.0	14.0	16.5	18.0	21.0
65–74	1,344	4,970	12.0	5.4	5.0	6.0	7.0	8.0	11.0	15.0	17.0	19.0	22.0
						BLACK							
	847	5,753	10.6	7.0	3.5	4.0	4.5	6.0	8.5	13.0	16.0	20.0	23.0
18–19	52	404	8.9	6.7	2.0	4.0	5.0	5.1	7.0	8.0	12.0	21.0	24.0
20–24	80	866	10.0	7.9	3.0	4.0	4.0	6.0	8.0	11.0	13.0	18.0	24.0
25–34	119	1,232	11.8	8.4	4.0	4.0	4.0	5.0	10.0	15.0	20.0	22.0	23.0
35–44	87	1,005	11.3	6.5	4.0	4.5	5.0	7.0	10.0	14.0	17.0	18.4	22.0
45–54	130	1,057	10.0	5.1	4.0	4.0	5.0	6.0	10.0	12.5	14.0	16.0	20.0
55–64	85	703	10.7	7.2	3.0	4.0	4.5	5.0	8.0	14.0	20.0	22.0	26.0
65–74	294	486	9.7	5.4	4.0	4.5	5.0	6.0	9.0	12.0	14.0	15.0	19.5

*Includes data for races that are not shown separately. Measurements are made in the right arm.

Source: National Center for Health Statistics, Department of Health and Human Services. See also Bishop CW, Bowen PE, Ritchey SJ. Norms for nutritional assessment of American adults by upper arm anthropometry. *Am J Clin Nutr* 34:2530, 1981.

TABLE 3–6 Subscapular Skinfold Thickness: Adult Men, United States, 1971–1974

Race and Age in Years	Number in Sample	Estimated Population in Thousands	Mean	SD	Percentile								
					5th	10th	15th	25th	50th	75th	85th	90th	95th
ALL RACES													
	5,261	61,180	15.9	7.7	6.0	7.0	8.0	10.0	14.5	20.0	24.0	26.0	30.5
18–19	260	3,673	12.3	7.1	6.0	6.5	7.0	8.0	10.0	13.0	18.0	23.5	28.5
20–24	513	8.110	13.7	7.4	6.0	7.0	7.0	8.0	12.0	17.0	20.5	24.0	30.0
25–34	804	13,003	15.9	8.1	6.5	7.0	8.0	10.0	14.0	20.0	24.5	26.0	30.5
35–44	664	10,676	16.8	7.2	7.0	8.0	10.0	11.5	16.0	21.0	24.0	26.0	30.5
45–54	765	11,150	17.5	7.9	7.0	8.0	9.0	12.0	16.5	22.0	25.0	29.0	32.0
55–64	598	9,073	16.5	7.5	6.0	7.0	8.5	11.0	15.5	21.0	24.5	27.0	30.0
65–74	1,657	5,496	15.9	7.2	6.0	7.5	9.0	10.5	15.0	20.0	23.0	25.0	30.0
WHITE													
	4,344	54,694	15.9	7.5	6.5	7.5	8.0	10.0	14.5	20.0	24.0	26.0	30.0
18–19	203	3,206	12.5	7.1	6.0	6.5	7.0	8.0	10.0	13.5	18.0	23.5	28.5

20–24	423	7,094	13.8	7.3	6.0	7.0	7.0	8.0	12.0	17.0	21.0	24.0	30.0
25–34	672	11,594	15.8	7.6	7.0	7.5	8.0	10.0	14.0	20.0	25.0	26.0	30.0
35–44	569	9,516	16.6	7.0	7.0	8.5	10.0	11.5	16.0	20.0	24.0	26.0	30.0
45–54	628	10,039	17.6	7.6	7.0	8.0	10.0	12.0	16.5	22.0	25.0	28.5	31.0
55–64	505	8,275	16.5	7.2	6.0	7.0	8.5	11.0	15.5	21.0	24.0	26.5	30.0
65–74	1,344	4,970	15.9	7.0	6.5	8.0	9.0	11.0	15.0	20.0	23.0	25.0	30.0
						BLACK							
	847	5,753	16.1	9.9	6.0	6.5	7.0	8.5	14.0	21.9	25.0	28.0	35.0
18–19	52	404	10.9	7.2	4.0	5.5	6.0	7.0	9.0	11.1	15.0	23.5	32.0
20–24	80	866	13.6	8.6	5.5	6.0	7.0	8.0	11.0	17.0	19.0	26.0	30.0
25–34	119	1,232	16.6	11.8	6.0	6.5	7.0	8.0	14.0	21.5	25.0	30.5	42.0
35–44	87	1,005	18.9	8.4	7.0	7.0	8.0	12.0	19.0	24.0	25.5	31.0	33.1
45–54	130	1,057	16.6	9.7	6.0	7.0	7.0	9.0	13.0	22.0	26.0	32.0	35.0
55–64	85	703	17.0	10.5	5.0	5.0	6.5	10.0	14.5	23.0	25.0	28.0	35.0
65–74	294	486	15.2	8.6	6.0	6.0	7.0	8.0	13.0	20.0	23.0	26.0	33.0

*Includes data for races that are not shown separately. Measurements are made in the right arm.

Source: National Center for Health Statistics, Department of Health and Human Services. See also Bishop CW, Bowen PE, Ritchey, SJ. Norms for nutritional assessment of American adults by upper arm anthropometry. *Am J Clin Nutr* 34:2530, 1981.

TABLE 3–7 Triceps Skinfold Thickness: Adult Women, United States, 1971–1974

Race and Age in Years	Number in Sample	Estimated Population in Thousands	Mean	SD	Percentile								
					5th	10th	15th	25th	50th	75th	85th	90th	95th
All Races													
	8,410	67,837	23.0	8.4	11.0	13.0	14.0	17.0	22.0	28.0	32.0	34.0	37.5
18–19	280	3,679	18.6	6.8	9.0	11.0	12.0	14.0	17.5	22.0	24.0	27.0	32.0
20–24	1,243	9,215	19.7	7.8	10.0	11.0	12.0	14.0	18.0	24.0	27.9	30.5	34.5
25–34	1,896	13,933	21.9	8.2	10.5	12.0	13.5	16.0	21.0	26.5	30.5	33.5	37.0
35–44	1,664	11,593	24.0	8.4	12.0	14.0	16.0	18.0	23.0	29.5	32.5	35.5	39.0
45–54	836	12,163	25.4	8.3	13.0	15.0	17.0	20.0	25.0	30.0	34.0	36.0	40.0
55–64	669	9,976	24.9	8.5	11.0	14.0	16.0	19.0	25.0	30.5	33.0	35.0	39.0
65–74	1,822	7,277	23.3	7.5	11.5	14.0	16.0	18.0	23.0	28.0	31.0	33.0	36.0
White													
	6,757	59,923	22.9	8.1	11.0	13.0	14.5	17.0	22.0	28.0	31.0	34.0	37.0
18–19	208	3,159	18.9	6.6	9.5	12.0	13.0	14.5	18.0	22.5	24.0	26.5	33.5

20–24	956	7,972	19.8	7.7	10.0	11.0	12.0	14.0	19.0	24.0	27.9	30.5	34.0
25–34	1,539	12,161	21.8	8.0	11.0	12.5	14.0	16.0	20.5	26.0	30.0	33.0	36.5
35–44	1,302	10,111	23.7	8.3	12.0	14.0	15.9	18.0	22.5	29.0	32.0	35.1	38.5
45–54	705	10,879	25.3	8.1	13.0	15.0	17.0	20.0	25.0	30.0	33.5	35.5	39.5
55–64	551	9,037	24.6	7.9	11.5	14.5	16.0	19.0	24.0	30.0	33.0	34.1	38.0
65–74	1,496	6,603	23.3	7.3	12.0	14.0	16.0	18.0	23.0	28.0	31.0	33.0	35.5
						BLACK							
	1,557	7,302	23.7	10.3	9.0	11.0	12.0	15.5	23.0	30.5	34.0	36.6	41.0
18–19	70	504	16.2	7.3	8.0	9.0	9.0	11.5	14.0	20.0	25.0	29.0	32.0
20–24	259	1,073	19.3	8.7	9.0	10.0	11.5	12.5	17.0	24.5	28.6	32.0	36.0
25–34	335	1,646	22.5	9.6	8.5	10.0	12.0	14.0	22.0	30.0	32.6	34.1	40.0
35–44	334	1,318	25.8	9.2	11.5	13.0	16.0	20.0	25.5	32.0	35.0	36.5	41.0
45–54	126	1,237	26.8	9.8	12.0	14.0	17.0	20.0	26.0	34.0	37.1	40.0	42.2
55–64	115	871	28.2	12.9	10.0	11.0	13.0	19.0	28.0	34.0	40.0	45.0	51.5
65–74	318	652	23.8	9.0	7.5	11.5	15.0	17.5	24.0	30.0	32.2	35.5	40.0

*Includes data for races that are not shown separately. Measurements are made in the right arm.

Source: National Center for Health Statistics, Department of Health and Human Services. See also Bishop CW, Bowen PE, Ritchey SJ. Norms for nutritional assessment of American adults by upper arm anthropometry. *Am J Clin Nutr* 34:2530, 1981.

TABLE 3–8 Subscapular Skinfold Thickness: Adult Women, United States, 1971–1974

Race and Age in Years	Number in Sample	Estimated Population in Thousands	Mean	SD	Percentile								
					5th	10th	15th	25th	50th	75th	85th	90th	95th
All Races													
	8,410	67,837	18.8	10.2	6.5	7.5	8.5	10.5	16.0	25.2	30.0	33.2	38.0
18–19	280	3,679	14.4	7.7	6.5	7.0	7.0	9.0	12.0	19.0	22.0	26.0	30.0
20–24	1,243	9,215	15.4	8.6	6.0	7.0	8.0	9.0	13.0	19.5	23.0	27.0	32.1
25–34	1,896	13,933	17.4	10.1	6.0	7.0	8.0	10.0	14.5	22.5	29.0	32.1	38.0
35–44	1,664	11,593	19.6	10.8	6.5	8.0	9.0	11.0	17.0	26.5	32.0	34.1	39.1
45–54	836	12,163	21.2	10.5	7.0	8.5	10.0	12.0	20.0	28.0	32.5	35.0	40.0
55–64	669	9,976	20.9	10.3	7.0	8.0	9.5	12.5	20.0	28.0	32.0	34.5	38.0
65–74	1,822	7,277	19.5	9.3	7.0	8.0	10.0	12.0	18.0	25.0	30.0	32.5	37.0
White													
	6,757	59,923	18.2	9.8	6.5	7.5	8.0	10.0	16.0	25.0	29.4	32.0	36.5
18–19	208	3,159	14.2	7.4	6.5	7.0	7.0	8.5	12.0	19.0	22.0	26.0	30.0

20–24	956	7,972	15.1	8.5	6.0	7.0	7.5	9.0	13.0	19.0	23.0	27.0	32.0
25–34	1,539	12,161	16.8	9.8	6.0	7.0	8.0	9.5	14.0	21.5	27.5	32.0	37.0
35–44	1,302	10,111	18.8	10.5	6.5	7.5	8.5	10.5	16.0	25.0	30.0	34.0	38.0
45–54	705	10,879	20.4	10.0	7.0	8.5	10.0	12.8	19.0	27.0	31.5	34.0	38.0
55–64	551	9,037	20.2	9.8	6.5	8.0	9.0	12.0	19.0	27.0	31.0	34.0	37.0
65–74	1,496	6,603	19.2	9.1	7.0	8.0	10.0	12.0	18.0	25.0	29.0	32.0	36.0
BLACK													
	1,557	7,302	23.4	12.0	7.0	9.0	10.0	13.0	28.0	31.5	36.1	39.0	44.1
18–19	70	504	14.9	9.4	6.5	7.0	7.5	9.0	12.0	19.0	20.0	26.0	38.0
20–24	259	1,073	17.6	9.3	7.0	8.0	9.0	11.0	15.0	22.5	28.0	30.5	35.1
25–34	335	1,646	21.7	11.3	6.5	8.0	10.0	12.0	20.0	30.0	33.1	36.0	41.0
35–44	334	1,318	26.0	11.0	9.0	10.0	12.0	17.0	26.5	34.0	38.0	40.1	42.4
45–54	126	1,237	28.5	12.0	10.5	11.5	14.0	17.5	30.0	37.1	40.0	43.1	46.0
55–64	115	871	27.5	13.4	7.5	9.5	12.0	19.0	27.0	35.5	40.0	47.0	55.0
65–74	318	652	22.8	10.5	6.0	8.0	10.0	14.0	24.0	31.0	34.0	35.5	39.0

*Includes data for races that are not shown separately. Measurements are made in the right arm.

Source: National Center for Health Statistics, Department of Health and Human Services. See also Bishop CW, Bowen PE, Ritchey SJ. Norms for nutritional assessment of American adults by upper arm anthropometry. *Am J Clin Nutr* 34:2530, 1981.

found to significantly under- or overestimate percentage fat compared to underwater weighing.[21,23] Another problem is that the ratio of intra-abdominal to subcutaneous fat is not consistent throughout the weight loss period, possibly violating the assumption of a constant ratio between skinfold thickness and total body fatness.[24]

Bioimpedance Analysis

Bioimpedance analysis (BIA) provides a simple, safe, affordable, and practical method of evaluating three body compartments: fat, fat-free body mass, and water. Surface electrodes are placed on the subject's upper and lower extremities. An electrical current is then passed through the distal electrodes, and a drop in current is detected by the proximal electrodes. The decrement in current or total body resistance is related to the complex interactions among a number of factors. These include distance between the electrodes, volume and composition of conducting tissues, anatomic factors, and frequency of electrical current discharged at the distal electrodes. In general, adipose tissue is a poor conductor and lean tissues, particularly the fluid compartments, are good conductors. The result is that good inverse correlations are observed between resistance and total body water and fat-free body mass, and high positive correlations are found between resistance and total body fat.[8] Although there are small measurement errors between instruments, most of the higher-quality BIA systems give similar and highly reproducible estimates of resistance.

Most commercial BIA machines come preprogrammed with body composition equations. Although equations vary, most require age, weight, and stature in addition to estimates of resistance. Some equations also include gender and levels of fatness.[25–28]

Most studies suggest that BIA improves the prediction of total body fat and water compared to body weight, height, or anthropometry used either alone or in combination.[25,26,29,30] The literature in this area is controversial, however, and new studies are appearing frequently. The following is a summary of observations related to BIA and obesity as of the preparation of this chapter:

Prediction of the deuterium dilution space, which is about 4% larger than total body water, is reliable in obese subjects both before and after long-term (several months) weight loss. Small changes in total body water are not reliably estimated by BIA.[20]

Fat-free body mass was overestimated using manufacturers' early equations compared to fat-free body mass derived by underwater weighing.[26–28,31] Most manufacturers now include new and improved equations in their BIA instruments.

Although fat- and sex-specific equations were developed,[26] recent studies by Gray[20] suggest that they offer little improvement in predicting fat-free body mass compared to general equations. None of the equations are very good predictors of fat-free body mass in very obese subjects (48% body fat).[29] Equations may also be inaccurate in specific population, ethnic, or racial groups, such as the Pima Indians.[31,32] Locally developed BIA equations may thus be needed for specific ethnic groups or obese subjects.

Short-term (several days) or small changes in the composition of weight loss as fat and fat-free body mass are not estimated accurately using BIA in individual patients.[33]

Total Body Electrical Conductivity

Similar in concept to BIA, total body electrical conductivity (TOBEC) systems rely on the concept that lean tissue is a better conductor of electrical energy than fat. The TOBEC system consists of a large coil driven by a 2.5-Hz radio frequency current and a computer that processes the various signals and provides a summary report of the subject's body composition.

The procedure begins by having the subject rest on a platform bed that moves into and out of the coil when the system is activated. A current is induced in the subject's body in proportion to the mass of conductive tissues and ion-containing fluids. The difference between the impedance of the empty coil and the impedance of the coil when it contains the subject is proportional to the total conductivity of the body.[34] The conductivity is then proportional to lean or fat-free body mass. Calibrations for TOBEC are usually done using reference methods for estimating total body water (e.g., dilution of tritiated water), fat, and fat-free body mass (e.g., underwater weighing) in appropriately selected subject groups. Once calibrated, TOBEC can provide estimates of fat, fat-free body mass, and total body water.

TOBEC has been validated and cross-validated in a number of studies, all of which show good results comparable to those achieved with other clinical methods. For example, Van Itallie et al.[35] found that TOBEC was the best predictor of fat-free body mass in 67 subjects who varied greatly in body fat content when compared to skinfolds, BIA, total body water, and total body potassium when fat-free body mass estimated by underwater weighing was used as the criterion method.[36–37,38] A similar study by Segal et al.[39] included 75 subjects who ranged in body fat from 4.9% to 54.9%. Estimates of fat by TOBEC correlated better ($r = 0.97$) than fat estimates from total body water, total body potassium, BIA, and skinfolds when hydrodensitometry was used as the reference method for deriving total body fat. Several studies have examined the between-day reproducibility of TOBEC in estimating total body fat, and the results consistently provide a coefficient of variation of $<2\%$.[39] Presta et al.[40] studied the use of TOBEC in 32 adults, many of whom were obese. Results showed that the reliability of TOBEC for a single trial was $r = 0.9991$, and for 10 trials it was $r = 0.9999$. TOBEC thus appears to be an accurate and reproducible method for estimating fat and fat-free body mass in both normal-weight and obese subjects.

TOBEC is a safe procedure that can be used in children and adults of all ages. The advantages of TOBEC are that it is rapid (1 min per study), requires minimal technical skill in making the measurement, and does not require patient cooperation in such techniques as underwater weighing.[40] The limitations of TOBEC are its relatively high initial cost, its lack of portability, and its need to be calibrated against other clinical methods such as hydrodensitometry.[41] In addition, a change in the water content of fat-free tissues could potentially alter TOBEC estimates of body composition.[42,43] However, in one study, Cochran et al.[34] found that in an experimental model using baby pigs, altering extracellular fluid volume did not affect the accuracy of TOBEC-derived estimates of fat-free body mass. Additional studies are needed to determine if and to what extent TOBEC estimates are influenced by hydration.

As with other clinical methods, short-term or small changes in body composition measured over several days or weeks cannot be reliably measured in individual patients with TOBEC. Large changes in body weight over long periods of time, particularly in groups rather than in individual patients, can be reliably evaluated using TOBEC. For example, Van Loan et al.[43] studied body composition in 11 overweight (120–130% ideal body weight) women who lost an average of 6.6 kg over 6 weeks, using combinations of diet and exercise to create an energy deficit. The investigators found good correlations between changes in total body water, fat, and fat-free body mass detected by TOBEC and reference methods such as deuterium and underwater weighing. However, some systematic differences were observed between TOBEC and the reference methods. The investigators concluded that TOBEC, with future refinements in software, has the potential to measure reliably changes in total body water, fat, and composition of fat-free body mass during weight loss.

Research Methods

As shown in Figure 3–4, human body composition can be described in terms of five levels ranging from elements to the whole body. Two have already been mentioned: the molecular (chemical) and tissue systems. The whole body level includes measurement levels such as body weight and density, skinfold thicknesses, and circumferences. Since methods needed to evaluate either fat (level II) or adipose tissue (level IV) are limited, those compartments are usually quantified indirectly by using other estimates at the same or different levels. Both direct and indirect research methods of evaluating body fatness are described in this section. Additional references are provided for the reader interested in more in-depth discussions of each topic.

Dual energy x-ray absorptiometry. The recent introduction of whole body dual energy x-ray absorptiometry (DEXA) is an important advance in body composition research. By using an x-ray system that generates two energy distributions, DEXA units enable the clinician or investigator to separate body weight into three chemical (level II) components: fat, fat-free soft tissue, and bone mineral. Regional measurements are also possible, and the usual whole body scan requires 15–20 min and delivers a minimal radiation dose. Obesity, osteoporosis, and other aspects of clinical nutrition can be investigated using DEXA. Additional information on DEXA is presented in the reviews of Mazess et al.,[44] Peppler and Mazess,[45] and Heymsfield et al.[46]

Underwater weighing. One of the oldest body composition methods, underwater weighing or hydrodensitometry, allows the investigator to divide body weight into two chemical (level II) compartments: fat and fat-free body mass. Subjects are immersed in a water-filled tank equipped with a scale for measuring weight during maximal exhalation and submersion.[47] Body density is then calculated after adjustments are made for residual lung volume.[48] The assumption is then made that fat and fat-free body mass have respective densities of 0.9 and 1.1 g/cm^3.[49] These assumptions are incorporated into the Siri equation, which allows calculation of percentage body weight as fat from body density. Siri's review gives an excellent description of the underwater weighing method and its underlying sources or error.[50]

Total body water. During weight stability in the adult, approximately 73% of fat-free body mass is water. Accordingly, if total body water is known, then this approximation allows calculation of fat-free body mass. Fat can then be calculated as the difference between body weight and fat-free body mass. Three isotopes of water can be used clinically to evaluate total body water: ^3H_2O, ^2H_2O, and $H_2{}^{18}O$. The total body water method is described in detail by Schoeller et al.[51–53]

Total body potassium. Potassium is mainly an intracellular cation that has a stable relationship to fat-free body mass in healthy subjects. For young adults, the ratio of total body potassium to fat-free body mass is about 68 mmol/kg, and this ratio tends to decrease with age. Reference values for the potassium content of fat-free body mass are available. Thus, measuring total body potassium can be used to calculate fat-free body mass and fat.[54]

Although total body potassium can be estimated using radioactive isotopes of potassium, the usual approach is to measure ^{40}K in a whole body counter. The naturally occurring radioactive ^{40}K is found in a constant proportion to total body potassium and is easily measured in research laboratories. As intracellular potassium is found under stable conditions at a concentration of 150 mmol/L, total body potassium can also be used to estimate intracellular fluid volume and body cell mass (level III, Figure 3–4).[54]

Neutron activation analysis. Interaction of neutrons with the elements in tissue results in the formation of unstable compounds that decay at varying rates. The decay products differ, but some can be quantified using appropriate detectors.

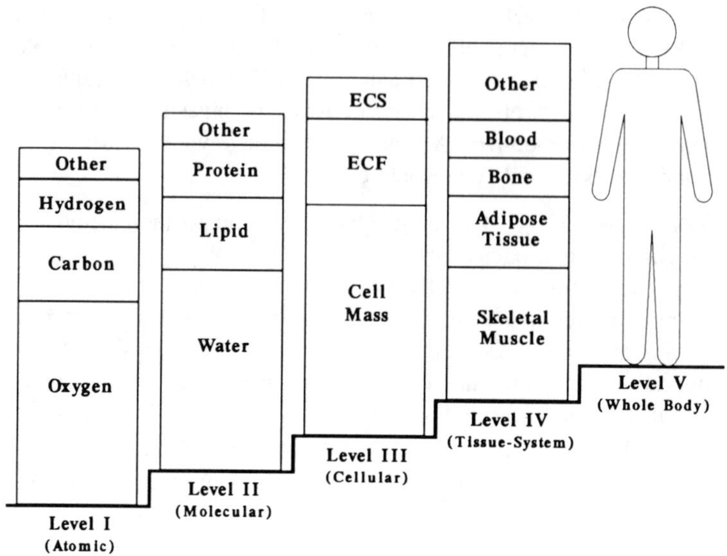

Figure 3–4. The five levels of body composition and the main compartments at each level. ECS, extracellular solids; ECF, extracellular fluid.

(Reprinted from Ref. 14 with permission)

Neutron activation systems contain a neutron source or generator and a detection unit. Exposure of the subject to neutron irradiation followed by counting the decay products allows quantification of at least 11 elements (level I), including carbon, nitrogen, oxygen, sodium, calcium, and hydrogen, which together account for over 95% of body weight. The elements can also be used to calculate chemical compartments such as fat, protein, and bone mineral. Neutron activation is an important research technique but is unavailable or impractical for clinical purposes.[55]

Imaging techniques. The introduction of computed tomography over the past 20 years and the more recent development of magnetic resonance imaging were not only major medical advances but were also important to investigators who study body composition. At present, both techniques are used due to their ability to generate high-resolution cross-sectional images. Magnetic resonance spectroscopy or, more precisely, nuclear magnetic resonance spectroscopy, eventually may also be capable of providing dynamic studies of important tissue substrates. The primary importance of the present imaging capability is that cross-sectional images can be used to assess regional or whole body tissue compartments such as skeleton, skeletal muscle, and adipose tissue (levels III and IV). It is also possible to determine the volume of visceral organs and the distribution of adipose tissue into visceral and subcutaneous components using imaging techniques. Additional information on imaging techniques in the study of body composition can be found in References 56 to 60.

Adipose Tissue Distribution

Adipose tissue is distributed into four main components: subcutaneous, visceral, interstitial, and yellow marrow. The topographic distribution of subcutaneous adipose tissue varies with gender, age, ethnicity, and degree of obesity. Visceral adipose tissue is also distributed into several subcompartments and varies among individuals in amount and location. Beginning in the 1940s, Vague[61,62] suggested that adipose tissue distribution in addition to total adiposity is an independent determinant of morbidity in obese patients. Although several classifications of adipose tissue distributions have been proposed, the one gaining most acceptance at present divides subjects into two categories: upper body, or android, and lower body, or gynoid.[63] Subjects with upper body obesity have a higher waist:hip ratio, increased deposition of visceral or mesenteric adipose tissue, increased circulating insulin levels, a higher degree of insulin resistance, increased serum levels of glucose, elevated blood pressure, and abnormalities of lipid metabolism compared to subjects with lower body adipose tissue distribution.[63,64] Further discussions of the pathophysiology related to upper body obesity are presented in later chapters. The primary concern related to patients with upper body obesity is that morbidity is increased at any level of fatness compared to subjects with lower body obesity.[63] This is shown in Figure 3–5 as the relation between the abdominal:gluteal (waist:hip) ratio, risk, and age for men and women. In addition, the waist:hip ratio may be related to behavioral character-

Figure 3–5. Risk associated with the waist:hip ratio (abdominal:gluteal ratio) for men (left) and women (right) by age groups.

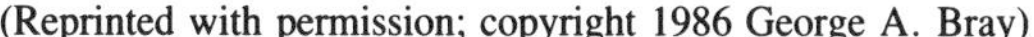
(Reprinted with permission; copyright 1986 George A. Bray)

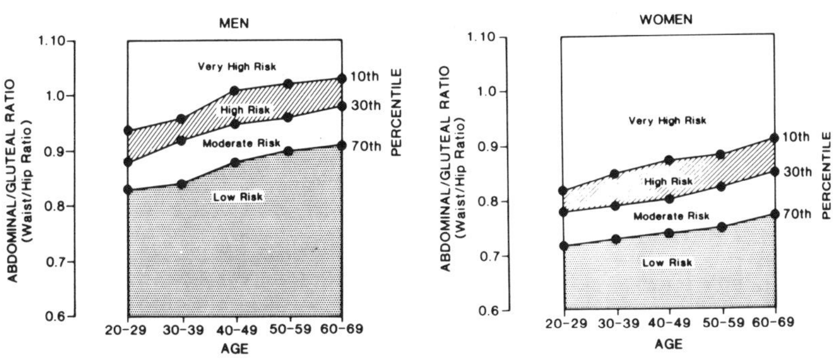

istics such as smoking, high alcohol consumption, sedentary lifestyle, and weight cycling.

Several methods are available for classifying adipose tissue distribution. These methods are in a continuing state of evolution. At present, the most widely accepted clinical measure is the waist:hip ratio.

The waist:hip ratio is easily measured with the use of a tape measure, although there is some variation in the definition of anatomic sites. Recommended sites include the minimal waist or lower border of the 10th rib for waist measurement and the maximal hip or iliac crest for the hip measurement. Whichever sites are chosen, it is important that they be easily identifiable anatomic landmarks and that the same sites be used for comparison over time. The cutoff points for defining upper body obesity vary among investigators as well, although the *Dietary Guidelines for Americans* suggest that men and women with a waist: hip ratio of over 0.95 and 0.80, respectively, are at increased risk.[5]

The waist:hip ratio increases with age and varies with gender. This ratio begins to rise in men in their twenties, while for women the increase begins in their forties. These sex differences continue until the age of 60. Above this age, gender differences are less marked, with increasing individual variability in the waist:hip ratio.[65] African-Americans and Native Americans appear to have a higher waist:hip ratio than their white counterparts.[5] Diabetic patients as a group also have a higher waist:hip ratio than nondiabetic patients of similar age, gender, and body weight.

Wadden et al.[66] studied the changes in waist:hip ratio with weight loss. Baseline results indicated that there was no significant correlation between initial weight, fat weight, or BMI and waist:hip ratio, leading Wadden and his colleagues to conclude that the waist:hip ratio is independent of the degree of obesity. The investigators found that with weight loss, patients with upper body obesity decreased their waist:hip ratio more than did patients with lower body obesity. Some of the difference was explained by regional variation in fat loss. The subjects with lower body obesity lost fat from both the upper and lower body, whereas those with upper body obesity lost fat almost exclusively from upper body stores. The two groups showed a similar decrease in waist circumference, although the group with lower body obesity lost significantly more in the hip measurement compared to the group with upper body obesity.

ENERGY EXPENDITURE

Clinical Relevance

The energy balance equation is well known:

$$\Delta \text{ Storage} = \text{intake} - \text{expenditure}$$

Since obesity involves the storage of excess energy intake as fat, intake and expenditure must be examined to establish whether the obese have a disorder of excessive intake or insufficient expenditure, or both, which results, over time, in the accumulation of excess fat stores. This section focuses on the expenditure term of the equation.

It is customary to divide total energy expenditure (TEE) into three major components (Figure 3–6): resting or basal energy expenditure (REE); thermic effect of food (TEF), also referred to as *dietary-induced thermogenesis;* and physical activity energy expenditure (AEE). The three energy expenditure terms typically account for about 60%, 10%, and 30%, respectively, of TEE in normal, moderately active persons.

Figure 3–6. Components of daily energy expenditure in humans. This example is an approximation for a 70-kg man (10% body fat) fed 3000 kcal/day.

(From Ravussin E, Bogardus C. Relationships of genetics, age, and physical fitness to daily energy expend, and fuel util. *Am J Clin Nutr* 1989; 49:968–975; reprinted with permission)

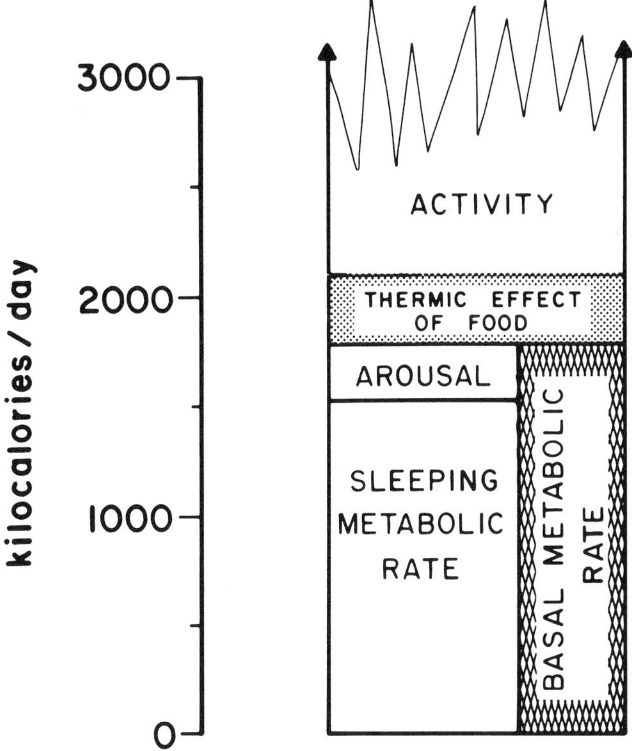

REE represents that portion of energy expended while at rest and after fasting for at least 12 hr (postabsorptive state). Four organs—the heart, liver, kidney, and brain—which comprise 5–6% of body weight, account for about 60–70% of REE.[67]

TEF is the increment in energy expenditure above REE that occurs after ingestion of food (postprandially) and represents the energy demands of digestive processes (biochemical reactions, peristalsis, etc.). Conventionally, TEF is determined over a period of 3–5 hr by subtracting REE measured on 1 day from postprandial energy expenditure measured on another day.

AEE is the increment in energy expenditure resulting from the action of skeletal muscle in performing physical work. It is the most difficult component of energy expenditure to measure accurately under natural conditions because of equipment limitations. A sedentary person may expend as little as 200–300 kcal/day in activity, whereas a world-class marathon runner will expend 2500 kcal during a 2-hr race.

Assessment

Resting energy expenditure. REE may be measured by direct or indirect calorimetry. Direct calorimetry is the measurement of heat given off by radiation, convection, or conduction and is accomplished by enclosing the patient in a special compartment such as a suit, box, or room and measuring heat transfer to the surroundings. Such equipment is usually available only in research settings.

Indirect calorimetry involves the measurement of CO_2, an endpoint of cellular oxidation. Since O_2 is utilized in known proportions during the oxidation of carbohydrate, protein, and fat, the measurement of O_2 intake and CO_2 production permits calculation of the caloric value of fuel oxidized during that period.[68] The sensors and recording instruments necessary to perform these measurements are widely available in an assembly known as a *metabolic cart*. There are a variety of devices for channeling inhaled and exhaled air through the appropriate O_2 and CO_2 sensors, including nose clamps and face masks, canopies, and ventilated hoods.

Many discrepancies in measurement results may be attributed to differences in factors such as the patient's state of relaxation, length of time over which measurements are made, time of day, single versus multiple measurement sessions, and length of fasting and resting periods. Obese patients should have a morning evaluation after an overnight fast of at least 12 hr and following at least 30 min of reclining comfortably in the testing location in a thermoneutral environment. Respiratory gases should be sampled for at least 20 min, with analysis of the O_2 and CO_2 during the last 10–15 min.

If calorimetry equipment is not available, there are equations for estimating REE from body weight, height, age, and sex. Several of these equations are presented in Table 3–9. Many of them will give reasonable results when applied to obese patients; however, estimates should not be mistaken for measured results because these estimates may have a large error in any individual case. These equations tend to overestimate the REE in obese patients, and the error is more significant in males than in females (possibly because the clinical sample of males is, on the whole, more obese). The best estimates for obese patients seem to be made by the Fleisch[69] and Robertson and Reid[70] equations.

Alternatively, REE may be estimated from measurements of fat-free body mass made as described earlier in this chapter. A convenient equation for this

TABLE 3–9 Equations for Estimating Resting Metabolic Rate (kcal/24 hr)

Bernstein et al.[71]	(F) 7.48 (w) − 0.42 (h) − 3.0 (a) + 844
	(M) 11.0 (w) + 10.2 (h) − 5.8 (a) − 1032
Cunningham[72]	501.6 + 21.6 (LBM)
	(F) LBM = (69.8 − 0.26 (w) − 0.12 (a)) × w $\sqrt{73.2}$
	(M) LBM = (79.5 − 0.24 (w) − 0.15 (a)) × w $\sqrt{73.2}$
Harris and Benedict[73]	(F) 655 + 9.5 (w) + 1.9 (h) − 4.7 (a)
	(M) 66 + 13.8 (w) + 5.0 (h) − 6.8 (a)
James[74]	(F) 18 − 30 yr: 487 + 14.8 (w)
	30 − 60 yr: 845 + 8.17 (w)
	>60 yr: 658 + 9.01 (w)
	(M) 18 − 30 yr: 692 + 15.1 (w)
	30 − 60 yr: 873 + 11.6 (w)
	>60 yr: 588 + 11.7 (w)
Mifflin et al.[75]	(F) 9.99 (w) + 6.25 (h) − 4.92 (a) − 161
	(M) 9.99 (w) + 6.25 (h) − 4.92 (a) + 5
Owen et al.[76, 77]	(F) 795 + 7.18 (w)
	(M) 879 + 10.2 (w)
Pavlou et al.[78] (a)	(M) −169.1 + 1.02 (pRMR)
(b)	(M) 2089.7 − 8.17 (h) + 16.8 (w) −8.9 (a) − 1.03 (%AIBW)
Equations using body surface area (BSA) and tabled values given in references	
	BSA (m^2) = 0.007184 $(w)^{0.425} \times h^{0.725}$
	RMR = BSA × 24 × tabled value
Aub and Dubois[79]	See tabled values
Boothby et al.[80]	See tabled values
Fleisch[69]	See tabled values
Robertson and Reid[70]	See tabled values

Abbreviations: F, female; M, male; w, weight (kg); h, height (cm); a, age (years); pRMR, predicted RMR by the Harris Benedict equation; %AIBW, percentage above ideal body weight; LBM, lean body mass, used here as equivalent to FFM.

purpose is REE = 370 + 21.6 × FFM.[81] Again, the standard error of the estimate tends to be large and may be significant when the equation is applied to an individual.

Thermic effect of food. TEF is assessed by measuring energy expenditure, in the manner described above, on 2 successive days. On one day, a series of standard REE measures are taken with gas samples at 30-min intervals in the morning after a 12-h fast. On another day, an identical series of measures is taken after ingestion of a standard meal. The standard meal is often a quantity (250–750 kcal) of a liquid food supplement, such as Sustacal (Mead Johnson Nutritional Division, Warswill, Ind) or Ensure (Ross Pharmaceutical, Columbus, Ohio), which consists of known standard proportions of carbohydrate, protein, and fat. The TEF is calculated from the increment in energy expenditure above the fasting metabolic rate following meal ingestion. It is important to continue measurements over an adequate time interval (3–5 hr) so that the effect is fully measured, that is, until the elevation in energy expenditure seen postprandially has returned to near baseline levels.

Here too, methodologic details are important and may lead to significant differences in results. Meal size (250–1200 kcal), meal state (liquid vs. solid), macronutrient composition (amount of protein, carbohydrate, fat, or proportions of these in a mixed meal), time of day, length of time over which measurements are taken (3–6 hr following ingestion), and specific food (e.g., content of glucose, fructose) may affect the magnitude of the TEF. Sources of error include day-to-day variation in baseline REE and subject fidgeting or dozing over the duration of the test.

Activity energy expenditure. AEE has been measured by indirect calorimetry by having subjects wear a mask and a portable gas sampling apparatus. However, such devices are cumbersome, interfere with normal activities, and distort the result.

For research purposes, subjects may be housed in special chambers that contain devices for measuring physical activity, such as ultrasonic or radar motion detectors, floor sensors, and photoelectric cells. These records of movements must eventually be converted to approximate energy equivalents.

In nonresearch settings, AEE may be measured by using accelerometers, pedometers, actometers, and similar devices. These detect acceleration/deceleration in one or more planes. They are worn affixed to a part of the body, and record the frequency and intensity of displacements of the body part to which they are attached. The records can then be used to estimate the amount of work performed and the AEE.[82] Alternatively, miniature heart rate recorders have long been used to monitor exercise training intensity, and the recent addition of memory capability enabling storage of heart rate data over a 24-hr period allows them to be used in estimating energy expenditure.[83] Data may be transferred from the device to a computer for analysis by software supplied by the manufacturer.

To obtain reasonable accuracies (e.g., standard deviation of differences from the doubly labeled water method = ±20%) with any of the above devices, they must be calibrated for each individual at several representative activity levels against an already validated energy expenditure measurement technique such as indirect calorimetry while on a graded treadmill. Equations based only on population average calibrations give poor estimates because of large individual differences in the relation of physical movement and heart rate to energy expenditure.[84] Even when calibrated for a particular individual, heart rate measures are prone to errors at low activity levels. Most accelerometers do not register in all three dimensions, and energy costs for movement in each plane may require different calibrations.

In the absence of mechanical records of physical activity, self-report diaries may be employed. Patients are asked to keep detailed records of activities in 15-min intervals over one or more 24-hr periods. These 15-min intervals are grouped into categories on the basis of intensity of activity, and the categories correspond to REE multipliers (Table 3–10). The measured or estimated REE can be used with these multipliers for each category of activity intensity and the products summed over a 24-hr period to get estimates of 24-hr energy expenditure.[85] The accuracy of the results depends to a great extent on the quality of record keeping, but there is a moderate correlation (r = 0.5–0.8) with values obtained by other methods.[86]

Total energy expenditure. At times it may be important to know simply what the TEE is, without regard to the contributions of the various components. If a person can be maintained at a stable weight on a known caloric intake, then, with certain caveats, the TEE must equal the energy intake. The caloric content of liquid meal replacement products is usually given, and the quantity consumed can be titrated to achieve weight stability. The procedure must be carried out over a relatively long time to ensure that weight loss or gain is not occurring at a very slow rate, since even small changes in fat stores represent large amounts of energy.

The caveats have to do with weight stability and changes in body composition. Hydration or dehydration may produce changes in body weight without changes in energy storage or, alternatively, may mask changes in energy stores. Similarly, the replacement of a unit weight of adipose tissue by an equal weight of skeletal muscle represents a change of about 5300 kcal of energy stores that will pass undetected by measures of body weight.

Although presently expensive, a very useful methodology for measuring free-living TEE that will be increasingly important in the future is that of doubly labeled water, $^{2}H_2{}^{18}O$, using stable isotopes of hydrogen (^{2}H) and oxygen (^{18}O).

TABLE 3–10 Activities, Energy Costs, and Corresponding Categorical Values

Categorical Value	Examples of Activities	Energy Cost in Mets from Various Studies		Median Energy Cost Used	
		Minimum	Maximum	Mets	kcal/kg/15 min
1	Sleeping, resting in bed	1.0		1.0	0.26
2	Sitting: eating, listening, writing, etc.	1.0	2.0	1.5	0.38
3	Light activity standing: washing, shaving, combing hair, cooking, etc.	2.0	3.0	2.3	0.57
4	Slow walk (<4 km/hr), driving, to dress, to shower, etc.	2.0	4.0	2.8	0.69
5	Light manual work: floor sweeping, window washing, driving a truck, painting, waiting on tables, nursing chores, several house chores, chores of electrician, or barman, walking at rate of 4–6 km/hr	2.3	5.0	3.3	0.84
6	Leisure activities and sports in a recreational environment: baseball, golf, volleyball, canoeing, rowing, archery, bowling, cycling (<10 km/hr), table tennis, etc.	3.0	8.0	4.8	1.2
7	Manual work at a moderate pace: mining, carpentry, house building, lumbering and wood cutting, snow shoveling, loading and unloading goods, etc.	4.0	8.0	5.6	1.4
8	Leisure and sport activities of higher intensity (not competitive): canoeing (5–8 km/hr), bicyling (>15 km/hr), dancing, skiing, badminton, gymnastics, swimming, tennis, horseback riding, walking, (>6 km/hr), etc.	5.0	11	6.0	1.5
9	Intense manual work, high-intensity sport activities, or sport competition: tree cutting, carring heavy loads, jogging and running (>9 km/hr), racquetball, swimming, tennis, cross-country skiing (>8 km/hr), hiking, mountain climbing, etc.	6.0	15	7.8	2.0

Sources: Reprinted from refs 85, 86 & Durnin J&GA, Passmore R. Energy, Work and Leisure. London: Heinemann Educ Books Ltd, 1967 with

Because hydrogen is eliminated from the body only as a component of H_2O, while oxygen is eliminated as both H_2O and CO_2, the difference in disappearance rates may be used to calculate CO_2 production and TEE. Measures can be taken over a period of 1 to 2 weeks. The technique is currently expensive due to the limited supply of isotopes and the need for mass spectrometry equipment for analysis.[87]

As a rule of thumb, TEE is about 1.7 times the REE for moderately active individuals.[88]

Significance of Energy Expenditure Measurement for Obesity Management and Weight Control

Obesity usually occurs gradually, developing over several years, and possibly resulting from only a small imbalance between intake and expenditure. Most of the methods described above have enough measurement error so that a small abnormality in energy expenditure would escape detection. Much recent work is aimed at obtaining more accurate measures of energy expenditure components over a longer period of time so that the question of disorders in thermogenesis can be definitively answered.

Are the obese different from the nonobese in the various components of energy expenditure? If they are, do these differences persist after weight reduction to near-normal weight? If so, do they also precede the onset of obesity and might they have caused it? And, finally, do these differences have implications for treatment, maintenance, or relapse prevention? The next section takes up some of these issues.

Resting energy expenditure. There is little doubt that the obese have higher REE values when matched for height and age than the nonobese. However, when adjusted for differences in body weight, the REE tends to be lower per unit weight for an obese person than would be expected for a nonobese person. This can be explained in terms of body composition. Fat-free mass, which is the more metabolically active compartment, is a smaller portion of the total weight of an obese person.

When standardized by fat-free mass, do the obese have REE values similar to those of the nonobese? The answer to this question is complicated by technical difficulties in measuring fat-free body mass in obese persons (e.g., more extracellular fluid in obese fat-free mass; ^{40}K, which is measured in whole body potassium counters, is attenuated by large fat deposits). Some older research reviews concluded that, once standardized for fat-free mass, lean and obese persons, both male and female, are similar to REE.[72] More recently, however, studies show an additional contribution to REE attributable to fat even after adjusting for fat-free mass.[71,72,89] This implies that once fat is lost, even if fat-free mass is maintained, the REE will necessarily be lower than before weight loss. Fortunately, the metabolic activity attributable to the fat stores is low, about one-third to one-fourth that of fat-free mass per unit weight. Consequently, the decrease in REE after fat loss should not be large and can be made up by small increases in fat-free body mass.

It is well known that REE decreases during severe caloric restriction, with a rapid decline before large amounts of weight have been lost, possibly through anatomic nervous system, hormonal, endocrine, and other mechanisms. The decrease in REE can be a source of frustration to a patient trying to lose weight through caloric restriction because the same degree of restriction that initially produced weight loss may become ineffective. The exact degree of deprivation that engages these various mechanisms is not known. There are reports of 1200-kcal diets in which REE is not significantly affected.[90] An important question for treatment, however, is whether these declines in REE during caloric restriction persist after weight reduction. This question can be answered only after a period of weight stability at the lower weight so that decreases in energy expenditure in response to caloric restriction sufficient to produce weight loss are clearly distinguished from an enduring decrease in energy expenditure after stabilization. The studies that exist are inconclusive. Some find no disproportionate decline,[91] while others do.[92,93]

On balance, however, after moderate amounts of weight loss, it seems that during maintenance, REE tends to return to levels near what would be expected for persons undergoing a given loss of fat-free body mass. If there is a remaining discrepancy, it may be due to decreased energy costs of fat storage[94] or to disproportionate loss of tissue in some of the more metabolically active organs.[95]

There is some evidence that REE differences may predate obesity. REE has been shown to have a heritable component. For example, it is more similar within families than between families;[96] in one prospective study, individuals who had lower REE values had a higher risk of developing obesity.[97] Also, infants who later became obese had a 20% lower TEE than those who did not, even at a point where they were indistinguishable with respect to body size and fatness.[98] This variation may be one of the mechanisms underlying the finding that obesity itself has a large heritable component.[99]

Why is REE lower in some individuals? Some recent work has found that the oxygen uptake of skeletal muscle may account for a significant part of the individual variation.[100] Although skeletal muscle has relatively low oxygen consumption in the resting state, it is a large compartment (about 50%) of adipose tissue free weight (level IV, Figure 3–4) and thus accounts for about 30% of resting metabolic rate. Another basis for REE differences may be sympathetic nervous system activation,[101] which could account for individual differences in heat production.

At present, little can be done to increase REE while holding fat-free body mass constant. Pharmacologic agents that increase the metabolic rate through sympathetic nervous system stimulation also tend to increase the heart rate and blood pressure. Thyroid supplements are sometimes given for a "sluggish" metabolism, but unless the patient is clearly hypothyroid, this may only serve to suppress endogenous production. Exercise will help build or conserve muscle mass, which contributes to enhanced REE, although any increase in muscle mass will reduce apparent weight loss.

Thermic effect of food. Many studies have suggested that obese people have a diminished TEF response. For example, in one study, lean and obese men matched for age, fat-free body mass, and fitness were given a 720-kcal liquid mixed meal (24% protein, 21% fat, and 55% carbohydrate). Over a 6-hr measurement period the TEF was 100 ± 12 kcal for the lean men and 69 ± 5 kcal for the obese.[102] The magnitude of the difference, about 30 kcal over 6 hr, is not large but could be significant over a long time.

There is some evidence that this difference in TEF may be related to impaired activity of the sympathetic nervous system. It has been shown that decreased sympathetic nervous system activity, as measured by fasting norepinephrine levels, is associated with increased amounts of body fat.[103] Another study showed that TEF in response to a meal, although lower in obese than in lean subjects, was made similar in both groups by administering a dose of ephedrine hydrochloride. The increase in TEF produced by the ephedrine was minor for the lean subjects but significant for the obese. Furthermore, in the obese group alone, the thermogenic effect of ephedrine was potentiated by aspirin.[104]

The research literature is by no means unanimous in finding a diminished TEF in the obese; many studies find no difference.[105] The lack of consistency may be the result of differences in methodology, differences in type of obesity, or poor reproducibility of measures of TEF.

A further issue is whether the diminished TEF is a cause of obesity or a consequence. Comparisons of postobese with matched lean controls showed no significant differences in TEF on a mixed meal,[105,106] and at least one researcher has claimed that TEF responses are not predictive of weight gain.[107]

Activity energy expenditure. An obvious questions is whether the obese are more sedentary and less active than nonobese. Although, as usual, there are conflicting results from many studies, on balance the answer is probably yes if activity is measured by actometers registering movements.[108] There is a known genetic component to the level of habitual physical activity.[109]

Part of the problem is how activity levels can be compared, since the added weight of the obese person will result in a greater energy cost for the same activity. One way of making activity levels approximately comparable is to use the ratio of TEE to REE, which indicates what proportion of an individual's energy expenditure comes from activity and TEF. Since TEF is usually small compared to AEE, the ratio is an approximate indicator of activity level.

A study of energy expenditure in obese and nonobese adolescents using doubly labeled water showed higher TEE and REE values in the obese subjects. However, the TEE:REE ratio was about 1.7 for males and females and did not differ for obese compared to nonobese subjects. Thus, differences in TEE did not appear to account for maintenance of obesity in adolescents.[110] A similar study of normal and overweight adult women also showed no differences in free-living energy expenditure.[88]

Does increased expenditure from activity result in a compensatory increase in food intake? This question has been intensively studied under metabolic ward conditions with normal and overweight women (mean, 167% of ideal body weight) and moderate levels of exercise (110% and 140% of REE).[111] The investigators concluded that normal-weight subjects adjusted their intake to match their level of expenditure and maintained their body weight, but that overweight women did not adequately compensate and lost weight.

Exercise conserves and replaces lean mass during weight loss, thus helping to maintain REE. In one study, moderately overweight men were randomized into a diet group or an exercise group. After 1 year both groups showed significant weight and fat mass loss compared to controls. However, the exercise group showed no change in energy expenditure, while the diet group showed a small decrease.[112]

Is difference in activity level a cause or a consequence of obesity? Some research suggests that, in children, reduced energy spent on activity may increase the susceptibility to obesity.[113]

With respect to its role in treatment, increased exercise seems desirable from several points of view (psychological and other health benefits independent of weight loss), but good data showing its efficacy for weight loss are lacking. Increased activity does not seem to enhance weight loss because it conserves or builds fat-free body mass, so that even though body composition is changing in a favorable direction, this is not readily apparent from measures of body weight alone.

SUMMARY

The assessment of body composition and energy expenditure is central to the evaluation and treatment of obesity. The intent of this chapter was to provide a broad overview of these areas and to give the practitioner with limited facilities guidelines on how to initiate clinical assessments of body composition and energy expenditure. In-depth texts and reviews, postgraduate courses, and seminars, as well as other chapters in this volume, provide additional sources of information on the techniques and application of body composition and energy expenditure assessments.

REFERENCES

1. Davenport CB. *Body Build and Its Inheritance*. Publication 329. Washington, DC: Carnegie Institute of Washington, 1923.
2. *1959 Build and Blood Pressure Study*. Society of Actuaries and Association of Life Insurance Medical Directors of America, 1960.
3. *1979 Build Study*. New York: Society of Actuaries and Association of Life Insurance Medical Directors of America, 1980.
4. Revicki D, Israel R. Relationship between body mass indices and measures of body adiposity. *Am J Pub Health* 76:992, 1986.
5. Cole TJ. Weight-stature indices to measure underweight, overweight, and obesity in anthropometric assessment of nutritional status, p. 83–111, 1991 Wiley Liss Inc. Ed. J. H. Hines, New York.
6. Womersley J, Durnin JVGA. A comparison of the skinfold method with extent of "overweight" and various weight–height relationships in the assessment of obesity. *Br J Nutr* 38:271, 1977.
7. Smalley KJ, Knerr AK, Kendrick ZV, et al. Reassessment of body mass indices. *Am J Clin Nutr* 52:405, 1990.
8. Gray DS. Diagnosis and prevalence of obesity, in Bray GA (ed), *The Medical Clinics of North America*. Philadelphia, Harcourt Brace Jovanovich, 1989, pp. 1–14.
9. Garn S, Leonard WR, Hawthorns VM. Three limitations of the body mass index. *Am J Clin Nutr* 44:996, 1986.
10. Norgan NG, Ferro-Luzz A. Weight–height indices as estimators of fatness in men. *Hum Nutr Clin Nutr* 36c:363, 1982.
11. Frisancho AR. *Anthropometric Standards for the Assessment of Growth and Nutritional Status*. Ann Arbor, University of Michigan Press, 1990, p. 47.
12. Frisancho AR, Flegel PN. Elbow breadth as a measure of frame size for United States males and females. *Am J Clin Nutr* 37:311, 1983.
13. Wang J, Pierson RN Jr. Disparate hydration of adipose and lean tissue require a new model for body water distribution in man. *J Nutr* 106:1687, 1976.
14. Wang Z, Pierson RN Jr, Heymsfield SB. The five level model: A new approach to organizing body composition research. *Am J Clin Nutr* 56:19–28, 1992.
15. Roche AF, Chumlea WMC. New approaches to the clinical assessment of adipose tissue, in Bjorntorp P, Brodoff BN (eds), *Obesity*. Philadelphia, JB Lippincott, 1992, pp. 55–66.
16. Bray GA, Greenway FL, Molitch ME, et al. Use of anthropometric measures to assess weight loss. *Am J Clin Nutr* 31:769, 1978.

17. Lohman TG, Roche AF, Martorell R (eds). *Anthropometric Standardization Reference Manual*. Champaign, Ill. Human Kinetics Books, 1988.

18. Roche A. Some aspects of the criterion methods for the measurement of body composition. *Hum Biol* 59:209, 1987.

19. Pollock, ML. Research progress in validation of clinical methods of assessing body composition. *Med Sci Sports Exerc* 16:606, 1984.

20. Gray DS. Changes in bioelectrical impedance during fasting. *Am J Clin Nutr* 48:1184, 1988.

21. Paijans I, Wilmore K, Wilmore J. Use of skinfolds and bioelectrical impedance for body composition assessment after substantial and rapid weight reduction. *Am Coll Nutr J* 11(2): 145–51, 1992.

22. Scherf J, Franklin BA, Lucas CP, et al. Validity of skinfold thickness measures of formerly obese adults. *Am J Clin Nutr* 43:128, 1986.

23. Barrows K, Snook JT. Effect of a high-protein, very-low-calorie diet on resting metabolism, thyroid hormones, and energy expenditure of obese middle-aged women. *Am J Clin Nutr* 15(2): 391–98, 1987.

24. Allen TH, Peng MT, Chen KP, Huang TF, Chang C, Fang HS. Prediction of total adiposity from skinfolds and the curvilinear relationship between external and internal adiposity. Metabolism 5:346–352, 1956.

25. Kushner R, Schoeller D. Estimation of total body water by bioelectrical impedance analysis. *Am J Clin Nutr* 44:417, 1986.

26. Segal KR, Van Loan M, Fitzgerald PI, et al. Lean body mass estimation by bioelectrical impedance analysis: A four site cross validation study. *Am J Clin Nutr* 47:7, 1988.

27. Segal KR, Burastero S, Chun, A, et al. Estimation of extracellular and total body water by multiple-frequency bioelectrical impedance measurement. *Am J Clin Nutr* 54:26, 1991.

28. Van Loan M, Mayclin P. Bioelectrical impedance analysis: Is it a reliable estimator of lean body mass and total body water? *Hum Biol* 2:299, 1987.

29. Lukaski HC, Johnson PE, Bolonchuk WW, et al. Assessment of fat-free mass using bioelectrical impedance measurements of the human body. *Am J Clin Nutr* 41:810, 1985.

30. Hodgdon J, Fitzgerald PI. Validity of impedance predictions at various levels of fatness. *Hum Biol* 59:281, 1987.

31. Ross R, Leger L, Martin P, et al. Sensitivity of bioelectrical impedance to detect changes in human body composition. *J Appl Physiol* 67:1643, 1989.

32. Rising R, Swinburn B, Larson K, et al. Body composition in Pima Indians: Validation of bioelectrical resistance. *Am J Clin Nutr* 53:594, 1991.

33. Deurenberg P, Weststrate JA, Hautvast JGAJ. Changes in fat-free mass during weight loss measured by bioelectrical impedance and by densitometry. *Am J Clin Nutr* 49:33, 1989.

34. Cochran WJ, Fiorotto ML, Sheng HP, et al. Reliability of fat-free mass estimates derived from total body electrical conductivity measurements as influenced by changes in extracellular fluid volume. *Am J Clin Nutr* 49:29, 1989.

35. Van Itallie TB, Segal KR, Yang M, et al. Clinical assessment of body fat content in adults: Potential role of electrical impedance methods, in Roche AF (ed), *Body Composition Assessment in Youth and Adults. Report of the Sixth Ross Conference on Medical Research.* Columbus, Ohio, Ross Laboratories, 1987, pp. 5–9.

36. Horswill CA, Geeseman R, Boileau RA, et al. Total body electrical conductivity (TOBEC): Relationship to estimates of muscle mass, fat-free weight, and lean body mass. *Am J Clin Nutr* 49:593, 1989.

37. Boileau RA. *Utilization of Total Body Electrical Conductivity in Determining Body Composition.* National Academy of Sciences, National Research Council, Board of Agriculture Symposium on The Measurement, Management and Modification of Nutritional Attributes of Animal Products, Woods Hole, Mass., August 14–15, 1986.

38. Harrison G. The measurement of total body electrical conductivity. *Hum Biol* 59:311, 1987.

39. Segal KR, Gutin B, Presta E, et al. Estimation of human body composition by electrical impedance methods: A comparative study. *J Appl Physiol* 58:1565, 1985.

40. Presta E, Segal KR, Gutin B, et al. Comparison in man of total body electrical conductivity and lean body mass derived from body density: Validation of a new body composition method. *Metabolism* 32:524, 1983.

41. Van Itallie TB. Recent developments in obesity research electromagnetic tools for measuring total body fat. *Alabama J Med Sci* 21:396, 1984.

42. Van Loan M, Segal KR, Bracco F, et al. TOBEC methodology for body composition assessment: A cross validation study. *Am J Clin Nutr* 46:9, 1987.

43. Van Loan M, Belko AZ, Mayclin PL, et al. Use of total-body electrical conductivity for monitoring body composition changes during weight reduction. *Am J Clin Nutr* 46:5, 1987.

44. Mazess RB, Peppler WW, Gibbons M. Total body composition by dual-photon (153 Gd) absorptiometry. *Am J Clin Nutr* 40:834, 1984.

45. Peppler WW, Mazess RB. Total body bone mineral and lean body mass by dual-photon absorptiometry 1: Theory and measurement procedure. *Calcif Tissue Int* 33:353, 1981.

46. Heymsfield SB, Wang J, Aulet M, et al. Dual photon absorptiometry: Validation of mineral and fat measurements, in Yasumura S (ed), *In Vivo Body Composition Studies*. New York, Plenum Press, 1990, pp. 327–38.

47. Akers R, Buskirk ER. An underwater weighing system utilizing *Force Cube* transducers. *J Appl Physiol* 26:649, 1969.

48. Wilmore J. A simplified method for determining residual lung volumes. *J Appl Physiol* 27:96, 1969.

49. Buskirk ER. Underwater weighing and body density: A review of procedures, in Brozek J, Henschel A (eds), *Techniques for Measuring Body Composition*. Washington, DC, National Academy of Sciences, National Research Council, 1981.

50. Siri WE. Body composition from fluid spaces and density: analysis of methods, in Brozek J, Henschel A (eds), *Techniques for Measuring Body Composition*. Washington, DC, National Academy of Sciences, National Research Council, 1961.

51. Schoeller DA, Kushner RF, Tayor P, et al. Measurement of Total Body Water: Isotope Dilution Techniques. Presented at the Sixth Ross Conference on Body Composition Assessments in Youth and Adults, Ross Laboratories, Columbus, Ohio, 1986.

52. Schoeller DA, Jones PJH. Measurement of total body water by isotope dilution: A unified approach to calculations, in Ellis KJ, Yasumura S, Morgan WD (eds), *In Vivo Body Composition Studies*. London, Institute of Physical Sciences in Medicine, 1987, pp. 138–143.

53. Schoeller DA, van Santen E, Peterson, DW, et at. Total body water measurement in humans with ^{18}O and ^{2}H labeled water. *Am J Clin Nutr* 33:2686, 1980.

54. Pierson RN Jr., Lin DHY, Phillips RA. Total body potassium in health: Effects of age, sex, height, and fat. *Am J Physiol* 226:206, 1974.

55. Keyhayias JJ, Heymsfield SB, Dilmanian FA, et al. Measurement of body fat by neutron inelastic scattering: Comments on installation, operation, and error analysis, in Yasumura S (ed), *In Vivo Body Composition Studies*. New York, Plenum Press, 1990. pp. 339–46.

56. Heymsfield SB, Noel RA. Radiographic analysis of body composition by computerized axial tomography, in Newell GR, Ellison NM (eds), *Nutrition and Cancer*. New York. Raven Press, 1981, pp. 161–172.

57. Heymsfield SB. Human body composition: Analysis by computerized axial tomography and nuclear magnetic resonance, in *AIN Symposium Proceedings*. Bethesda, MD, American Institute of Nutrition, 1987, pp. 92–96.

58. Sjcstrom L, Kvist H, Cederblad, A et al. Determination of total adipose tissue and body fat in women by computed tomography, ^{40}K, and tritium. *Am Physiol Soc* 250:E736, 1986.

59. Lewis DS, Rollwitz WL, Bertrand HA, et al. Use of NMR for measurement of total body water and estimation of body fat. *J Appl Physiol* 60:836, 1986.

60. Gumby P. The new wave in medicine: Nuclear magnetic resonance. *JAMA* 247:151, 1982.

61. Vague J. Les obesities etude biometrique. *Biol Med* 36:1, 1947.

62. Vague J. The degree of masculine differentiation of obesities: A factor determining predisposition to diabetes, atherosclerosis, gout, and uric calculous disease. *Am J Clin Nutr* 4:20, 1956.

63. Kissebah AH, Freedman DS, Peiris AN. Health risks of obesity, in Bray GA (ed), *The Medical Clinics of North America*. Philadelphia, Harcourt Brace Jovanovich, 1989, pp. 111–38.

64. Seidell JC, Bakx JC, De Boer E, et al. Fat distribution of overweight persons in relation to morbidity and subjective health. *Int J Obes* 9:363, 1985.

65. Forbes GB. The abdomen:hip ratio. Normative data and observations on selected patients. *Int J Obes* 14:149, 1990.

66. Wadden T, Stunkard A, Johnston F, et al. Body fat deposition in adult obese women. II. Changes in fat distribution accompanying weight reduction. *Am J Clin Nutr* 47:229, 1988.

67. Grande F. Energy expenditure of organs and tissues, in Kinney J (ed), *Assessment of Energy Metabolism in Health and Disease, Ross Conference on Medical Research*. Columbus, Ohio, Ross Laboratories, 1980, pp. 88–91.

68. Weir JB de V. New methods for calculating metabolic rate with special reference to protein metabolism. *J Physiol* 109:1, 1949.

69. Fleisch A. Le metabolisme basal standard et sa determination au moyen du Metabo-calculator. *Helv Med Acta*. 1:23, 1951.

70. Robertson JD, Reid DD. Standards for the basal metabolism of normal people in Britain. *Lancet* 1:940, 1952.

71. Bernstein RS, Thornton JC, Yang MU, et al. Prediction of the resting metabolic rate in obese patients. *Am J Clin Nutr* 37:595, 1983.

72. Cunningham JJ. A reanalysis of the factors influencing basal metabolic rate in normal adults. *Am J Clin Nutr* 33:2372, 1980.

73. Harris JA, Benedict FG. *Biometric Studies of Basal Metabolism in Man*. Pub. No. 297. Washington, DC. Carnegie Institute of Washington, 1919.

74. James WPT. Dietary aspects of obesity. *Postgrad Med J* 60 (Suppl 3):50, 1984.

75. Mifflin MD, St Jeor ST, Hill LA, et al. A new predictive equation for resting energy expenditure in healthy individuals. *Am J Clin Nutr* 51:241, 1990.

76. Owen OE, Holup JL, D'Alessio DA, et al. A reappraisal of the caloric requirements of men. *Am J Clin Nutr* 46:875, 1987.

77. Owen OE, Kavle E, Owen RS, et al. A reappraisal of caloric requirements in healthy women. *Am J Clin Nutr* 44:1, 1986.

78. Pavlou KN, Hoeffer MA, Blackburn GL. Resting energy expenditure in moderate obesity: Predicting velocity of weight loss. *Ann Surg* 203:136, 1986.

79. Aub JC, DuBois EF. The basal metabolism of old men. *Arch Intern Med* 19:823, 1917.

80. Boothby WM, Berkson J, Dunn HL. Studies of the energy metabolism of normal individuals: A standard for basal metabolism with a nomogram for clinical application. *Am J Physiol* 116:468, 1936.

81. Cunningham JJ. Body composition as a determinant of energy expenditure: A synthetic review and a proposed general prediction equation. *Am J Clin Nutr* 54:963, 1991.

82. Tryon WW. *Activity Measurement in Psychology and Medicine*. New York, Plenum Press, 1991.

83. Livingstone MRE, Prentic AM, Coward WA, et al. Simultaneous measurement of free living energy expenditure by the doubly labeled water method and heart rate monitoring. *Am J Clin Nutr* 52:59, 1990.
84. Haskell WL, Yee MC Evans A, Irby PJ. Simultaneous measurement of heart rate and body motion to quantitate physical activity. *Med Sci Sports Exerc* 25:109, 1993.
85. Bouchard C, Tremblay A, Leblanc C, et al. A method to assess energy expenditure in children and adults. *Am J Clin Nutr* 37:461, 1983.
86. Schulz S, Westerterp KR, Brück K. Comparison of energy expenditure by the doubly labeled water technique with energy intake, heart rate and activity recording in man. *Am J Clin Nutr* 49:1146, 1989.
87. Schoeller DA. Measurement of energy expenditure in free-living humans using doubly labeled water. *J Nutr* 118:1278, 1988.
88. Welle S, Forbes GB, Statt M, et al. Energy expenditure under free-living conditions in normal-weight and overweight women. *Am J Clin Nutr* 55:14, 1992.
89. Garby L, Garrow JS, Jorgensen B, et al. Relation between energy expenditure and body composition in man: Specific energy expenditure in vivo of fat and fat-free tissues. *Eur J Clin Nutr* 42:301, 1988.
90. Wadden TA, Foster GD, Letizia KA, et al. Long-term effects of dieting on resting metabolic rate in obese outpatients. *JAMA* 264:707, 1990.
91. Dore C, Hesp R, Wilkins D, et al. Prediction of energy requirements of obese patients after massive weight loss. *Hum Nutr Clin Nutr* 36C:41, 1982.
92. Elliot DL, Goldberg L, Kuehl KS, et al. Sustained depression of the resting metabolic rate after massive weight loss. *Am J Clin Nutr* 49:93, 1989.
93. Leibel RL, Hirsch J. Diminished energy requirements in reduced-obese patients. *Metabolism* 33:164, 1984.
94. Heshka S. Yang MU, Wang J, et al. Weight loss and change in resting metabolic rate. *Am J Clin Nutr* 52:981, 1990.
95. Burrin DG, Ferrell CL, Briton RA, et al. Level of nutrition and visceral organ size and metabolic activity in sheep. *Br J Nutr* 64:439, 1990.
96. Bogardus C, Lillioja S, Ravussin E, et al. Familial dependence of the resting metabolic rate. *N Engl J Med* 315:96, 1986.
97. Ravussin E, Lillioja S, Knowler WC, et al. Reduced rate of energy expenditure as a risk factor for body-weight gain. *N Engl J Med* 318:467, 1988.
98. Roberts SB, Savage J, Coward WA, et al. Energy expenditure and intake in infants born to lean and overweight mothers. *N Engl J Med* 318:461, 1988.
99. Stunkard AJ, Sorensen TIA, Hanis C, et al. An adoption study of human obesity. *N Engl J Med* 314:193, 1986.
100. Zurlo F, Larson K, Bogardus C, et al. Skeletal muscle metabolism is a major determinant of resting energy expenditure. *J Clin Invest* 86:1423, 1990.
101. Dulloo A, Miller DS. Obesity: A disorder of the sympathetic nervous system. *World Rev Nutr Diet* 50:1, 1988.

102. Segal KR, Edano A, Thomas MB. Thermic effect of a meal over 3 and 6 hours in lean and obese men. *Metabolism* 38:985, 1990.
103. Peterson HR, Rothschild M, Weinberg CR, et al. Body fat and the activity of the autonomic nervous system. *N Engl J Med* 318:1077, 1988.
104. Horton TJ, Geissler CA. Aspirin potentiates the effect of ephedrine on the thermogenic response to a meal in obese but not lean women. *Int J Obesity* 15:359, 1991.
105. Bukkens S, McNeill G, Smith JS, et al. Post-prandial thermogenesis in post-obese women and weight-matched controls. *Int J Obesity* 15:147, 1991.
106. Thorne A, Naslund I, Wahren J. Meal induced thermogenesis in previously obese patients. *Clin Physiol* 10:99, 1990.
107. Matthews D, Heymsfield SB. ASPEN 1990 Research Workshop on Energy Metabolism. *J Parenter Enter Nutr* 15:3, 1991.
108. Shah M, Jefferey RW. Is obesity due to overeating and inactivity or to a defective metabolic rate? A review. *Ann Behav Med* 3:73, 1991.
109. Perusse L, Tremblay A, Leblanc C, et al. Genetic and environmental influences on the level of habitual physical activity and exercise participation. *Am J Epidemiol* 129:1012, 1989.
110. Bandini LG, Schoeller DA, Dietz WH. Energy expenditure in obese and nonobese adolescents. *Pediatr Res* 27:198, 1990.
111. Woo R, Pi-Sunyer FX. Effect of increased physical activity on voluntary intake in lean women. *Metabolism* 34:836, 1985.
112. Frey-Hewitt B, Vranizan KM, Dreon DM, et al. The effect of weight loss by dieting or exercise on resting metabolic rate in overweight men. *Int J Obes* 14:327, 1990.
113. Gortmaker SL, Dietz WH Jr, Cheung LWY. Inactivity, diet, and the fattening of America. *J Am Diet Assoc* 90:1247, 1990.

CHAPTER 4

Metabolic Abnormalities of Obesity

Claudia S. Plaisted, M.S., R.D.
and Nawfal W. Istfan, M.D., Ph.D.

INTRODUCTION

Although epidemiologic studies[1–4] indicate elevated rates of morbidity and mortality in the obese population, the actual mechanisms by which these abnormalities become manifest are incompletely understood. As suggested recently by Grundy and Barnett[5] and previously by Wooley and Wooley,[6] obesity may pose a significant risk only to those individuals who have an underlying metabolic abnormality—a risk that exists on a continuum: Defects may be due to the complications of overnutrition and obesity even at the high end of the generally desirable body mass index (BMI) range of 19 to 27 kg/m^2.[4,5,7] In this respect, obesity is not a uniform disease but brings about a set of conditions uniquely expressed in each individual.[5,8]

Indeed, Fontbonne and Eschwege[9] postulate that a constellation of mild abnormalities linked to obesity increases the cardiovascular disease risk. The altered metabolism generally resulting from overnutrition and obesity, including hyperglycemia, hyperinsulinemia, hypertriglyceridemia, hypercholesterolemia, elevated rates of fatty acid synthesis, and insulin resistance, can contribute to the development of the actual disease states of hypertension, dyslipidemia, diabetes, and possibly certain cancers in susceptible individuals. Thus, underlying defects may be exacerbated to life-threatening severity when the metabolic picture is complicated by excess weight.

Obesity has been related to abnormalities of the cardiovascular and endocrine systems, cholecystitis, infertility, cancer, and arthritis. It is the interrelationship with the cardiovascular and endocrine systems that remains the major concern for public health and that is most reliably documented. In addition to the functional impact of obesity, its effect on these two systems will serve as the focus of this discussion.

PHENOTYPIC EXPRESSION OF OBESITY AND FUNCTIONAL CARDIOVASCULAR EFFECTS

The adverse effects of excess weight on the cardiovascular system are in part functional, with the metabolic abnormalities imposed on these functional disturbances. Obesity severely burdens the left ventricle, impairing left ventricular filling regardless of arterial pressure.[10,11] Additionally, obesity typically increases blood volume, which increases stroke volume and hence cardiac output, ultimately raising arterial blood pressure.[12] Chronic hypercaloric consumption generally brings with it increased sodium intake, as well as other dietary factors that lead to hyperglycemia and hyperinsulinemia. A vicious cycle ensues: High sodium consumption promotes increased intravascular volume, while the hyperinsulinemia promotes additional sodium retention, further raising intravascular volume.[5,13] The complicated relationship between insulin resistance, hyperinsulinemia, and cardiovascular disease in obesity will be addressed later in this chapter. Because these metabolic abnormalities coexist with this hemodynamic picture, the physiologic problem may lie in an inability to reduce vascular resistance in the face of rising blood volume and cardiac output.[14,15]

The unique implications of obesity in a patient are likewise associated with the type of excess weight.[8,16] A strong family history of obesity may indicate a different set of risks than those for obesity induced by hyperphagia or a disordered endocrine system (e.g., Prader-Willi syndrome). In general, obesity results from five basic etiologies. As mentioned above, hyperphagia and reduced physical activity are two common routes. Endocrine disorders involving adrenal glucocorticosteroids affect a smaller proportion of other patients. The sympathetic nervous system may also predispose to the development of obesity (Bray's Mona Lisa hypothesis).[17] Finally, impairment of insulin action may direct enhanced adipose deposition. The activity of these systems, and their response to changes in diet and physical activity level, affect nutrient partitioning among fat, protein, and carbohydrate stores.

Recent evidence suggests that the effects of obesity may be related less to the degree of obesity and more to its regional distribution.[8,13,18] Indeed, body fat patterning may be an integral part of the cardiovascular risk profile. Metabolically, upper body adiposity (abdominal or android) may lead to more adverse alterations in metabolism or hormone regulation than lower body adiposity (gluteal or gynoid),[18,19] as upper body fat is strongly associated with cardiovascular disease, stroke, diabetes mellitus, hypertension, and hyperlipidemia.[8,13,16,20,21] Men are considered to be at increased risk if their waist:hip ratio (WHR) exceeds 0.95 and women if their ratio exceeds 0.80.

Although women are generally considered at less risk than men for the same degree of fatness, Wing et al.[22] found that android obesity in postmenopausal women was associated with elevated systolic blood pressure and higher levels of cholesterol, triglycerides (TG), and apolipoprotein B (apo B). These women also showed lower levels of high density lipoprotein (HDL) subfractions 2 and 3, even after adjusting for BMI. In fact, this effect of upper body fat may increase the cardiovascular risk more than lack of fitness. In a 14-month study of weight loss through exercise in women, Despres et al.[23] showed that reduction of body fat and deep abdominal fat mass but not improved maximum oxygen consumption (VO_2max) correlated with improvements in the insulinogenic index, plasma cholesterol, low density lipoprotein (LDL), apo-B,[23] and HDL. However, other studies[24] have shown a relationship between short-term exercise training and improvements in insulin action with diminished peripheral and hepatic insulin resistance.

RELATIONSHIP TO DYSLIPIDEMIA

Some of the more common metabolic abnormalities of obesity are the dyslipidemias. Although not all obese patients present with hypertriglyceridemia or hypercholesterolemia, Ramierez et al.[25] and others[22] have found that both blood pressure and blood lipids are strongly associated with most, if not all, indices of body size and adiposity, including WHR, BMI, subscapular skinfold measure, and relative fat pattern.[2,5,25,26]

Two basic mechanisms exist for the hypertriglyceridemia of obesity: overproduction of very low density lipoprotein (VLDL) triglycerides and defective lipolysis of the triglyceride (TG)-rich liproproteins.[5] It is known that excess caloric intake in obese patients results in an overproduction of VLDL-TG. In general, as production of these lipids increases, clearance capacity follows, thus maintaining lipemic equilibrium. Since lipolytic capacity varies among individuals, the expression of dyslipidemia is not consistent across populations. Although this is in part genetically determined, the mechanisms responsible for this variability remain unknown. When an underlying defect in adaptation exists or when chronic excess production of VLDL-TG begins to overwhelm the production of lipoprotein lipase, overt hypertriglyceridemia results.[5]

Many patients with primary hypertriglyceridemia are also resistant to the peripheral action of insulin, which itself is common in obesity.[27–34] Peripheral resistance to glucose uptake may stimulate hepatic overproduction of VLDL by delivery of excess substrate to the liver. However, it remains unclear whether the primary site of the defect is related to this peripheral insulin resistance or to liver function itself.[5]

Hypercholesterolemia is also common in obesity. Hypercholesterolemia usually consists of elevated serum LDL concentrations. Although polygenic in origin, it usually results from LDL overproduction or insufficient clearance. LDL originate from the breakdown products of the VLDL remnants, themselves products of VLDL catabolism. The serum LDL concentration is determined by this rate of conversion, as well as by the rate of LDL and VLDL clearance from the blood. In some cases, a defect in the primary structure of apo-E will cause a reduced affinity of VLDL for LDL receptors. Most circulating LDL particles are removed by hepatic LDL receptors, although the peripheral tissues can contribute to LDL removal as well. As with the VLDL concentrations, defects in production or clearance may be responsible for hypercholesterolemia, and these defects may remain unexpressed in the nonobese condition[5,35,36] and may be exacerbated by obesity.

Yamori[37] has highlighted the potency of dietary factors in the development of atherosclerosis. They have shown that a diet high in cholesterol alone will produce fatty deposits in mesenteric and cerebrobasal arteries within a few weeks in spontaneously hypertensive rats (SHR) and stroke-prone SHR rats. Clearly, dietary factors compound the existing metabolic abnormalities manifested by the condition of obesity. This is of particular importance when the incidence of hypertension in obesity is considered. When underlying abnormalities are compounded, such as when an overweight, hypertensive individual consumes a diet rich in saturated fats and cholesterol, the potential harm to the cardiovascular system is quite potent. Caloric excess will raise hepatic synthesis rates for lipoproteins, particularly VLDL. As detailed above, elevated VLDL levels will, in turn, affect LDL levels. Although the hyperinsulinemia of overconsumption may serve to stimulate the LDL receptors and thus help to mitigate hypercholesterolemia,[5] insulin resistance in peripheral tissues may shunt carbohydrate substrate into hepatic VLDL production, thus continuing the cycle. Further studies have supported a link between abnormalities in lipoprotein metabolism associated with obesity and insulin resistance,[38] and the relationships among hyperlipemias, glucose intolerance, hyperinsulinemia, and insulin resistance are so strong that they were grouped to comprise syndrome X by Reaven in his Banting Award Lecture in 1988.[39]

HDL cholesterol is currently thought to play a protective role in the development of cardiovascular diseases and is characteristically depressed in obese individuals.[5] Much remains unknown about HDL. Its exact origins and endpoints are not well established, and the specific mechanisms by which overnutrition or obesity reduces HDL also remain unknown. Grundy and Barnett[5] speculate that HDL may be lowered in obese patients, either through direct removal of HDL from the circulation by the adipose tissue or through separation of the lipid from its apo A–1 transport protein or its cholesterol ester. However, conclusions must be carefully drawn, since it is likely that the removal of excess adipose mass will be required for HDL levels to rise to normal in these patients.[5,23] A detailed review of the relationship between dyslipidemias and obesity is published elsewhere.[5]

RELATIONSHIP TO HYPERINSULINEMIA AND INSULIN RESISTANCE

Although hyperinsulinemia and insulin resistance appear to be independent metabolic derangements, clearly they are closely interrelated.[5,27,29,33,40–43] Their separation is difficult in that current in vivo measurements of resistance to this hormone do not differentiate between hyperinsulinemia and the actual cellular defect responsible for diminished glucose metabolism. In both the insulin clamp procedure[38,43,44] and Bergman et al.'s minimal model,[44,45] circulating insulin levels are artificially elevated. This methodologic gap is partially responsible for the confounding of the terms *insulin resistance* and *hyperinsulinemia* that is common in current literature.[39,47,48]

It is important to note that although obesity is commonly recognized as causing insulin resistance, evidence also exists to suggest that a genetic defect in skeletal muscle metabolism contributes to the development of this condition.[28] Regardless of which comes first—obesity or insulin resistance—hyperinsulinemia serves as a hallmark of hypertension and non-insulin-dependent diabetes mellitus (NIDDM) in the obese patient population.[5,27,40,49] Hyperinsulinemia commonly occurs with dyslipidemias as well.[5,50]

As an adaptive mechanism, insulin resistance may develop through receptor site down regulation after prolonged hyperinsulinemia.[5,41,42] On the other hand, hyperinsulinemia may evolve through progressive development of insulin resistance, possibly due to post–receptor site abnormalities.[42,43,51–53] Compensation for ineffective insulin leads to hyperinsulinemia and may contribute to dyslipidemia and further atherogenesis, although glucocorticoids likely play a role as well.[5] Hyperinsulinemia and insulin resistance compound each other, causing another cycle of abnormal metabolism.[42,54] The effects of genetics and age on islet cell function and insulin secretion cannot be ignored and may account for the possibility of variable insulin secretion in the presence of insulin resistance.

Finally, exercise training has been shown to influence hepatic glucose production and insulin sensitivity of hepatic and peripheral tissues,[24] and may therefore need to be considered in a clinical picture.

According to Landsberg and Young,[55] the insulin resistance of obesity may serve to limit weight gain and restore energy balance. The authors reason that insulin resistance at the level of the adipocyte antagonizes further synthesis and storage of triglycerides. On the other hand, Caro et al.[28] postulate that obesity must be viewed as a genetic condition, with insulin resistance developing as a mutation promoting survival, since insulin affects fat storage and sodium and water retention, all important in times of famine or drought. In this scenario, obesity is promoted and maintained by insulin resistance rather than impeded by it. The studies by Caro et al. of adipocytes, hepatocytes, and skeletal muscle tissues demonstrate far more profound insulin resistance in the muscle than in adipose tissue, and this condition becomes exaggerated in NIDDM. Caro et al. theorizes that euglycemia is promoted through the participation of the adipocytes in postprandial glucose clearance that shunts nutrients toward fat accumulation. They propose that this primary defect in skeletal muscle tissue is predictive of the development of future obesity.

Our studies[56] of hyperinsulinemia and insulin resistance in over 90 patients indicate that the two are separate but related. We measured insulin sensitivity index (Si) by the minimal model of Bergman,[44,45] which uses an intravenous glucose-tolbutamide tolerance test (IVGTTT) to quantify the resistance to peripheral glucose uptake. This model plots the rate of glucose disappearance versus tolbutamide-stimulated insulin concentration after a glucose load. The Bergman model expresses Si scores between 0 (highly-insulin-resistant or diabetic state) and roughly 9×10^{-4} (highly insulin-sensitive state). As expected, we found that obesity and age are linearly and inversely related to insulin action on glucose uptake,[56] as shown in Figure 4–1. The apparent nonlinearity in the relationship between Si and body fat is due to inclusion of both female and male subjects. Separation of the data according to gender results in linear relationships with a slope of -0.18 (SE 0.042, $n = 38$, $r = 0.58$) in female subjects and a slope of -0.25 (SE 0.035, $n = 31$, $r = -0.81$) in males.

By using these relationships, it is possible to calculate the percentage of body fat associated with abnormal insulin action, defined through our studies as a value of Si equal or less than 3.52×10^{-4}. Thus, women are resistant to insulin action at an average percentage body fat of 37.7% (SE 2.03), while men develop an equivalent condition at an average percentage body fat of 23.9% (SE 1.5). Figure 4–2 shows the linear regression lines for body fat against BMI for men and women ($r = 0.75$ and 0.88, respectively). As seen here, the mean values of body fat associated with the decrease in Si defined above correspond to a BMI of approximately 30 kg/m^2 for both men and women.

To assess hyperinsulinemia, we estimated insulin secretion via measurement

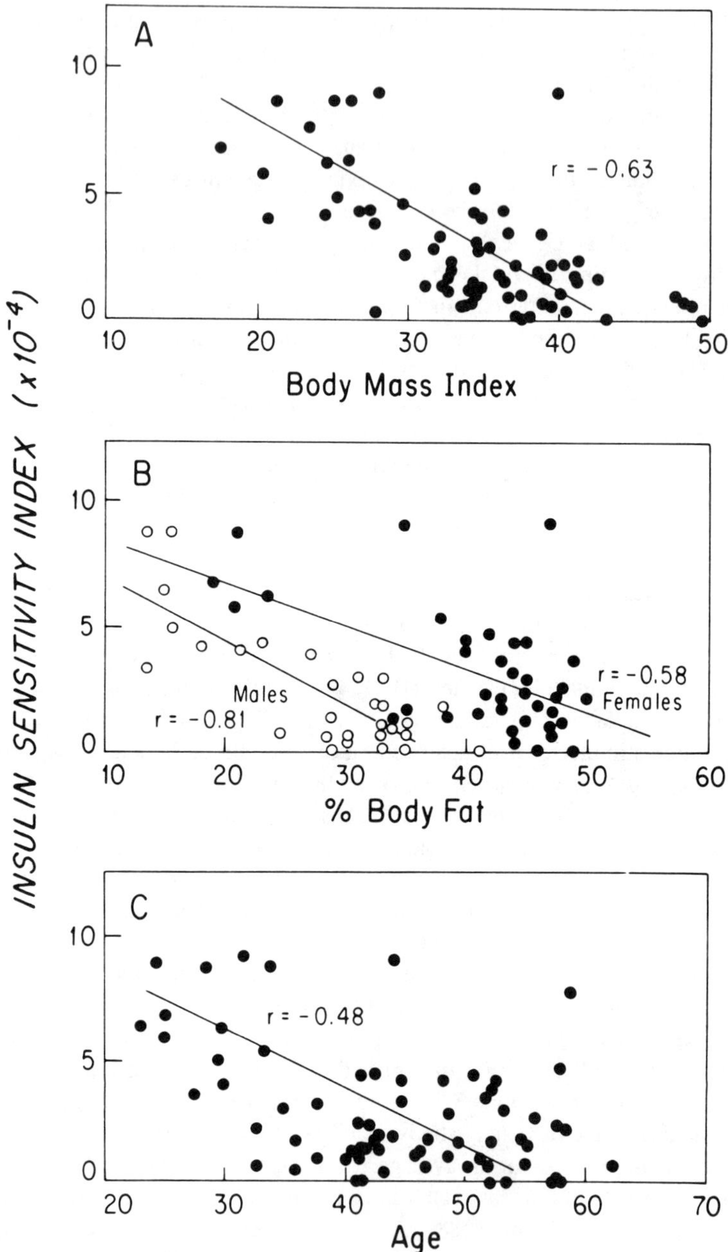

Figure 4–1. Relationship between insulin sensitivity index (Si in 10^{-4} min/[microunits/ml], calculated according to Bergman's minimal model) and each of BMI percent fat, and age. The relationship between Si and body fat is shown separately for males and females.

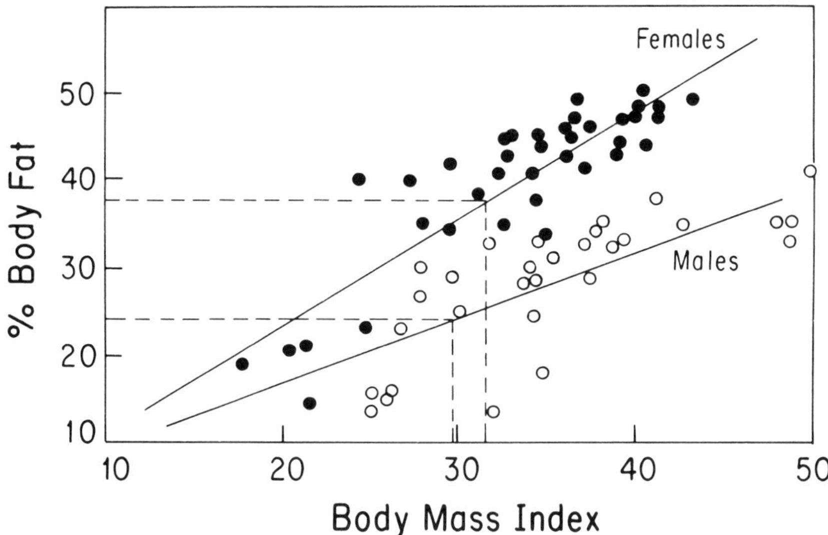

Figure 4–2. Relationship between percent body fat and mass index BMI in males and females. Dotted lines indicate the level of body fat at which Si equals 3.52 × 10–4 (23.9% in males; 37.7% in females, as determined by regression analysis) in both sexes. This figure indicates that at a BMI of approximately 30, subjects of either sex begin to exhibit significant reduction in insulin action.

of 12-hr meal stimulated c-peptide (MSCP) excretion. Despite the strong relationships between both insulin resistance and insulin secretion with obesity, our studies supported the independence of these two abnormalities from one another.[56] Correlations between Si and MSCP excretion did not achieve statistical significance ($r = 0.23$, $n = 55$, $p =$ NS) in our trials, implying that elevated baseline insulin levels in obesity are related to diminished clearance[57] and that factors other than insulin resistance are important determinants of insulin secretion.

RELATIONSHIP TO HYPERTENSION

Obesity serves as a strong early predictor for the development of hypertension.[31] According to Stamler,[58] only about 20% of middle-aged Americans have optimal systolic and diastolic blood pressures, with a strong relationship between body weight and blood pressure beginning in adolescence, if not earlier. Hypertension is a multifactorial disorder that itself increases the risk of cardiovascular disease. Like the dyslipidemias, hypertension is characterized by fundamental metabolic as well as additional hemodynamic abnormalities.[5,31,49] Some suggest that obesity may protect against the effects of hypertension and cardiovascular disease;[59,60]

however, since 30–50% of hypertension in the United States has been attributed to obesity,[5,58,61] these aggregate effects must be considered. For example, whereas the risk of stroke and atherosclerosis is heightened in the obese patient, Yamori has demonstrated that severe hypertension may predispose to the development of these usually lipid-related disorders.[37] There is some controversy about whether obese hypertension may be less malignant than essential hypertension,[12] but the majority of researchers consider the health risks to be compounded,[5,61,62] as the obese are at greater risk for the development of end-organ disease than are normotensive individuals.[5]

Although the mechanisms by which obesity raises blood pressure have not been fully elucidated, hypercaloric intake, hyperinsulinemia, insulin resistance, enhanced metabolic activity of visceral adipose tissue, enhanced sympathetic activity, and even the greater lean body mass present in obese subjects are all held suspect.[5,30–31,58,62–68] Modan and Halkin[54] hypothesize that two primary types of obese hypertension occur: one based on insulin action and the other on the effects of the sympathetic nervous system.

Strong evidence supports the role of hyperinsulinemia in hypertension,[66,69] either in the presence or absence of obesity.[63] Some researchers allow that hyperinsulinemia, developing through insulin resistance, may accentuate or even cause hypertension,[40] while others argue the opposite: Insulin resistance, through an unknown mechanism, is associated with an elevated pressor response.[29,33] In support of the latter position, Flack and Sowers[33] maintain that insulin resistance, not hyperinsulinemia, is the primary insulin-related abnormality operating in human hypertension, with adipocytes serving as a site of this resistance.[33,35] Rocchini agrees,[29] demonstrating that insulin resistance plays a predominant role in obese hypertension. It may be this tissue and pathway specificity that permits the expression of hypertension in genetically at-risk obese individuals.

Our results confirm the the importance of insulin resistance. For the same degree of obesity (measured by BMI), hypertensive patients are more insulin resistant and secrete more insulin than do nonhypertensive patients.[56] We have also demonstrated that meal-stimulated c-peptide excretion is significantly increased in hypertensive but not in normotensive obese individuals. Thus, insulin resistance (measured by Bergman's minimal model) and c-peptide excretion are both independent determinants of blood pressure levels in our obese patient population. Despite significant correlations between fasting insulin and Si, circulating insulin levels were not significantly associated with blood pressure. The increase in basal circulating insulin levels in obese patients may be determined by a decrease in clearance rather than in an actual increase in secretion.[57,70] Our results support this hypothesis, since the correlation between meal-stimulated c-peptide excretion and fasting insulin was also not statistically significant. Therefore, hyperinsulinemia, as defined by elevated systemic insulin concentrations, does not accurately reflect insulin secretion, and we feel that it is an insensitive measure of insulin resistance.

Modan and Halkin[54] acknowledge the contribution of the sympathetic nervous system to pressor regulation. Hyperinsulinemia may increase the activity of the sympathetic nervous system,[5,50,54,71,72] further promoting elevations in pressure. Borderline hypertension is characterized by a decreased parasympathetic tone, as well as an increased cardiac sympathetic drive and an increased sympathetic tone to the kidneys, arterioles, and veins. Normal-weight individuals with borderline hypertension are at risk for a neurogenically based elevated cardiac output but with a normal vascular resistance. In established hypertension, the opposite occurs[73]: Vascular resistance is elevated, and cardiac output remains normal. The previously detailed effects of obesity on cardiovascular volume and cardiac output are superimposed on these derangements when the two health risks coexist.[13]

Modan and Halkins' two theories come together at the level of prostaglandin synthesis. Adipose tissue, one of the largest organs in the body, is a major producer of prostaglandin I_2 (PGI_2) and PGE_2. Physiologic concentrations of insulin impede the catecholamine-induced production of these potent vasodilators. Thus, as Alexrod suggests, hyperinsulinemia increases peripheral vascular resistance and blood pressure by inhibiting the stimulatory effect of adrenergic agonists on the production of PGI_2 and PGE_2.[63] If insulin does partially regulate PGI_2 and PGE_2 released by adipose and other tissues, a wide range of physiologic as well as clinical consequences are possible in obesity when insulin resistance is overcome by hyperinsulinemia.

This pathway through which hyperinsulinemia influences hypertension may further involve the hyperinsulinemic impairment of sodium excretion, thus accentuating peripheral pressor resistance,[27,62] although this theory is not without its skeptics.[33] Expansion of blood volume would have similar pressor effects. As hyperinsulinemia can develop into insulin resistance, there could be an adverse affect on the distribution of intracellular and extracellular potassium, possibly promoting vasoconstriction and raising blood pressure.[5] An impaired cellular response to insulin is also associated with increased vascular smooth muscle contraction, which may result in the hemodynamic and metabolic derangements underlying hypertension, diabetes, and atherosclerotic cardiovascular disease.[18]

Sowers et al.[31] note that insulin appears to attenuate the vascular response to both receptor-mediated and voltage-mediated calcium-induced contractions. The hormone increases renal tubular absorption of Na^+ as well[5]; the Na^+, $K(^+)$-ATPase and $Ca(2^+)$-ATPase pumps are insulin sensitive. Thus, when insulin resistance is present, the activity of these pumps in the smooth muscle of the arterial wall could be reduced, as vascular smooth muscle may be sensitized to the intracellular accumulation of these ions. This abnormal handling of calcium and other ions and the exaggerated vascular contraction may be shown to be intimately related to insulin resistance.[5,31,74] In concert with these adaptations, secondary hyperinsulinemia will occur, furthering the cycle of elevated pressor responses.

RELATIONSHIP TO NIDDM

The association between obesity and NIDDM is well documented.[43] Indeed, 70–80% of NIDDM patients are obese, and 40–60% of markedly obese patients can be expected to develop diabetes.[5] Although it is popularly believed that obesity contributes independently to the pathogenesis of NIDDM, three possible relationships between the two exist. First, obesity may predispose to NIDDM. Alternatively, obesity may serve as an additional physiologic stress that allows the expression of an inherent underlying abnormality in glucose metabolism.[5] Finally, functional deficits may occur, such as acquired impaired insulin production, that are coincident with but not the result of excess weight or nutrition.

As a causative factor, obesity acts to promote hyperinsulinemia and insulin resistance, interfering with the peripheral action of the hormone,[5,8,16,28,31,33,39,68] regardless of the state of glucose homeostasis. Although the adipose tissue of obese subjects has been demonstrated to be insulin resistant,[55] this defect occurs mainly in the skeletal muscle.[28,75] Worsening insulin resistance, which is common in NIDDM,[43] may be related to a reduction in the number of insulin receptors synthesized in peripheral tissues, making the system inadequate to meet the needs for glucose uptake.[5,41,42]

Prolonged hypercaloric intake and obesity may contribute to the development of NIDDM in that chronic hyperglycemia could produce an irreversible defect in insulin secretion. As hypothesized by Modan et al.,[76] glycosylation of key proteins in beta or islet cells could impair insulin production, with subsequent deterioration in glycemic control. Hepatic glucose production is also increased in NIDDM, contributing to further hyperglycemia,[5] which may be either a primary defect or secondary to insulin resistance.[24] The inability of insulin to counterregulate hepatic glucose output[24] may be superimposed on a decrease in insulin-stimulated glucose uptake by muscle.[5,74] In this way, long-term obesity may play a direct role in the etiology of NIDDM.

However, obesity may not serve as an initiator of NIDDM but may act to tip the balance of metabolism. The independence of NIDDM from obesity is supported by the view that a progressive impairment in beta-cell insulin production is a likely candidate for the primary defect in this disease. Although the degree and duration of overweight likely influence the degree of hyperglycemia and its persistance,[5] some research demonstrates normal beta-cell function when glucose tolerance is maintained, despite the degree of obesity.[32] Independence from obesity is also supported by the work of Johnson et al.,[77] who found no relationship between obesity and the activation of skeletal muscle glycogen synthetase in NIDDM. Moreover, as noted earlier, obesity is not universally recognized to cause insulin resistance.[48]

NIDDM appears to be comprised of several defects rather than a single defect. Each step in the regulation of carbohydrate metabolism serves as a potential site for irregularities to occur[53]—irregularities that could lead to the development of NIDDM.[5,43,77–79] These potential sites likely involve the primary structure of the insulin receptor[78,79] or the secondary postreceptor cellular mechanisms involved in glucose uptake and utilization.[5,42,51,52,74] Though scientific confirmation is lacking, genetic deficiencies of other key enzymes involved in glucose oxidation may play a role here as well.[5] There may also be a role for an acquired defect in glucose oxidation. The Randle effect[80,81] postulates the preferential oxidation of fatty acids over glucose by the muscle tissue,[82] which would seemingly be related to the resistance to peripheral glucose uptake[28] but not necessarily to the development of obesity.

In general, nutritional intake of the obese provides high levels of free fatty acids. This dietary load, combined with excess adipose tissue and increased catabolism of VLDL triglycerides, may promote the preferential use of fatty acids as substrate at the expense of glucose[5,28,80–82] and thus antagonize hyperglycemia. The vicious cycle previously described once again comes into play here. The preferential oxidation of fatty acids results in hyperglycemia, which stimulates hyperinsulinemia. This, in turn, affects peripheral resistance to insulin, possibly through down regulation of receptor sites. Insulin resistance promotes hyperglycemia, which itself can impair insulin secretion through glycosylation of membranes and other proteins.[76] Subsequently, glucose intolerance or NIDDM becomes manifest.

A third possible etiology presents obesity in a concomitant but acausal relationship to NIDDM. Approximately 20–30% of patients with this type of diabetes are within their normal weight range.[5] In more severe forms of NIDDM, insulin secretion is actually decreased,[83] although the particular defect remains undetermined. Slow, progressive degeneration of beta cells or pancreatic function may be completely unrelated to weight. Similarly, abnormalities in the handling or storage of glucose may manifest at any body weight range and are not related to the metabolic abnormalities of obesity. Inherent abnormal tendencies toward the preferential use of fatty acids as substrate or even outright defects in glucose uptake may exist. There may be abnormalities in the structure of the muscle tissue itself,[28] which influence glucose tolerance and NIDDM development. With different muscle groups containing various proportions of fiber types and levels of capillary perfusion,[53] rates of glucose oxidation could differ markedly and thus promote hyperglycemia.[5] Inactivity, present in both obese and lean individuals, tends to decrease capillary perfusion of muscle tissue and promote insulin resistance.[5,53] These functional considerations could discourage the system from glucose utilization.

CONCLUSIONS

Although many generalities can be drawn regarding the metabolic abnormalities of obesity, each patient is unique. A standard set of challenges to normal function will be met by a varying set of adaptive mechanisms in each individual. The expression of dyslipidemias will be based largely on the capacity of the system to clear the excess lipids from the bloodstream. The manifestation of hyperinsulinemia and insulin resistance will depend in part on the types of muscle fibers and the response of tissues to the stress of chronic hyperphagia and/or chronic inactivity and the resultant changes in glucose concentration. Hypertension may be present or absent in the obese patient, despite the known contributions of hyperinsulinemia, insulin resistance, enhanced sympathetic tone, renal mineral reabsorption, and the effect of obesity on the structural function of the cardiovascular system. Similarly, the etiology of NIDDM is polygenic, with even severe obesity not always associated with abnormal glucose tolerance. Nevertheless, obese patients are likely to manifest several metabolic abnormalities affecting their cardiovascular and endocrine systems. Where one aberration of metabolism alters the normal homeostasis or functioning of the body, it is likely to work in concert with others. Patients must therefore be evaluated for additional metabolic complications and risk factors. Hence, the concern for the increased health risks of obesity is not unfounded, and the benefits of weight loss in ameliorating or correcting metabolic aberrations should be emphasized.

REFERENCES

1. *Build Study 1979*. Chicago, Society of Actuaries and Association of Life Insurance Medical Directors, 1980.
2. Body weight, health, and longevity: Conclusions and recommendations of the workshop. *Nutr Rev* 43:61, 1985.
3. Hubert HB, Feinleib M, McNamara PM, et al. Obesity as an independent risk factor for cardiovascular disease; a 26-year follow-up of participants in the Framingham heart study. *Circulation* 67:968, 1983.
4. Kuczmarski RJ. Prevalence of overweight and weight gain in the United States. *Am J Clin Nutr* 55:495S, 1992.

5. Grundy SM, Barnett JP. Metabolic and health complications of obesity. *Disease-a-Month* 36:645, 1990.
6. Wooley SC, Wooley OW. Should obesity be treated at all?, in Stunkard AJ, Stellar E (eds), *Eating and Its Disorders*. New York, Raven Press, 1984, pp. 185–92.
7. National Institutes of Health, Technology Assessment Conference Statement Methods for Voluntary Weight Loss and Control, Mar 30–Apr 1, 1992.
8. Pi-Sunyer FX. Health implications of obesity. *Am J Clin Nutr* 53:1595S, 1991.
9. Fontbonne AM, Eschwege EM. Insulin and cardiovascular disease. Paris Prospective Study. *Diabetes Care* 14:461, 1991.
10. Grossman E, Oren S, Messerli FH. Left ventricle filling in the systemic hypertension of obesity. *Am J Cardiol* 68:57, 1991.
11. Lauer MS, Anderson KM, Kannel WB, et al. The impact of obesity on left ventricular mass and geometry. The Framingham Heart Study. *JAMA* 266:231, 1991.
12. Guyton AC. Personal views on mechanisms of hypertension, in Genest J, Koiw E, Kuchel O, et al. (eds), *Hypertension, Physiopathology and Treatment*. New York, McGraw-Hill, 1977, pp 566–575.
13. Benotti PN, Bistrian B, Benotti JR, et al. Heart disease and hypertension in severe obesity: The benefits of weight reduction. *Am J Clin Nutr* 55:586S, 1992.
14. Dustan HP. Hypertension and obesity. *Prim-Care* 18:495, 1991.
15. Dustan HP. Obesity and hypertension. *Diabetes Care* 14:488, 1991.
16. Bray GA. Pathophysiology of obesity. *Am J Clin Nutr* 55:488S, 1992.
17. Bray GA. Obesity, a disorder of nutrient partitioning: The Mona Lisa hypothesis. *J Nutr* 121:1146, 1991.
18. Kaplan NM. The deadly quartet. *Arch Intern Med* 149:1514, 1989.
19. Haffner SM, Katz MS, Dunn JF. Increased upper body and overall adiposity is associated with decreased sex hormone binding globulin in postmenopausal women. *Int J Obes* 15:471, 1991.
20. Sjostrom L. Morbidity and mortality of severely obese subjects. *Am J Clin Nutr* 55(Suppl):508S, 1992.
21. Bouchard C., Bray GA, Hubbard VS. Basic and clinical aspects of regional fat distribution. *Am J Clin Nutr* 52:946, 1990.
22. Wing RR, Matthews KA, Kuller LH, et al. Waist to hip ratio in middle-aged women. Associations with behavioral and psychosocial factors and with changes in cardiovascular risk factors. *Arterioscler Thromb* 11:1250, 1991.
23. Despres JP, Pouliot MC, Moorjani S, et al. Loss of Abdominal fat and metabolic response to exercise training in obese women. *Am J Physiol* 261(2 pt 1): E159, 1991.
24. DeFronzo RA, Sherwin RS, Kraemen N. Effect of physical training on insulin action in obesity. *Diabetes* 36:1379, 1987.
25. Ramierez ME, Hunt SC, Williams RR. Blood pressure and lipids in relation to body size in hypertensive and normotensive adults. *Int J Obes* 15:127, 1991.

26. National Research Council. *Diet and Health: Implications for Reducing Chronic Disease Risk.* Washington, DC, National Academy Press, 1989.

27. Kaplan NM. Hypertension and hyperinsulinemia. *Prim Care* 18:483, 1991.

28. Caro JF, Sinha MK, Dohm GL. Insulin resistance in obesity, in Bray GA, Ricquier D, Spiegelman BM (eds), *Obesity: Toward a Molecular Approach.* New York, Alan R Liss, 1990, pp 203–217.

29. Rocchini AP. Insulin resistance and blood pressure regulation in obese and nonobese subjects. Special lecture. *Hypertension* 17:837, 1991.

30. Daly PA, Landsberg L. Hypertension in obesity and NIDDM. Role of insulin and sympathetic nervous system. *Diabetes Care* 14:240, 1991.

31. Sowers JR, Standley PR, Ram JL, et al. Insulin resistance, carbohydrate metabolism, and hypertension. *Am J Hypertens* 4(7 pt 2):466S, 1991.

32. Shiraishi I, Iwamoto Y, Kuzuya T, et al. Hyperinsulinemia in obesity is not accompanied by an increase in serum proinsulin/insulin ratio in groups of human subjects with and without glucose intolerance. *Diabetologia,* 34:737, 1991.

33. Flack JM, Sowers JR. Epidemiologic and clinical aspects of insulin resistance and hyperinsulinemia. *Am J Med* 91(1A):11S, 1991.

34. Eaton RP, Hye HR. The relationship between insulin secretion and triglyceride concentration in endogenous lipemia. *J Lab Clin Med* 81:682, 1973.

35. Stryer L. *Biochemistry,* ed. 2. San Francisco, WH Freeman, 1981.

36. Krause MV, Mahan LK. *Food, Nutrition, and Diet Therapy,* ed 7. Philadelphia, WB Saunders, 1984.

37. Yamori Y. Predictive and preventive pathology of cardiovascular diseases. *Acta Pathol Jpn* 39:683, 1989.

38. Abbott WGH, Lillioja S, Young AA, et al. Relationships between plasma lipoprotein concentrations and insulin action in an obese hyperinsulinemic population. *Diabetes* 36:897, 1987.

39. Reaven GM. Banting Lecture 1988. Role of insulin resistance in human disease. *Diabetes* 37:1595, 1988.

40. Sechi LA, Melis A, Poda A, et al. Serum insulin, insulin sensitivity, and erythrocyte sodium metabolism in normotensive and essential hypertensive subjects with and without overweight. *Clin Exp Hypertension* 13:261, 1991.

41. Bar RS, Harrison LC, Muggeo M, et al. Regulation of insulin receptors in normal and abnormal physiology in human beings. *Adv Intern Med* 24:23, 1979.

42. Unger RH, Grundy SM. Hyperglycemia as an inducer as well as a consequence of impaired islet cell function and insulin resistance: implications for management of diabetes. *Diabetoligia* 28:119, 1985.

43. Smith U. Insulin action—biochemical and clinical aspects. *Acta Med Scand* 222:7, 1987.

44. Bergman R, Finegood DT, Ader A. Assessment of insulin sensitivity in vivo. *Endocrine Rev* 6:45, 1985.

45. Bergman RN, Prager R, Volund A, et al. Equivalence of insulin sensitivity index in man derived by the minimal model method and euglycemic glucose clamp. *J Clin Invest* 79:790, 1987.
46. Cobelli C, Pacini G, Toffolo G, et al. Estimation of insulin sensitivity and glucose clearance from minimal model: new insights from labeled IVGTT. *Am J Physiol* 250(*Endocrinol Metab* 13):E591, 1986.
47. Modan M, Halkin H, Almog S, et al. Hyperinsulinemia, a link between hypertension, obesity, and glucose intolerance. *J Clin Invest* 75:809, 1985.
48. Hollenbeck CB, Chen Y-DI, Reaven GM. A comparison of the relative effects of in vivo insulin-stimulated glucose utilization. *Diabetes* 33:622, 1984.
49. Smith U, Gudbjornsdottir S, Landin K. Hypertension as a metabolic disorder—an overview. *J Intern Med Suppl* 735:1, 1991.
50. Ferrannini E, Haffner SM, Stern MP, et al. High blood pressure and insulin resistance: influence of ethnic background. *Eur J Clin Invest* 21:280, 1991.
51. Gravey WT, Huechsteadt TP, Matthaei S. Role of glucose transporters in cellular insulin resistance. *J Clin Invest* 81:1528, 1988.
52. Olefsky JM, Gravey WT, Henry RR, et al. Cellular mechanisms of insulin resistance in non-insulin dependent diabetes. *Am J Med* 85:86, 1988.
53. Lillioja S, Bogardus C. Obesity and insulin resistance: Lessons learned from the Pima Indians. *Diabetes/Metab Rev* 4:517, 1988.
54. Modan M, Halkin H. Hyperinsulinemia or increased sympathetic drive as links for obesity and hypertension. *Diabetes Care* 14:470, 1991.
55. Landsberg L, Young J. Obesity and the sympathetic nervous system, in Bray GA, Ricquier D, Spiegelman BM (eds), *Obesity: Toward a Molecular Approach*. New York, Alan R Liss, 1990, pp. 81–93.
56. Istfan NW, Plaisted CS, Bistrian BR, et al. Insulin resistance versus insulin secretion in the hypertension of obesity. *Hypertension* 19:385, 1992.
57. Meistas MT, Margolis S, Kowarski A. Hyperinsulinemia of obesity is due to decreased clearance of insulin. *Am J Physiol* (*Endocrinol Metab* 8):E155, 1983.
58. Stamler J. Blood pressure and high blood pressure. Aspects of risk. *Hypertension* 18(3 Suppl):I95, 1991.
59. Bloom E, Reed D, Yano K, et al. Does obesity protect hypertensives against cardiovascular disease? *JAMA* 256:2972, 1986.
60. Barrett-Connor E, Khaw KT. Is hypertension more benign when associated with obesity? *Circulation* 72:53, 1985.
61. Van Itallie TB. Health implications of overweight and obesity in the United States. *Ann Intern Med* 103:983, 1985.
62. Blair D, Habicht J-P, Sims EAH, et al. Evidence for an increased risk for hypertension with centrally located body fat and the effect of race and sex on this risk. *Am J Epidemiol* 119:526, 1984.
63. Axelrod L. Insulin, prostaglandins, and the pathogenesis of hypertension. *Diabetes* 40:1223, 1991.

64. Christlieb AR, Krolewski AS, Warram JH, et al. Is insulin the link between hypertension and obesity? *Hypertension* 7(Suppl II):II–54, 1985.
65. O'Hare JA. The enigma of insulin resistance and hypertension. Insulin resistance, blood pressure, and the circulation. *Am J Med* (3JU) 84(3 Pt 1):505, 1988.
66. Weinsier RL, Norris DJ, Birch R, et al. Serum insulin and blood pressure in an obese population. *Int J Obes* 10:11, 1986.
67. Ferrannini E, Buzzigoli G, Bonadonna R, et al. Insulin resistance in essential hypertension. *N Engl J Med* 317:350, 1987.
68. Shen DC, Shieh SM, Fuh MMT, et al. Resistance to insulin stimulated glucose uptake in patients with hypertension. *J Clin Endocrinol Metab* 66:580, 1986.
69. Horswill CA, Zipf WB. Elevated blood pressure in obese children: Influence of gender, age, weight, and serum insulin levels. *Int J Obes* 15:453, 1991.
70. Mbanya JC, Thomas TH, Wilkinson R, et al. Hypertension and hyperinsulinemia: A relation in diabetes but not essential hypertension. *Lancet* 2:733, 1988.
71. Forbes GB, Brown MR, Welle SL, et al. Hormonal response to overfeeding. *Am J Clin Nutr* 49:608, 1989.
72. Olefsky J, Crapo PA, Ginsberg H, et al. Metabolic effects of increased caloric intake in man. *Metabolism* 24:495, 1975.
73. Julius S. Autonomic nervous dysfunction in essential hypertension. *Diabetes Care* 14:249, 1991.
74. Resnick LM. Hypertension and abnormal glucose homeostasis. *Am J Med* 87:6A 17S, 1989.
75. Defranzo RA, Gunnarsson R, Bjorkman O, et al. Effects of insulin on peripheral and splanchnic glucose metabolism in non-insulin dependent (type II) diabetes mellitus. *J Clin Invest* 76:149, 1985.
76. Modan M, Karasik A, Halkin H, et al. Effect of past and concurrent body mass index on prevalence of glucose intolerance and type 2 (non-insulin-dependent) diabetes mellitus. *Diabetologia* 29:82, 1986.
77. Johnson AB, Argyraki M, Thow JC, et al. Impaired activation of skeletal muscle glycogen synthase in non-insulin-dependent diabetes is unrelated to the degree of obesity. *Metabolism* 40:252, 1991.
78. Taira M, Taira M, Hashimoto N, et al. Human diabetes associated with a deletion of the tyrosine kinase domain of the insulin receptor. *Science* 245:63, 1989.
79. Odawara M, Kadowaki T, Yamamoto R, et al. Human diabetes associated with mutation in the tyrosine kinase domain of the insulin receptor. *Science* 245:66, 1989.
80. Randle PJ, Garland PB, Newsholme EA, et al. The glucose fatty acid cycle in obesity and maturity onset diabetes mellitus. *Ann NY Acad Sci* 131:324, 1965.
81. Randle PJ, Newsholme EA, Garland PB. Regulation of glucose uptake by muscle: Effects of fatty acids, ketone bodies, and pyruvate, and of alloxan-diabetes and

starvation of the uptake and metabolic fate of glucose in rat heart and diaphragm muscles. *Biochem J* 93:652, 1964.

82. Felber JP, Ferrannini E, Golay A, et al. Role of lipid oxidation on pathogenesis of insulin resistance of obesity and type II diabetes. *Diabetes* 36:1341, 1987.
83. Ward WK, Bolgiano DC, McKight B, et al. Diminished B-cell secretory capacity in patients with non-insulin-dependent mellitus. *J Clin Invest* 74:1318, 1984.

CHAPTER

5

The Endocrinology of Obesity

David Heber, M.D., Ph.D.

INTRODUCTION

The endocrine system is critical in translating lifestyle factors such as overnutrition and underactivity into the excess adiposity associated with obesity. In the obese patient, changes in hormone secretion and action result both from the effects of ongoing positive caloric balance and from excess adiposity. In the course of weight reduction, the levels of many hormones are decreased in a biphasic manner, with an initial decrease secondary to caloric restriction over the first 1 to 2 weeks of dieting followed by a further decline as weight reduction progresses over several months. A number of hormones can promote obesity, and some hormones have been utilized in the treatment of obesity. It is clear that changes in endocrine function can affect both the assessment and treatment of obesity. In this chapter, the endocrine aspects of obesity, including syndromes promoting obesity, endocrine changes secondary to obesity, and hormones used in the treatment of obesity, will be considered.

ENDOCRINE SYNDROMES PROMOTING OBESITY

It is a common misconception that obesity is most often a glandular disorder resulting from a deficiency of a particular hormone that promotes normal nutrient metabolism. Obese patients frequently request a complete endocrinologic examination to exclude this possibility. While the vast majority of obese patients do not have an endocrine disorder, the most common syndromes and hormones promoting obesity are discussed below.

Cushing's Syndrome

This is the endocrine syndrome most often associated with obesity.[1] It presents with central adiposity often accompanied by a "buffalo hump" fat deposit in the intrascapular area. It is common for this diagnosis to be entertained in an obese patient with mild kyphosis or kyphoscoliosis even when peripheral muscle and fat wasting are not present. However, such patients do not usually have an adrenal disorder. Obesity results in an increased rate of cortisol production together with enhanced cortisol clearance and excretion, resulting in normal circulating cortisol levels.[2] A dexamethasone suppression test and a 24-hr urine collection for urinary free cortisol corrected for creatinine excretion will usually determine whether true Cushing's syndrome is present.[3] While true Cushing's syndrome due to adrenal hyperplasia secondary to increased secretion of adrenocorticotropic hormone (ACTH) from the pituitary gland is a rare cause of obesity, iatrogenic Cushing's syndrome due to administration of glucocorticoids for the treatment of connective tissue disorders, chronic lung disease, chronic liver disease, and some hematologic disorders can lead to obesity with peripheral wasting.[4] Since this syndrome is treatable by elimination of unnecessary glucocorticoid medication, its recognition is important. In those patients in whom glucocorticoids are required for control of underlying disease activity, dietary therapy can be pursued to prevent further weight gain.

Hypothalmic Syndromes

Destruction of the hypothalamus in humans by trauma, infections, or malignancy can lead to hyperphagia and obesity.[5] Genetic hypothalamic syndromes in which hypogonadism, hypomentia, hypotonia, and obesity occur together include Prader-Lambhardt-Willi syndrome and Lawrence-Moon-Bardet-Biedl syndrome.[6] These syndromes are analogous to the obesity that can be produced in rodents with experimental lesions in the ventromedial hypothalamus.[6]

Hypothyroidism

In clinical practice, hypothyroidism is rarely a cause of mild hypometabolism promoting obesity.[7] The early weight gain seen in hypothyroidism is usually due to water retention, as evidenced by edema.[8] This edema results from the decrease in renal free water clearance that occurs in hypothyroidism. Unfortunately, the use of pharmacologic doses of thyroid hormone to accelerate weight loss is not unusual. The use of pharmacologic amounts of thyroid hormone clearly leads to loss of lean body mass.[9,10] Homeopathic doses of thyroid hormone appear to be harmless but impose on the patient a lifelong unnecessary medication. Such patients often report being told that their thyroid hormone levels were in the lower range of normal prior to the prescription of thyroid hormone. Discontinuing this medication can result in transient symptoms of hypothyroidism, which may lead to decreased patient compliance with dietary therapy or may dissuade the patient from discontinuing the thyroid medication.

Hyperinsulinemia

Hyperinsulinemia is seen in several conditions and has been implicated in the etiology of associated obesity. The most important association of obesity in this regard is with non-insulin-dependent (type II) diabetes mellitus. Most, but not all, patients with this type of diabetes are obese,[11] and these patients comprise the vast majority of the approximately 15 million diabetics in this country.[12] Obese nondiabetic subjects may also have hyperinsulinemia.[13] This has been shown to be secondary to both increased insulin secretion from the pancreas and decreased hepatic clearance of insulin,[14] especially in individuals with abdominal or central obesity. In addition, obese patients are resistant to the effects of insulin on glucose metabolism, with lesser effects on lipid and protein metabolism.[15] Therefore, higher insulin levels result in part from the abnormal control of glucose metabolism. These higher insulin levels promote lipogenesis via increased activity of lipoprotein lipase, the enzyme that catalyzes the hydrolysis of circulating triglycerides into fatty acids and glycerol for uptake by the adipocyte to synthesize stored triglyceride intracellularity.[16] In the obese population hyperglycemia is uncommon, but the exact size of the latent diabetic population or the population that might benefit from weight reduction by an amelioration or delay in the development of obesity remains to be determined.

Iatrogenic hyperinsulinemia can result from the administration of excessive insulin in an attempt to regulate blood glucose levels in diabetic patients who do not adhere to dietary therapy. In these patients, increased insulin administration is associated with increased hunger and weight gain. The same phenomenon can be observed with excessive use of oral hypoglycemic agents.

Hyperinsulinemia at different levels of blood glucose achieved using the euglycemic insulin clamp technique is associated with increased hunger, heightened perceived pleasantness of the sweet taste, and increased food intake.[17]

Polycystic Ovarian Syndrome (Stein-Leventhal Syndrome)

This heterogeneous syndrome is characterized by infertility, dysmenorrhea, hirsutism, and insulin resistance.[18] Insulin resistance in these patients has been associated with both increased ovarian androgen and pituitary gonadotropin secretion in this syndrome.[18]

Reproductive Hormones and Weight Gain

Following the onset of puberty, women have increased adiposity compared to men. Obese women have higher levels of circulating estrogens than lean women due to conversion of adrenal androgens to estrogens by an aromatase enzyme found in the adipose stromal cells.[19] Premenopausal women develop gluteofemoral fat as well as abdominal fat, while men develop primarily abdominal fat.[20–22] The gluteofemoral fat is a useful store of energy for lactation and increases during each pregnancy. However, in our society, women rarely breastfeed their infants to the extent found in more primitive societies, so that the gluteofemoral fat is not lost effectively.[23] In fact, food intake can increase after pregnancy, and postpregnancy weight gain is an important factor in the epidemiology of obesity in American women.[24] Premenopausal women have two significant sources of estrogen: ovaries and fat tissue. Following menopause, the gluteofemoral fat depots decrease in size in many women, and adiposity increases in the abdominal and breast fat depots. The use of pharmacologic amounts of estrogens by males who impersonate females leads to gynoid fat distribution, while the use of anabolic androgens by female weight lifters leads to male fat patterns. While these data suggest that the gluteofemoral fat deposits are estrogen dependent, estrogen receptors have not been found in cells isolated from gluteofemoral fat.[25]

The activity of lipoprotein lipase (LPL) in gluteofemoral fat is affected by reproductive endocrine status. Gluteofemoral fat in premenopausal women has higher levels of LPL activity than abdominal fat when normalized per surface area.[26] During early pregnancy (up to 10 weeks), this difference in LPL activity is more pronounced. In late pregnancy, LPL activity begins to decrease in the femoral adipocytes. During lactation, LPL activity declines further in the femoral adipocytes until there is little difference from the levels found in the abdominal adipocytes. These changes parallel the storage and subsequent mobilization of fat from the gluteofemoral fat stores. In early pregnancy and in nonpregnant premenopausal women, the abdominal adipocytes, with lower LPL activity, are found to release fatty acids more readily in response to stimulation by norepinephrine than the gluteofemoral adipocytes.[27] In late pregnancy and during lactation, triglycerides are as easy to mobilize from gluteofemoral as from abdominal fat, providing energy and fat for lactation.

Women report craving fatty and sweet foods during the last 10 days of the menstrual cycle, when circulating progesterole levels are significantly elevated compared to the follicular phase; this has been documented in nutritional studies of premenopausal women.[28] A progestational steroid drug, megestrol acetate, has been shown to increase appetite in malnourished cancer and AIDS patients, with resultant significant weight gain.[29]

Approximately 80% of all patients in weight reduction programs are women. The effects of reproductive hormonal status on fat accumulation and mobilization are critical issues in the understanding of the pathogenesis of obesity in women.

Hypogonadism

Hypogonadism is associated with increased body fat in both men and women.[30] The exact mechanism underlying the accumulation of eunuchoid fat is not known, but the low level of testosterone relative to estrogen is a possibility. In men, the low levels of circulating estrogen result primarily from peripheral aromatization of adrenal androgens by fat tissue. Finally, growth hormone deficiency is associated with an accumulation of body fat.[31] Approximately a 2.5-kg average weight gain is observed at the time of menopause in women.[32] It has not been determined whether the observed weight gain is due to a metabolic effect of the loss of estrogen and progesterone, decreased physical activity, or simply increased food intake at the time of menopause.

ENDOCRINE CHANGES SECONDARY TO OBESITY

Endocrine function is markedly affected by obesity. In some cases, the differences observed in obese compared to lean subjects have clear implications for the etiology of obesity, as discussed above for insulin and estrogen secretion. In other cases, the differences in function do not have clear consequences for the physiologic changes observed in obese subjects. However, abnormalities secondary to obesity are important to differentiate from actual endocrine disorders presenting with weight gain. A patient who presents with amenorrhea and weight gain may have a primary weight gain due to undiagnosed acromegaly. Realizing that suppressed, not elevated, growth hormone levels are characteristic in obesity is important in differentiating endocrine disorders from changes secondary to obesity. The major endocrine changes are discussed below.

Insulin Resistance

As discussed above, obese patients commonly have hyperinsulinemia. However, despite the high levels of insulin observed, such patients do not become hypoglycemic, suggesting that they are resistant to the hypoglycemic effects of insulin. Exogenous insulin administration leads to a subnormal drop in blood glucose levels in obese patients.[33] This insulin resistance is most pronounced at physiologic and submaximal doses of insulin. The response to maximal doses of insulin infused under euglycemic conditions appears to be normal. In addition, the resistance to insulin effects on amino acid metabolism and lipogenesis appears to be insignificant. The latter point is important since insulin stabilizes LPL posttranslationally, promoting lipogenesis in the adipocyte and promoting obesity in the presence of insulin resistance. Once glucose homeostasis fails, subjects with insulin resistance develop non-insulin-dependent diabetes mellitus, as already discussed. The interrelationships of hyperinsulinemia, insulin resistance, and the etiology of obesity are closely intertwined, and it is not possible to state which is primary and which is secondary.

Decreased Growth Hormone Secretion

Growth hormone secretion is blunted in obese patients when determined in the fasting state or over a 24-hr period.[34] Increases in growth hormone secretion in response to a number of stimuli including administration of growth hormone-releasing hormone (GHRH),[35] sleep,[36] fasting,[37] protein-containing meals,[38] and exercise.[39] Growth hormone secretion can be increased in obese patients by administration of thyroid hormone,[40] by fasting,[41] or by pulsatile administration of GHRH.[42]

It is likely that the defects in growth hormone secretion are secondary to obesity but are not involved in the etiology of obesity. First, lean subjects who are overfed develop impaired growth hormone responses to a number of stimuli, including sleep, exercise, hypoglycemia, and GHRH administration.[43] Second, when obese subjects lose weight, normal growth hormone responsiveness is usually restored.[44] Finally, the degree of impairment of growth hormone responsiveness appears to be related to the degree of obesity.[45]

In many tissues, growth hormone promotes growth indirectly through stimulation of somatomedin or (insulin-like growth factor 1 (IGF–1) secretion. In obese subjects, IGF–1 levels are normal or elevated in the face of reduced growth hormone levels, explaining why normal growth is maintained in obese children despite low levels of growth hormone.[46] The mechanism by which IGF–1 is maintained at normal or elevated levels has not been established.

It is not known whether the abnormalities in growth hormone secretion or responsiveness to physiologic and pharmacologic stimuli have important consequences for the obese patient or are merely epiphenomena to be considered in the endocrine evaluation of these patients.

Blunted Prolactin Responsiveness

The serum levels and 24 integrated serum prolactin levels are normal in obese subjects.[47] However, prolactin responses to standard stimuli including insulin, thyrotropin-releasing hormone, and dopamine blockers are subnormal in obese patients.[48] The responses are improved by weight loss,[49] but some abnormalities may persist, such as the response to insulin-induced hypoglycemia,[50] suggesting some underlying hypothalamic abnormality. The significance of this abnormality is not established.

Hyperparathyroidism

Obese patients have elevated levels of parathyroid hormone compared to lean subjects,[51] and the elevation correlates with the degree of obesity.[52] Primary hyperparathyroidism due to a parathyroid adenoma or parathyroid gland hyperplasia is associated with elevated levels of both serum calcium and parathyroid hormone. In obese patients in whom calcium levels are normal or low, secondary hyperparathyroidism occurs by definition. In this situation, the elevated parathyroid hormone levels are presumed to be secondary to a primary deficiency of body stores of calcium or some other regulatory hormone such as vitamin D. The cause of the elevated parathyroid hormone levels in obese patients remains unknown, as is the significance of this observation.

Decreased Serum Testosterone

Obese men have been shown to have normal libido, secondary sexual characteristics, potency, and testicular size in spite of low or borderline low levels of total serum testosterone.[53] This discrepancy is explained by the fact that approximately 98% of circulating testosterone is bound to serum proteins, primarily sex hormone-binding globulin (SHBG). In obese men, SHBG levels are reduced, leading to a reduced total serum testosterone level with normal free levels of testosterone.[54] Since free testosterone is the biologically active form, there are no associated abnormalities of reproductive hormonal function in obese men without other reproductive disorders.

HORMONES USED IN THE TREATMENT OF OBESITY

Given the impression that obesity is a disorder of the endocrine system, a number of drugs have been used in the treatment of this disorder. None have been successful, and there are clear dangers in the use of some of them.

Thyroid Hormone

A number of studies have indicated that excessive use of thyroid hormone increases muscle catabolism. This can lead to excessive muscle loss and cardiac arrhythmias. This medication is both prescribed by certain physicians and self-administered by patients desperate to lose weight. If such patients are taking thyroxine, the level of triiodothyronine may be low relative to the level of thyroxine. This disorder is called *thyrotoxicosis factitia* when the hormone is taken secretly. Health professionals with access to medications should be suspected when symptoms of hyperthyroidism such as tachycardia, thinning hair, and nail changes are found in obese subjects. The most celebrated case in which thyroid hormone was prescribed for weight loss involved Muhammad Ali while in preparation for a fight he subsequently lost. He complained that he lost the strength in his punch due to the hormone treatment. The diagnosis can be established by measuring thyroid hormone levels.

In physiologic doses, thyroid hormone administration results in adjustments in the output of endogenous thyroid hormones, and a euthyroid state is maintained after some initial adjustment. These doses of thyroid hormone have been used to promote weight loss, without either proven efficacy or side effects.[55]

Human Chorionic Gonadotropin (hCG)

The Simeons diet is a plan that combines the use of hCG injections with a 500-calorie diet. It is claimed that the hCG promotes fat mobilization during weight loss. Carefully controlled studies have shown that hCG has no measurable effect on weight loss resulting from a 500-calorie diet compared to a control vehicle such as sesame oil.[56] It is generally assumed that the injection promotes adherence to the diet, and this treatment continues to be the basis of medically supervised weight loss programs in some commercial clinics.

Dehydroepiandrosterone

In some animal studies this adrenal hormone, which is a very weak androgen, has been shown to reduce food intake.[57] However, in humans there is no evidence that this hormone promotes weight loss. It has been sold in health food stores for this purpose. With prolonged or high-dose use, it has the potential problem of being converted into other biologically active steroids. Its safety for human use is not established.

CONCLUSION

Clearly, the endocrine system plays an integral role in the etiology and maintenance of obesity. Many of the changes observed in the obese patient are epiphenomena of unknown significance. However, abnormalities in insulin secretion and action are central to many of the observed metabolic changes in the obese patient and may play a role in the etiology and maintenance of obesity. Similarly, reproductive hormonal abnormalities appear to be closely related to obesity and may have special significance for understanding obesity in women throughout the various stages of development and during pregnancy. In designing strategies to address obesity in the population and in individual patients, an understanding of the role of the endocrine system is useful for both prevention and treatment.

REFERENCES

1. Copinschi G, DeLaet MH, Brion JP. Simultaneous study of cortisol, growth hormone, and prolactin nyctohemeral variations in normal and obese subjects: Influence of prolonged fasting in obesity. *Clin Endocrinol* 9:15, 1978.
2. Dunkelman SS, Fairhurst B, Plager J. Cortisola metabolism in obesity. *J Clin Endocrinol Metab* 24:832, 1964.
3. Strain GW, Zumoff B, Strain JJ, et al. Cortisol production in obesity. *Metabolism* 29:980, 1980.
4. Bray GA. Classification and evaluation of the obesities, in Bray GA (ed), *Obesity Med Clin North Am.* 73:170, 1989.
5. Bray GA. Syndromes of hypothalamic obesity in man. *Pediatr Ann* 13:525, 1984.
6. Bray GA, York DA. Hypothalamic and genetic obesity in experimental animals: An autonomic and endocrine hypothesis. *Physiol Rev* 59:719, 1979.
7. deRosa G, Della Casa S, Corsello M, et al. Thyroid function in altered nutritional state. *Exp Clin Endocrinol* 82:173, 1983.
8. Carlson HE, Drenick EJ, Chopra IJ. Alterations in basal and TRH-stimulated serum levels of thyrotropin, prolactin, and thyroid hormones in obese starved men. *J Clin Endocrinol Metab* 45:707, 1977.
9. Kyle LH, Ball MS, Doolan PD. Effect of thyroid hormone on body composition in myxedema and obesity. *N Engl J Med* 275:12, 1966.
10. Bray GA, Melvin KEW, Chopra IJ. Effect of triiodothyronine on some metabolic responses of obese patients. *Am J Clin Nutr* 26:715, 1973.
11. West KM. *Epidemiology of Diabetes and Its Vascular Complications.* New York, Elsevier, 1978, p. 231.
12. West KM, Kalbfleisch JM. Influence of nutritional factors on prevalence of diabetes. *Diabetes* 20:99, 1971.
13. Bagdade JD, Bierman EL, Porte D. The significance of basal insulin levels in the evaluation of the insulin response to glucose in diabetic and nondiabetic subjects. *J Clin Invest* 46:1549, 1967.
14. Faber OK, Christensen K, Kehlet H, et al. Decreased insulin removal contributes to hyperinsulinemia in obesity. *J Clin Endocrinol Metab* 53:618, 1981.

15. Howard BV, Klimes I, Vasquez B, et al. The antilipolytic action of insulin in obese subjects with resistance to its glucoregulatory action. *J Clin Endocrinol Metab* 58:544, 1984.
16. Ong JM, Kirschgessner TG, Schotz MC, et al. Insulin increases the synthetic rate and messenger RNA level of lipoprotein lipase in isolated rat adipocytes. *J. Biol. Chem* 263:1293, 1988.
17. Rodin J. Insulin levels, hunger, and food intake: An example of feedback loops in body weight regulation. *Health Psychol* 4:1, 1985.
18. Hartz AJ, Barboriak PH, Wong A, et al. The association of obesity with infertility and related menstrual abnormalitites in women. *Int J Obes* 3:57, 1987.
19. Nimrod A, Ryan KH. Aromatization of androgens by human abdominal and breast fat tissue. *J Clin Endocrinol Metab* 40:367, 1975.
20. Vague J. The degree of masculine differentiation of the obesities: A factor determining predisposition to diabetes, atherosclerosis, gout, and uric calculous disease. *Am J Clin Nutr* 4:20, 1956.
21. Kissebah AH, Evans DJ, Peiris A, et al. Endocrine characteristics in regional obesities: Role of sex steroids, in Vague J, Bjorntorp P, Guy-Grand B, et al (eds), *Metabolic Complications of Human Obesities*. Amsterdam, Excerpta Medica, 1985, p 115.
22. Spain DM, Nathan DJ, Gellis M. Weight, body type, and the prevalence of coronary atherosclerotic heart disease in males. *Am J Med Sci* 245:63, 1963.
23. Rebuffe-Scrive M, Eldh J, Hafstrom LO, et al. Metabolism of mammary, abdominal, and femoral adipocytes in women before and after the menopause. *Metabolism* 35:792, 1986.
24. Kerr MG. Significance of weight gain in pregnancy. *Lancet* 1:663, 1969.
25. Rebuffe-Scrive M. Metabolic differences in fat depots, in Bouchard C, Johnston FE (eds), *Fat Distribution during Growth and Later Health Outcomes*. New York, Alan R Liss, 1988, p 175.
26. Rebuffe-Scrive M, Enk L, Crona N, et al. Fat cell metabolism in different regions in women. *J Clin Invest* 75:1973, 1985.
27. Leibel RH, Hirsch J. Site and sex-related differences in adrenoreceptor status of human adipose tissue. *J Clin Endocrinol Metab* 64:1205, 1987.
28. Lyons PM, Truswell AS, Mira M, et al. Reduction of food intake in the ovulatory phase of the menstrual cycle. *Am J Clin Nutr* 49:1164, 1989.
29. Tchekmedyian NS, Hickman M, Heber D. Treatment of anorexia and weight loss in patients with cancer or acquired immunodeficiency syndrome. *Semin Oncol* 18:35, 1991.
30. Smals AGH, Kloppenberg PWC, Benraad TJ. Body proportions and androgenicity in relation to plasma testosterone levels in Klinefelter's syndrome. *Acta Endocrinol* 77:387, 1974.
31. Odell WD. Isolated deficiencies of anterior pituitary hormones: Symptoms and diagnosis. *JAMA* 197:1006, 1966.

32. Vermeulen A, Verdonck L. Sex hormone concentrations in postmenopausal women. Relation to obesity, fat mass, age, and years postmenopause. *Clin Endocrinol* 9:59, 1978.
33. Arendt EC, Pattee CJ. Studies on obesity. I. The insulin–glucose tolerance curve. *J Clin Endocrinol* 16:367, 1956.
34. Meistas MT, Foster GV, Margolis S, et al. Integrated concentrations of growth hormone, insulin, C-peptide and prolactin in human obesity. *Metabolism* 31:1224, 1982.
35. Kopelman PG, Noonan K, Goulton R, et al. Impaired growth hormone response to growth hormone releasing factor and insulin in obesity. *Clin Endocrinol* 23:87, 1985.
36. Kalucy RS, Crisp AH, Chart T. Nocturnal hormonal profiles in massive obesity, anorexia nervosa and normal females. *J Psychosom Res* 20:595, 1976.
37. Beck P, Koumans JHT, Winterling CA, et al. Studies of insulin and growth hormone secretion in human obesity. *J Lab Clin Med* 64:454, 1964.
38. Rabinowitz D, Merimee T, Nelson JK. The hormonal profile in obesity. *Trans Assoc Am Physicians* 80:190, 1967.
39. Hansen AP. Serum growth hormone response to exercise in nonobese and obese normal subjects. *Scand J Clin Lab Invest* 31:175, 1973.
40. Londono JH, Gallagher TF, Bray GA. Effect of weight reduction, triiodothyronine, and diethylstilbestrol on growth hormone in obesity. *Metabolism* 18:986, 1969.
41. Kelijman M, Frohman LA. Enhanced growth hormone responsiveness to GH-releasing hormone after dietary manipulation in obese and non-obese subjects. *J Clin Endocrinol Metab* 66:489, 1988.
42. Loche S, Cappa M, Berrelli P, et al. Reduced growth hormone response to growth hormone releasing hormone in children with simple obesity: Evidence for somatomedin-C mediated inhibition. *Clin Endocrinol* 27:145, 1987.
43. Sims EAH, Horton ES. Endocrine and metabolic adaptation to obesity and starvation. *Am J Clin Nutr* 21:1455, 1968.
44. Crockford PM, Salmon PA. Hormones and obesity: Changes in insulin and growth hormone secretion following surgically induced weight loss. *Can Med Assoc J* 103:147, 1970.
45. Williams T, Berelowitz M, Joffe SN, et al. Impaired growth hormone responses to growth hormone releasing factor in obesity: A defect reversed with weight reduction. *N Engl J Med* 331:1403, 1984.
46. Rosskamp R, Becker M, Soetadji S. Circulating somatomedin-C levels and the effect of growth hormone releasing factor on plasma levels of growth hormone and somatostatin-like immunoreactivity in obese children. *Eur J Pediatr* 146:48, 1987.
47. Wilcox RG. Triiodothyronine, TSH, and prolactin in obese women. *Lancet* 1:1027, 1977.
48. Cavagnini F, Maraschini C, Pinto M, et al. Impaired prolactin secretion in obese patients. *J Endocrinol Invest* 4:149, 1981.

49. Kopelman PG, White N, Pilkington TRE. Impaired hypothalamic control of prolactin secretion in massive obesity. *Lancet* 1:747, 1979.
50. Kopelman PG, Pilkington TRE, White N, et al. Persistence of defective hypothalamic control of prolactin secretion in some obese women after weight reduction. *Br Med J* 281:358, 1980.
51. Atkinson RL, Dahms WT, Bray GA, et al. Parathyroid hormone levels in obesity: Effects of intestinal bypass surgery. *Min Electr Metab* 1:315, 1978.
52. Bell NH, Epstein S, Greene A, et al. Evidence for alteration of the vitamin D-endocrine system in obese subjects. *J Clin Invest* 76:370, 1985.
53. Glass AR, Swerdloff RS, Bray GA, et al. Low serum testosterone and sex hormone binding globulin in massively obese men. *J Clin Endocrinol Metab* 45:1211, 1977.
54. Amatruda JM, Harman SM, Pourmotabbed G, et al. Depressed plasma testosterone and fractional binding of testosterone in obese males. *J Clin Endocrinol Metab* 47:268, 1978.
55. O'Brien JT, Bybee DE, Burman KD, et al. Thyroid hormone homeostasis in states of relative caloric deprivation. *Metabolism* 29:721, 1980.
56. Greenway FL, Bray GA. Human chorionic gonadotropin (HCG) in the treatment of obesity. A critical assessment of the Simeons method. *West J Med* 127:461, 1977.
57. Schwartz AT, Lewbart ML, Pashko U. Novel dehydroepiandrosterone analogues with enhanced biological activity and reduced side effects in mice and rats. *Cancer Res* 48(17):4817, 1988.

CHAPTER

6

Mechanisms of Appetite and Body Weight Regulation

Adam Drewnowski, Ph.D.

INTRODUCTION

Human obesity is a disease of multiple origin resulting from an interaction between genetic predisposition and diverse environmental variables, including diet.[1,2] Human obesities may therefore resemble animal models, ranging from those that are familial in nature to those that are largely diet-induced.[3] The expression of obesity is modified by caloric intake and expenditure, and may depend further on the macronutrient composition of the habitual diet.[4–6] In addition to diet-related factors, other psychological and sociocultural variables may contribute in different ways to the development and maintenance of the obese state.[7]

Dietary factors clearly play a major role in the regulation of body weight. Given genetic predisposition, the extent of obesity seems to be determined by long-term exposure to a given diet.[1] In animal studies, the most effective obesity-promoting diets were generally those that were high in fat, sugar, or both.[3,8–10] Laboratory rats responded to sweet taste or the oral sensation of fat and overconsumed calorie-dense sweet or fat-rich foods.[8] Although human data are still scarce, recent dietary intake studies suggest that the habitual diet of obese men and women may also be rich in fat.[4–6] The wide availability of fat-containing foods in the typical American diet[11] may be an important risk factor, promoting the expression of obesity among susceptible individuals.

Several studies have attempted to show that abnormalities in appetite and food selection have a direct impact on the development of obesity and the regulation of body weight. For example, increased preferences for sweet taste or a "sweet tooth" were once thought to lead to overconsumption of sweet desserts, resulting in weight gain.[12,13] Similarly, centrally induced cravings for a single macronutrient, carbohydrate, were thought to promote excessive intake of carbohydrate-rich snacks.[14,15] However, for a number of reasons, it has proved difficult to link human obesity with excess consumption of calories, let alone macronutrients or individual foods. Obese people do not appear to share a common profile of taste responsiveness and do not necessarily prefer the same kinds of foods. In most studies of taste preference or food consumption, intersubject variability was greater than any obese/lean distinctions.[16]

Given the heterogeneity of human obesity syndromes, it may be that some obese men and women are more susceptible than others to the effects of diet.[1] Specifically, it may be that a genetic predisposition to obesity is reflected in increased vulnerability to dietary challenge.[17] One type of challenge may involve exposure to palatable sweet or high-fat foods. Animal studies have already shown that various strains of rats are differentially susceptible to the effects of sugar- or fat-supplemented diets.[9] Osborne-Mendel rats are far more susceptible than the Sprague-Dawley strain to prolonged feeding with a high-fat diet.[3,9] Similarly, increased appetite for sweet or high-fat foods may be one behavioral mechanism by which susceptible individuals gain body weight.

Another possibility is that past cycles of weight loss and weight regain lead to improved metabolic efficiency and enhanced fat storage.[18] Loss and regain of body weight in laboratory rats was found to lead to an increased selection of a high-fat diet.[19] Although comparable human data are scarce, recent studies suggest that preferences and cravings for sweet, fat-rich desserts may be an important behavioral factor preventing dietary compliance and promoting subsequent weight regain.[17,20]

The study of sensory preferences and the appetite for sweet or high-fat foods has therefore acquired new importance in obesity research. According to some reports, elevated sensory preferences for ice cream, chocolate, pastries, and other sweet desserts among weight cyclers ("yo-yo" dieters) have been associated with weight regain.[21] Elevated taste responses to sugar/fat stimuli have been observed in obese men and women characterized by large fluctuations in body weight compared to obese individuals whose weights were more stable.[17,20] Taste preferences for sugar- and fat-containing stimuli may predict patterns of food selection. Taste preference profiles may also help distinguish between potentially different subgroups of obese individuals.

Potential subgroups may be characterized by an elevated familial risk of obesity, early age at onset, or a history of unsuccessful past attempts at weight reduction. Familial risk, thought to be a measure of genetic predisposition to obesity, is defined as the proportion of first-degree relatives (parents and siblings) who are also obese. At least two studies[17,22] have linked childhood-onset (<10 years) obesity with higher familial risk, suggesting that early age at onset may be a useful marker for genetic predisposition to the obese state.

This chapter will address the mechanisms of appetite and food preference and their impact on diverse subgroups of obese individuals.

Sensory Studies

The role of appetite and dietary choices in human obesity can be inferred from the study of taste preferences. Taste preferences are a major determinant of food selection, and taste data have been used to predict food choices in both humans and rats.[23, 24] Preferences for sweet taste are thought to predict the consumption of sweet, calorie-dense foods. While past research on taste preferences in obesity was largely restricted to sugar solutions in water,[25,27] more recent studies have focused on taste responsiveness to more complex food-like stimuli containing both sugar and fat.[28–30] Among such stimuli were milkshakes, cream cheese, cake frostings, and ice cream.[31–33]

Early studies on obesity and sweet taste failed to show that obese patients overrespond to the taste of intensely sweet solutions.[25,26] While some investigators reported an increased liking for sweetness among moderately obese subjects,[27] others did not find a consistent relationship between sweet taste preferences and overweight.[12,16,25,26] Still others found that massively obese patients disliked intensely sweet tastes in water, lemonade, or KoolAid.[31] Large-scale consumer studies found no relationship between body weight and sensory preferences for different levels of sugar in apricot nectar, canned peaches, lemonade, or vanilla ice cream.[32,33] Intersubject variability was generally far greater that any observed obese/normal differences.[33]

Later clinical studies examined sensory preferences for mixtures of milk, cream, and sugar among obese and anorectic women and age-matched normal-weight controls.[31] Massively obese women gave highest preference ratings to stimuli that were relatively low in sugar but rich in fat. In contrast, emaciated, anorectic patients liked an intensely sweet taste but showed an aversion to the oral sensation of fat.[34] These studies allowed us to link relative taste preferences for sugar versus fat with a measure of overweight. Figure 6–1 shows a negative relationship between hedonic preferences for sweet taste (expressed as the optimal sugar:fat ratio) and the degree of overweight expressed in terms of body mass index ($r = -0.43$). Increasing overweight was linked with elevated preferences for dietary fat. Other investigators have now confirmed that sensory preferences

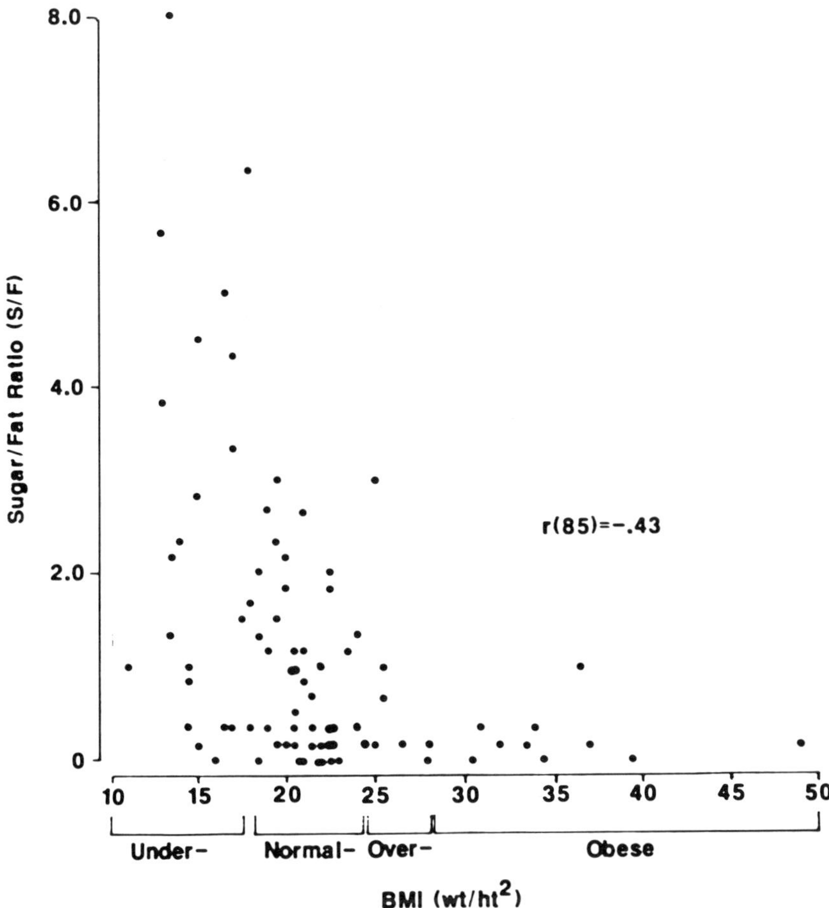

Figure 6–1. Relationship between the optimally preferred sugar:fat ratios and body mass indices of anorectic, normal-weight, and obese subjects. Low sugar:fat ratios denote a preference for fat over sugar in stimulus mixtures, while high ratios denote a preference for sugar over fat.

for a given level of fat in foods (though not fat consumption) are linked to the subjects' own percentage of body fat.[35]

Other studies have shown that a past history of weight loss and weight regain has a direct impact on sensory preferences for sweet, high-fat foods. In one recent study,[17] a representative community-based sample of 61 obese and 31 lean adults tasted and rated nine taste stimuli resembling cake frostings. The stimuli were composed of butter, sucrose, polydextrose, and water, and contained between 20% and 70% sucrose, weight by weight, and between 15% and 35%

fat. No significant differences in sweetness, fat content, or preference ratings were initially observed between groups of obese and lean subjects.

Obese subjects were then divided into subgroups based on the age of onset of obesity and past fluctuations in body weight. Age at onset of obesity (<10 years), though associated with elevated familial risk, had no effect on taste preference profiles. In contrast, obese subjects characterized by high restraint scores and large fluctuations in body weight showed elevated sensory preferences for the frosting-like stimuli compared to obese subjects whose weights were more stable. These data are consistent with anecdotal reports that elevated preferences for fat-rich desserts are typical of weight cyclers.[21]

Another study[20] makes a similar point. A group of 37 obese women was divided into low-flux and high-flux subgroups according to the magnitude of past fluctuations in body weight. Variability in body weight coupled with high maximal weight during adult life is thought to be indicative of the weight cycling syndrome. The subjects tasted and rated a range of sucrose solutions in water, as well as nine ice creams of varying sugar (12–18% wt/wt) and fat content (10–20% wt/wt). The high-flux and low-flux groups did not differ in their perceptions of preferences for sweet solutions. In contrast, the high-flux group gave significantly higher hedonic preference ratings for ice cream than did the low-flux group. Variability in body weight seems to be associated with elevated sensory preferences for calorie-dense foods.

Food Preferences

Preferences for sweet, high-calorie foods are thought to play a major role in the development of human obesity. However, enhanced responsiveness to sugar/fat mixtures does not necessarily lead to increased preferences for and overeating of all sweet desserts. Although taste factors may influence appetite and food preference, attitudes toward body weight and dieting often override physiologic and metabolic signals.[36,37] In other words, taste is often tempered by cognitive factors, including prior learning and prior experience.

One important point is that people think in terms of foods, not macronutrients. Food preferences and food acceptance are typically assessed with regard to a specific food item rather than a macronutrient—carbohydrate, protein, or fat. Yet the literature on food choices in human obesity has been dominated by reports of cravings for a single macronutrient, carbohydrate.[14,15] A majority of obese people reportedly showed a specific appetite for carbohydrate-rich foods, selecting carbohydrates as meals or snacks even though other foods were available.[15,38] Cravings for carbohydrates among obese patients were reputed to be widespread,[38,39] and excess carbohydrate intake was viewed as an important contributor to the obese state.[14]

In contrast, other studies have suggested that dietary fat plays a major role in human obesity. Dietary intake studies have shown that obese women consumed more fat calories than did lean women and had a lower dietary carbohydrate:fat ratio.[40] In taste preference studies with sugar/fat mixtures, obese women preferred sensory stimuli that were relatively low in sugar but high in fat.[28] In other studies, high levels of body fat have been correlated with the amount of fat in the diet[41].

A systematic study of the food preferences of obese men and women should help us to distinguish between preferences for carbohydrates versus fat-rich foods. However, past reports of food preferences in human obesity were largely restricted to preferences for carbohydrates or sweet desserts, thus reinforcing the persistent notion that sugars and starches are the characteristic food choices of obese individuals.[14]

In one recent study,[42] 93 obese male and 386 obese female patients were asked to generate lists of their 10 favorite foods. These lists were then analyzed, not according to whether the foods were high in carbohydrate or fat, but according to whether they were major contributors of carbohydrate or fat calories to the typical American diet. If food preference questionnaires are to predict the consumption of a given nutrient, they should be based on foods that are major sources of that nutrient in the population's diet. Preferences for frequently eaten foods should be weighted more heavily than preferences for rarely eaten foods, since the latter are less likely to affect the nutritional status of the population or influence the development of obesity. Thus, if human obesity is indeed caused largely by carbohydrate cravings and excessive carbohydrate consumption, then obesity should be associated with heightened preferences for major sources of carbohydrate in the U.S. diet. Conversely, consistent selection of a fat-rich diet should be reflected in more widespread preferences for chief nutrient sources of fat.

Foods that are the top sources of calories in the American diet are listed in Table 6–1. The category of white bread, rolls and crackers contributes 9.6% of total daily calories, followed by doughnuts, cookies, and cake (5.7%) and by alcoholic beverages (5.6%). Together these 10 foods or food categories contribute a cumulative total of almost 46% calories in the typical U.S. diet.

The top 10 sources of carbohydrate calories are listed in Table 6–2. These foods contribute a cumulative total of 76.3% of carbohydrate calories to the diet. According to NHANES II data,[11] the largest single source of carbohydrate is the category of white bread, rolls and crackers, followed by nondiet soft drinks and doughnuts, cookies, and cake.

More than half (56.2%) of obese women named at least one item from the "doughnuts, cookies, or cake" category among their favorite foods. Similarly, over half of the women (54.4%) named as favorites at least one instance of white bread, rolls, or crackers, or listed ice cream (51.3%) as a favorite food. Named less frequently were pasta dishes (39.1%), chocolate candy (32.4%), potatoes (29.5%), and salty snacks (23.8%).

Men tended to list carbohydrate sources among their favorite foods less often

TABLE 6-1 Chief Nutrient Sources of Calories in the U.S. Diet

Food Type	% of Caloric Intake	Cumulative % of Caloric intake
1. White bread, rolls	9.6	9.6
2. Doughnuts, cookies, cake	5.7	15.3
3. Alcoholic beverages	5.6	20.9
4. Whole milk	4.7	25.6
5. Hamburger, cheeseburger	4.4	30.0
6. Beefsteaks, roasts	4.1	34.1
7. Regular soft drinks	3.6	37.7
8. Hot dogs, ham, lunch meats	3.2	40.9
9. Eggs	2.5	43.5
10. French fries	2.5	46.0

Source: Data are based on the NHANES II survey, 1976–80.[11]

than did women. Fewer men than women named white bread, doughnuts, chocolate candy, salty snacks, and soft drinks among their favorite foods. In contrast, there was no difference between men and women in their preferences for ice cream, pasta dishes, potatoes, and french fries.

Among carbohydrate sources, such foods as doughnuts, white bread, ice cream, pasta dishes, french fries, and salty snacks are also major sources of fat. In addition, doughnuts, pies, and ice cream are generally sweet. Preferences for

TABLE 6-2 Obese Respondents' Preferences for Foods that are Major Sources of Carbohydrate in the U.S. Diet

Food Type	% of Carbohydrate Intake	Percentage of	
		Women (n=386)	Men (n=93)
1. White bread, rolls	15.0	54.4	37.6
2. Regular soft drinks	8.6	7.3	1.1
3. Doughnuts, cookies, cake	7.5	56.2	39.8
4. Sugar	3.5	0.3	—
5. Whole milk	3.5	6.0	6.5
6. French fries, fried potatoes	3.3	14.2	18.3
7. Alcoholic beverages	3.3	4.1	4.3
8. Whole wheat, dark breads	3.1	1.6	1.1
9. Orange juice	3.0	1.0	—
10. Potatoes, excl. fried	2.3	29.5	26.9

Source: Food list based on the National Health and Nutrition Examination Survey (NHANES II), as cited by Block et al. (11). Preference data are based on Drewnowski et al.[42]

these foods far outweighed preferences for carbohydrate sources that did not contain fat, such as cereals, rice, fruit juices, or sugar itself. These findings suggest that preferences for carbohydrate/fat sources are far more common than preferences for carbohydrate sources. Furthermore, preferences for sweet, fat-rich foods such as doughnuts or ice cream appear to be far more common among obese women than among obese men.

Major nutrient sources of fat in the American diet are summarized in Table 6–3. According to NHANES II data,[11] the category of hamburgers, cheeseburgers, and meatloaf contributes the largest percentage of fat calories to the diet (7.0%); followed by hot dogs, ham, lunch meat (6.4%), and whole milk and milk beverages (6.0%). Together the 25 foods contribute a cumulative total of 81.6% of fat calories.

As many as 72% of the men but only 41.2% of the women listed steak or roast among their favorite foods. Preferences for other sources of fat were also more marked than preferences for sources of carbohydrate. Some gender differences were also observed. More men than women expressed preferences for hot dogs, bacon and sausage, eggs, and salad and cooking oils. On the other hand, women listed cheese more often than did men.

While obese men named more fat and fat/protein sources (i.e., meats) among their favorite foods, obese women named more carbohydrate/fat sources and more foods that were sweet. Thus selective preferences for carbohydrate-rich foods do not appear to be a characteristic feature of human obesity. On the contrary, it seems that the favorite foods of obese men and women were those

TABLE 6-3 Obese Respondents' Preferences for Foods that are Major Sources of Fat in the U.S. Diet

		Percentage of	
Food Type	% of Fat Intake	Women (n=386)	Men (n=93)
1. Hamburgers, cheeseburgers, meatloaf	7.0	18.4	25.8
2. Hot dogs, ham, lunch meat	6.4	9.3	25.8
3. Whole milk, milk beverages	6.0	6.0	6.5
4. Doughnuts, cookies, cake	6.0	56.2	39.8
5. Beef steaks, roasts	5.4	41.2	72.0
6. White bread, rolls	4.9	54.4	37.6
7. Eggs	4.6	11.7	23.7
8. Cheeses, excl. cottage cheese	4.5	37.6	26.9
9. Margarine	4.5	—	—
10. Mayonnaise, salad dressings	4.3	6.5	2.2

Source: Food list based on the National Health and Nutrition Examination Survey (NHANES II), as cited by Block et al. (11). Preference data are based on Drewnowski et al.[42]

that were major nutrient sources of fat. Carbohydrates were listed less frequently, and only if they were also major sources of fat or were sweet.

Obesity and Caloric Intake

The question of whether obesity is associated with excess caloric intake has a long, controversial history. Clinical studies have generally found that obese men and women consumed no more calories than lean controls.[43] Of course, the accuracy of dietary recall among the obese population has been questioned, and the common assumption is that obese patients underreport daily caloric intakes by one-third or more.[44]

Analysis of large-scale NHANES I data based on 24-hr food recalls actually found a negative correlation between overeating and overweight.[45] The most obese women appeared to be consuming the fewest calories. It is questionable whether the measure of a single day's recall is suitable for use with a chronically dieting population. However, in another study involving obese men, greater obesity was associated with lower caloric intake.[46] Only one study, conducted with a large patient population in a Paris hospital, demonstrated a positive relationship between the extent of obesity (as measured by body mass index) and dietary intake.[47]

Early epidemiologic studies focused on the supposed connection between obesity and excessive sugar consumption. However, in a nationwide study of almost 1000 adolescents aged 5–18, no significant link was found between self-reported intakes of sweet snacks and body fatness.[48] Data from the Ten State Nutrition Survey showed no relationship between triceps skinfolds of teenagers and reported intakes of sugar-containing foods including jams, honey, candies, and soft drinks.[49]

By contrast, there is increasing evidence that the diet of obese individuals is relatively rich in fat.[40,41,47,50] In one recent study, percentage of calories from fat, as estimated from 7-day food records, was linked to percentage of body fat in 155 adult men.[41] However, another study[35] which linked sensory preferences for fat in foods with percentage of body fat in men and women, failed to find a significant relationship between percentage of body fat and percentage of fat calories in the diet.

Additional studies showed that men and women who derived a higher proportion of energy intake from fat weighed more than those who consumed a lower-fat diet.[50] Fat intake, adjusted for total caloric intake, was positively correlated with adiposity, as measured by the sum of skinfolds technique. The available data suggest that the habitual diet of obese individuals is not characterized by overeating and excessive caloric intake. On the other hand, there are indications that their diet may be rich in fat.

CONCLUSIONS

Both genetic and dietary factors contribute to the expression of human obesity. However, there is still little evidence that selective appetites for macronutrients or individual foods lead directly to overeating and overweight. Indeed, only a few studies have managed to link obesity with excess caloric intake: In most cases, obese subjects appear to eat no more than lean controls. However, there is preliminary evidence that the habitual diet of obese men and women is relatively rich in fat.

Some of these discrepancies may be solved by methodologic improvements. Obtaining accurate dietary intake data from obese patients is notoriously difficult. However, it should also be noted that not all obese people are alike and that human obesity represents a range of syndromes. Obesity need not always be associated with overeating. Elevated preferences for fat and sugar are by no means characteristic of all obese people. As noted above, significant differences in taste responsiveness were found among obese individuals of comparable body weight but different weight history. Continued comparisons of obese and lean subjects may no longer be the research strategy of choice. There is no reason to expect obese people with different familial predispositions and past weight histories to resemble each other in terms of taste responsiveness, food preference, or food consumption.

Further research should aim to classify human obesities into potential sub-

TABLE 6-4 Subcategories of Human Obesity

Criteria	Possible Options		
	I	II	III
Taxonomic			
Overweight	Mild : 120–150 IBW	Moderate: 150–200% IBW	Massive: >200% IBW
Obese (fat %)	Mild	Moderate	Massive
Fat distribution	Lower body	Upper body	
Familial			
Family history	Neither parent obese	One parent obese	Both parents obese
Age of onset	Adult >20 years	Juvenile 10–20 years	Childhood <10 years
Environmental			
Body weight status	Net loss	Stable	Weight gain
Weight cycling	None	1–3 cycles	>3 cycles

groups on the basis of genetic, metabolic, and behavioral variables. Past criteria in classifying human obesities have been such taxonomic variables as the extent of obesity, body composition, and the amount and distribution of body fat. Additional criteria may include familial risk of obesity, age at onset, and history of weight loss and weight regain. One possible scheme is summarized in Table 6–4. However, as far as we know, these criteria do not seem to predict success at therapy or the likelihood of sustained weight loss. The present studies suggest that classification of obesity should be supplemented with behavioral variables, notably taste preference profiles, food preferences, and dietary intake measures. Such behavioral variables may predict vulnerability to the effects of diet and thus help characterize different types of human obesity.

REFERENCES

1. Stunkard AJ. Some perspectives on human obesity: its causes. *Bull NY Acad Med* 64:902, 1988.
2. Dept of Health and Human Services. *The Surgeon General's Report on Nutrition and Health*. DHHS Pub. (PHS) 88–50210. Washington, DC; US Government Printing Office, 1988.
3. Sclafani A. Animal models of obesity: Classification and characterization. *Int J Obes* 8:491, 1986.
4. Lissner L, Levitsky DA, Strupp BJ, et al. Dietary fat and the regulation of energy intake in human subjects. *Am J Clin Nutr* 46:886, 1987.
5. Romieu I, Willett WC, Stampfer M, et al. Energy intake and other determinants of relative weight. *Am J Clin Nutr* 47:406, 1988.
6. Tremblay A, Plourde G, Despres JP, et al. Impact of dietary fat content and fat oxidation on energy intake in humans. *Am J Clin Nutr* 49:799, 1989.
7. Drewnowski A. Taste and food preferences in human obesity, in Capaldi ED, Powley TL (eds), *Taste, Experience and Feeding*. Washington, DC, American Psychological Association, 1990, pp. 227–240.
8. Lucas F, Sclafani A. Hyperphagia in rats produced by a mixture of fat and sugar. *Physiol Behav* 47:51, 1990.
9. Schemmel R, Mickelson O, Gill JL. Dietary obesity in rats: Body weight and body fat accretion in seven strains of rats. *J Nutr* 100:1041, 1970.
10. Kanarek RB, Hirsch E. Dietary induced overeating in experimental animals. *Fed Proc* 36:154, 1977.
11. Block G, Dresser CM, Hartman AM, et al. Nutrient sources in the American diet: Quantitative data from the NHANES II survey. *Am J Epidemiol* 122:27, 1985.
12. Rodin J, Moskowitz HR, Bray GA. Relationship between obesity, weight loss, and taste responsiveness. *Physiol Behav* 17:591, 1976.

13. Rodin J. Implications of responsiveness to sweet taste in obesity, in Weiffenbach JM (ed), *Taste and Development: The Genesis of Sweet Preference*. DHEW Pub (NIH) 77–1068. Washington, DC, US Government Printing Office, pp. 295–308, 1977.
14. Wurtman JJ. The involvement of brain serotonin in excessive carbohydrate snacking by obese carbohydrate cravers. *J Am Diet Assoc* 84:1004, 1984.
15. Wurtman JJ, Wurtman RJ, Growdon JH, et al. Carbohydrate craving in obese people: Suppression by treatments affecting serotoninergic transmission. *Int J Eating Disorders* 1:2, 1981.
16. Witherly SA, Panghorn RM, Stern J. Gustatory responses and eating duration of obese and lean adults. *Appetite* 1:53, 1980.
17. Drewnowski A, Kurth CL, Rahaim JE. Taste preferences in human obesity: Environmental and familial factors. *ASM J Clin Nutr* 54:635, 1991.
18. Yost TJ, Eckel RH. Fat calories may be preferentially stored in reduced obese women: A permissive pathway for resumption of obese state. *J Clin Endocrinol Metab* 67:259, 1988.
19. Reed DR, Contreras RJ, Maggio C, et al. Weight cycling in female rats increases dietary fat selection and adiposity. *Physiol Behav* 42:389, 1988.
20. Drewnowski A. Holden-Wiltse J. Taste responses and food preferences in obese women: Effects of weight cycling. *Int J Obes* 16:639, 1992.
21. Anonymous. Could I be addicted to sweets? *Lose Weight Naturally* 4:10, 1990.
22. Price RA, Stunkard AJ, Ness R, et al. Childhood onset (age < 10) obesity has high familial risk. *Int J Obes* 14:185, 1990.
23. Beidler LM. Biological basis of food intake, in Beidler LM (ed.), *The Psychobiology of Human Food Selection*. Westport, Conn., AVI, 1983, pp. 3–15.
24. Drewnowski A. Sensory preferences for fat and sugar in adolescence and in adult life. *Ann NY Acad Sci* 561:243, 1989.
25. Thompson DA, Moskowitz HR, Campbell R. Effects of body weight and food intake on pleasantness ratings for a sweet stimulus. *J Appl Psychol* 41:77, 1976.
26. Underwood PJ, Belton JE, Hulme P. Aversion to sucrose in obesity. *Proc Nutr Soc* 32:93a, 1973.
27. Cabanac M, Duclaux R. Obesity: Absence of satiety aversion to sucrose. *Science* 170:496, 1970.
28. Drewnowski A, Brunzell J, Sande K, et al. Sweet tooth reconsidered: Taste responsiveness in human obesity. *Physiol Behav* 35:617, 1985.
29. Drewnowski A, Schwartz M. Invisible fats: Sensory assessment of sugar/fat mixtures. *Appetite* 14:203, 1990.
30. Drewnowski A. Fats and food texture: Sensory and hedonic evaluations, in Moskowitz HR (ed), *Food Texture*. New York, Marcel Dekker, 1983, pp 629–633.
31. Drewnowski A. Sweetness and obesity, in J. Dobbing (ed), *Sweetness*. ILSI-Nutrition Foundation Symposium. Berlin, Springer-Verlag, 1987, pp 177–192.

32. Pangborn RM, Simone M. Body size and sweetness preference. *J Am Diet Assoc* 34:924, 1958.
33. Pangborn RM. Individuality in responses to sensory stimuli, in Solms J, Hall RL (eds), *Criteria* of Food Acceptance: How a Man Chooses What He Eats. Zurich, Foster Verlag AG, 1981, p. 177.
34. Drewnowski A, Halmi KA, Gibbs J, et al. Taste and eating disorders. *Am J Clin Nutr* 46:442, 1987.
35. Mela DJ, Sacchetti DA. Sensory preferences for fats: Relationships with diet and body composition. *Am J Clin Nutr* 53:908, 1991.
36. Drewnowski A. Fats and food acceptance: Sensory, hedonic and attitudinal aspects, in Solms J, Booth DA, Pangborn RM, et al (eds), *Food Acceptance and Nutrition*. New York, Academic Press, 1987, pp. 189–204.
37. Drewnowski A, Pierce B, Halmi KA. Fat avoidance in eating disorders. *Appetite* 10:119, 1988.
38. Lieberman HR, Wurtman JJ, Chew B. Changes in mood after carbohydrate consumption among obese individuals. *Am J Clin Nutr* 44:772, 1986.
39. Heraief E, Burckhardt P, Wurtmann JJ, et al. Tryptophan administration may enhance weight loss by some moderately obese patients on a protein-sparing modified fast (PMSF) diet. *Int J Eating Disorders* 4:281, 1985.
40. Romieu I, Willett WC, Stampfer MJ, et al. Energy intake and other determinants of relative weight. *Am J Clin Nutr* 47:406, 1988.
41. Dreon DM, Frey-Hewitt B, Ellsworth N, et al. Dietary fat:carbohydrate ratio and obesity in middle-aged men. *Am J Clin Nutr* 47:995, 1988.
42. Drewnowski A, Kurth CL, Holden-Wiltse J, et al. Food preferences in human obesity: Carbohydrates versus fats. *Appetite* 18:207, 1992.
43. Gates JC, Huenemann RL, Brand RJ. Food choices of obese and non-obese persons. *J Am Diet Assoc* 76:339, 1975.
44. Lansky D, Brownell KD. Estimates of food quantity and calories: Errors in self-report among obese patients. *Am J Clin Nutr* 35:727, 1984.
45. Braitman LE, Adlin EV, Stanton JL. Obesity and caloric intake: The National Health and Nutrition Examination Survey of 1971–75. *J Chronic Dis* 38:727, 1985.
46. Kromhout D. Energy and macronutrient intake in lean and obese middle-aged men (the Zutphen study). *Am J Clin Nutr* 37:295, 1983.
47. Fricker J, Fumeron F, Clair D, et al. A positive correlation between energy intake and body mass index in a population of 1312 overweight subjects. *Int J Obes* 13:663, 1989.
48. Morgan KJ, Johnson SR, Stampley GL. Children's frequency of eating, total sugar intake and weight/height stature. *Nutr Res* 3:635, 1983.
49. Garn SM, Solomon MA, Cole PE. Sugar-food intake of obese and lean adolescents. *Ecol Food Nutr* 9:219, 1980.
50. George V, Tremblay A, Despres JP, et al. Effect of dietary fat content on total and regional adiposity in men and women. *Int J Obes* 14:1085, 1990.

Obesity and Exercise

CHAPTER

7

Janet E. Whatley, Sc.D.
and Eric T. Poehlman, Ph.D.

INTRODUCTION

Historically, exercise has not been included in weight loss programs for the treatment of obesity. A review by Wing and Jeffrey[1] reported that less than 6% of all weight loss studies included exercise as a component of obesity treatment. Today, however, the Scientific Affairs Council of the American Medical Association[2] and the American Dietetic Association[3] have recognized exercise as one of the three basic modalities necessary for effective treatment of obesity, along with caloric restriction and behavior modification. The combination of exercise and caloric restriction is based on the hypothesis that exercise will accelerate fat loss, preserve fat-free mass (FFM), and prevent or decelerate the decline in resting metabolic rate (RMR) more effectively than caloric restriction alone.

Dr. E.T. Poehlman is supported by the National Institute of Aging (AG07857) and the American Association of Retired Persons Andrus Foundation (AARP). This work was partially supported by the General Clinical Research Center at the University of Vermont (RR–109).

Relationships between caloric restriction, exercise, weight loss, fat loss, FFM preservation, and alterations in RMR are complex and multifactorial. First, the ability of the body to spare FFM during caloric restriction is dependent on numerous dietary factors, including the magnitude of the energy deficit; the quality and quantity of protein; and the presence of adequate vitamins, electrolytes, and minerals.[4] Second, initial body fat status appears to be inversely related to the amount of FFM lost during caloric restriction, with a greater initial body fat content associated with a smaller proportion of FFM lost.[5] In addition, the greater the magnitude of weight loss, the greater the proportion of FFM lost during caloric restriction.[5] Finally, genotype may affect an individual's ability to spare FFM during caloric restriction.[6]

Certain exercise programs have been shown to result in body weight and fat loss, but the magnitude of these losses is less dramatic than that achieved by caloric restriction alone.[7] The ability of exercise to elicit positive body composition changes is affected by numerous factors, including mode of exercise, length of exercise training, and initial fitness level.[8] In addition, there may be a genetic influence in an individual's response to exercise training.[6] The American College of Sports Medicine suggests that for body weight and fat loss to occur, an endurance exercise threshold exists that consists of a frequency of at least 3 days per week, a duration of at least 20 min, and an intensity sufficient to expend approximately 300 kcal per exercise session.[8]

Although a plethora of studies have examined the combined influence of exercise and caloric restriction on changes in body composition and energy expenditure, no definitive conclusions regarding their optimal combination have emerged. The majority of studies employed a research design that compares fixed caloric restriction alone, of various adequate and inadequate nutrient composition, to caloric restriction in combination with endurance exercise. In general, the energy cost of exercise when combined with caloric restriction results in a greater energy deficit compared to the energy deficit created by caloric restriction alone. Thus, it is unclear (1) if the variation in the magnitude of the deficit state created by these conditions can be compared and (2) if the body adapts similarly to an energy deficit created by low versus very low caloric restriction, various exercise routines, or some combination of the two.

This chapter will briefly examine data derived from studies that employed both exercise and caloric restriction in their treatment of obesity. Only those studies that measured body composition will be examined, since the relative contribution of FFM and fat weight to total weight loss is a critical issue.

This chapter will relate changes in body weight, fat, FFM, and RMR to energy deficits created by caloric restriction, either alone or in combination with exercise. Possible explanations for inconsistent results in the literature are discussed, and methodologic considerations for future studies are considered.

ENDURANCE EXERCISE, CALORIC RESTRICTION, AND BODY COMPOSITION

The additional energy cost of exercise, when combined with caloric restriction, has been shown to increase body weight and fat loss compared to diet alone. For example, Hagan et al.[9] reported a significantly greater weight loss in 48 obese males and females after a 12-week, 1200 kcal/day diet combined with exercise compared to diet alone (−11.4 kg vs. −8.4 kg in males; −7.5 kg vs. −5.5 kg in females; $p < .05$). Exercise consisted of 30 min of walking or running for 5 days per week. Exercise intensity was not reported. Body composition, estimated by hydrostatic weighing, showed that for both males and females, the weight lost as fat in the exercise-plus-diet group was significantly greater than that of the diet-only group (−7.9 kg vs. −5.9 kg; $p < 0.05$). The energy cost of exercise was reported to create a 700- to 900-kcal/session deficit for the males and a 500- to 600-kcal/session deficit for the females. The authors suggested that this additional energy deficit created by exercise explained the difference in body weight and fat loss between the groups. These results are consistent with those of Hill et al.,[10] who evaluated 40 obese females consuming an average diet of 1200 kcal/day, with or without exercise, over a 12-week period. Exercise consisted of a supervised walking program five times per week, progressing from 20 to 50 min per session at an intensity of 70% of the maximum heart rate (HR max). Results showed that the exercising groups lost significantly more weight than the nonexercisers (−8.6 ± 0.9 kg vs. −6.5 ± 0.9 kg; $p < 0.5$). Although the energy cost of exercise was not reported, body composition, estimated by hydrostatic weighing, showed that for exercisers 86% of the weight loss came from fat mass and 14% from FFM, but that for the nonexercisers, 73% of the weight loss came from fat mass and 27% from FFM.

Several studies report similar total weight loss with exercise plus caloric restriction compared to caloric restriction alone. However, a greater proportion of fat loss and preservation of FFM are found when exercise is added to caloric restriction. Pavlou et al.[11] investigated 72 obese males consuming an average of 800 kcal/day, with or without exercise, over an 8-week period. Exercise was conducted 3 days per week and consisted of a walk/jog program progressing from 2.4 to 8.9 km at an intensity of 70 to 85% HR max. Body weight loss was not significantly different between the exercising and nonexercising groups (−11.8 ± 0.6 kg vs. −9.2 ± 0.3 kg). Body composition changes, estimated by whole body potassium (^{40}K), showed that FFM for the exercisers remained relatively unchanged (−0.6 ± 0.9 kg), whereas the nonexercisers lost a significant amount of FFM (−3.3 ± 1.0 kg). The composition of weight lost was 5% as FFM for the exercisers compared to 36% as FFM for the non-exercisers. The estimated energy cost of the exercise program was 12,000 kcal.

In a metabolic ward study, Hill et al.[12] investigated body composition changes estimated by hydrostatic weighing in eight obese females over 5 weeks consuming an 800-kcal/day diet. Five subjects participated in a daily progressive walking program (2.3 to 5.7 km/day), while three subjects remained sedentary. Total weight loss did not differ significantly between the groups (−8.2 ± 0.7 kg vs. −8.0 ± 1.2 kg). However, the exercisers lost 74% of their weight as fat and 26% as FFM, whereas the nonexercisers lost 57% of their weight from fat and 43% from FFM. The energy cost of exercise, which was estimated to be 10,101 ± 830 kcal, accounted for the greater energy lost in the exercise group.

The above studies collectively show that the additional energy cost of exercise combined with caloric restriction results in a greater proportion of fat loss compared to caloric restriction alone. The lack of difference in total body weight loss found in some studies may be explained by the greater energy lost when a greater proportion of fat is lost, assuming that 1 kg of fat equals 7000 kcal and 1 kg of FFM is equivalent to 900 kcal.[13] In addition, it appears that an exercise threshold deficit of greater than 10,000 kcal is necessary to observe a measurable difference in body composition changes between caloric restriction plus exercise versus caloric restriction alone.

In contrast, other studies report similar body weight loss, fat loss, and FFM loss with exercise plus caloric restriction compared to caloric restriction alone. Phinney et al.[14] investigated the use of a 720 kcal/day diet with 12 obese subjects for 4–5 weeks, with or without exercise. Exercise was conducted 5 days per week and consisted of a cycle ergometry protocol progressing from 30 min to 2 hr daily at an intensity of 50% maximum oxygen consumption (VO_2 max). Total weight loss was not significantly different between the two groups (−6.9 ± 0.7 kg vs. −6.5 ± 0.7 kg). No differences were reported in the average daily nitrogen balance data between the groups, suggesting a similar proportion of FFM and thus of fat loss. The authors indicate that the cost of exercise should have resulted in an additional loss of 1 kg of fat during the first 3 weeks of the study protocol; however, this effect was not observed.

Krotkiewski et al.[15] investigated 18 obese subjects following a 500 kcal/day diet for 3 weeks when subjects either exercised 3 days per week for 55 min/session, using a variety of endurance exercises, or remained sedentary. Body weight loss was not significantly different between the exercise and nonexercise groups (−6.8 ± 2.6 kg vs. −6.2 ± 1.7 kg). FFM and body fat loss, as estimated by ^{40}K total body potassium, showed no differences between groups. The cost of exercise was estimated to be approximately 5000 kcal over the 3-week study period, too small an increase to result in significantly different weight or fat loss compared to the nonexercisers.

Van Dale et al.[16] studied 12 obese women on a diet alone or on a diet plus exercise program. A 700 kcal/day diet was consumed for 5 weeks, followed by an 820 kcal/day diet for 8 weeks. Exercise was conducted 4 days per week for

1 hr, consisting of aerobic dance and calisthenics. No significant differences were found between the exercise and nonexercise groups in total weight loss (-13.2 ± 1.5 kg vs. -12.2 ± 4.7 kg). Body composition, estimated by hydrostatic weighing, showed no significant differences in loss of fat or FFM. Although the cost of exercise was estimated at 11,520 kcal over the 3-month study protocol and accounted for the additional 1.5 kg of fat lost in the exercise group, it was not a measurable difference compared to the non-exercise group.

The above findings demonstrate the inability of endurance exercise in combination with caloric restriction to produce a significantly greater fat loss and a preservation of FFM compared to caloric restriction alone in obese individuals.

POSSIBLE EXPLANATIONS FOR THE INCONSISTENT FINDINGS

Reasons for the discrepant findings in body composition changes during caloric restriction combined with exercise are not completely understood. Table 7–1 presents a summary of the studies reviewed. Methodologic differences and/or flaws, as well as lack of adequate documentation of both diet and exercise protocols, make it difficult to interpret and compare studies. Discrepant results among studies may be a function of differences in the following areas:

1. *Magnitude of caloric restriction:* The ability of exercise to elicit a positive effect on body composition during caloric restriction may be dependent on the level of caloric restriction, with the effect of exercise diminishing as caloric restriction becomes more severe.[12,17] With severe caloric restriction, the protein content of the diet may be the most critical factor for preserving FFM.[18]
2. *Duration of exercise training:* Physiologic adaptations to endurance exercise such as improved cardiorespiratory function and increased skeletal muscle mitochondria occur over time. A minimum of 15 to 20 weeks of training may be necessary for changes to occur; therefore, short-term studies may be limited in their ability to observe exercise training adaptations.[8] These training adaptations could result in changes in substrate utilization. For example, endurance exercise after adequate adaptation (3–5 weeks) may preserve FFM by causing an increase in the oxidation of lipid, which, in turn, would spare muscle glycogen stores and reduce the need to deaminate amino acids for synthesis of glycogen.[19,20]
3. *Initial body fat status:* The large fat stores in obese individuals increase their ability to retain FFM during caloric restriction.[5,21] Thus, it is important to take into account the degree of obesity when comparing results regarding preservation of FFM in weight loss studies.
4. *Heterogeneity of obesity:* Morphologically distinct subgroups of obesity may exist that respond differently to exercise. Individuals with hypertrophic obesity display

TABLE 7-1 Comparison of Body Composition Changes Among Studies

Study	Caloric Intake (kcal/day)	Weeks	Weight Loss (kg)		FFM Loss (kg)	
			Diet	Diet and Exercise	Diet	Diet and Exercise
Hagan et al.[9]	1200	12	8.4 (M)	11.4 (M)*	3.5 (M)	2.5 (M)
			5.5 (F)	7.5 (F)*	1.6 (F)	0.6 (F)
Hill et al.[10]	1200	12	6.5	8.6*	1.8	1.6
Pavlou et al.[11]	800	8	9.2	11.8	3.3	0.6*
Hill et al.[12]	800	5	8.0	8.2	3.5	2.2*
Van Dale et al.[16]	720–800	13	12.2	13.2	2.8	2.3
Krotkiewski et al.	500	3	6.2	6.8	2.0	2.8

*Significant difference diet versus diet and exercise.

M, males; F, females.

a reduction in body fat following exercise, whereas those with hyperplastic obesity may show no change in body fat with exercise.[19]

5. *Activity during nonexercising time:* It is presently unclear if caloric restriction versus caloric restriction plus exercise causes individuals to become more or less active during nonexercising time. Variation in this component of energy expenditure could partially account for variation in the change in body composition.

RESISTANCE EXERCISE, CALORIC RESTRICTION, AND PRESERVATION OF FFM

A relatively unexplored area of research concerns the effect of resistance exercise on the preservation of FFM during caloric restriction. Ballor et al.[17] studied obese females over an 8-week period when caloric intake was reduced from baseline by 1000 kcal/day (averaging 1200 kcal/day). Weight training was conducted three times per week by one group, while the other group remained sedentary. Comparisons between the diet-only and diet-plus-weight-training groups show that there was no significant difference between the groups for body weight loss (−4.47 kg vs. −3.89 kg). However, the diet-plus-weight-training group significantly increased its FFM compared to the diet-only group (+0.43 kg vs. −0.91 kg).

In contrast, Lemons et al.[22] investigated 60 obese subjects consuming a 405 kcal/day diet for 8 weeks followed by an additional 8 weeks of a 1500 kcal/day diet. Subjects were divided into the following groups: (1) diet only, (2) diet and weight training, (3) diet and cycling, (4) diet and cycling for 6 weeks followed by 8 weeks of weight training, (5) weight training only, and (6) cycling only. The majority of weight loss occurred during the first 8 weeks during the 405 kcal/day diet, with no significant changes noted during the 8 weeks of the 1500 kcal/day diet. At 16 weeks, body weight loss and body composition changes were similar for all groups.

Donnelly et al.[23] examined the effects of a 520 kcal/day diet and diet combined with endurance exercise only; weight training only; and both endurance and weight training over a 13-week period in 69 obese females. No significant differences between groups were seen in body weight loss (−20.4 to −22.9 kg) or body composition changes, as estimated by hydrostatic weighing. Similar contributions of fat mass (~77%) and FFM (~23%) to total weight loss was also similar between the groups. However, the authors suggest that the most favorable body composition changes were found in the group that combined endurance exercise and weight training with caloric restriction.

The mechanisms of resistance exercise to potentially preserve FFM during caloric restriction have not been fully explored. Body composition changes associated with resistance training for 6 to 24 weeks include increased FFM and decreased fat mass.[24] Resistance exercise is associated with muscle hypertrophy through synthesis of contractile proteins and increases in the size of ligaments and tendons. The energy needs of the body, however, must be met before the body can synthesize protein for muscular development and repair. Thus, during caloric restriction, the ability of resistance-type exercise to cause muscle hypertrophy may diminish. However, maintaining an appropriate percentage of FFM rather than increasing muscle mass during weight loss should perhaps be the goal of adding resistance exercise to weight loss programs.

In contrast to endurance-type exercise, resistance exercise generally relies on anaerobic metabolism for the energy supply and is therefore a less "costly" exercise. Therefore, it may not contribute to an energy deficit created by caloric restriction, which causes the body to adapt by conserving energy.

Despite the failure to clearly demonstrate an independent effect of resistance exercise to elicit a better preservation of FFM during caloric restriction, this is an area where more research is needed. Future research should be directed to determining the mechanisms and rationale for utilizing resistance exercise during caloric restriction for preservation of FFM. In addition, further investigation is needed to determine if a combination of endurance and resistance exercise during caloric restriction resulting in substantial weight loss may achieve the most favorable body composition changes in obese individuals.

RESTING METABOLIC RATE

Resting metabolic rate (RMR) constitutes 60–70% of total energy expenditure and is defined as the energy expenditure required to maintain normal physiologic processes during rest in a postabsorptive state.[25] Age, sex, body surface area, nutritional state, exercise, and various thermogenic hormones have been shown to influence RMR.[26–28] In addition, RMR has a strong genetic influence and a familial resemblance.[29] The most meaningful data are obtained when RMR is normalized to FFM.[30]

Evidence clearly shows that RMR declines with caloric restriction,[21] with the magnitude of this decline dependent on numerous factors. The magnitude of short-term reductions in RMR may be proportional to the caloric restriction.[12,21] Smaller declines in RMR may be found if initial RMR levels are abnormally low.[21] Variations in the response of RMR to caloric restriction may also be affected by genetics[6] and by changes in sympathetic nervous system activity.[25] In addition, reductions in RMR have been attributed to changes in FFM concomitant with weight loss, since FFM has been established as the primary determinate of RMR.[30] However, under conditions of severe caloric restriction, the decrease in RMR is greater than can be explained by changes in FFM alone.[31] Under such conditions, there appears to be increased energy efficiency of the existing tissues.[32]

Acute and chronic exercise training has been reported to affect RMR and has been reviewed.[25,32] Both cross-sectional and exercise intervention studies have been used to examine the effect of exercise on RMR. It appears that intense, prolonged exercise must be performed to affect energy expenditure significantly beyond the exercise period itself.[32] In comparing trained with untrained individuals, it is likely that only highly trained individuals (VO_2 max > 60 ml/kg/min) exhibit a higher RMR per kilogram of FFM.[33] Evidence also suggests a genetic influence in the response of RMR to exercise training.[6]

The inclusion of exercise in weight loss programs has been based on the hypothesis that exercise may offset or attenuate the decline in RMR indirectly by its energy cost and indirectly by its potential to preserve FFM during caloric restriction. However, the response of RMR during a combination of caloric restriction and exercise has been inconsistent. Studies report that exercise either offsets, has no effect on the diet-induced decline in RMR, or in some cases during severe caloric restriction exercise exacerbates the decline in RMR.[14]

RESTING METABOLIC RATE, CALORIC RESTRICTION, AND EXERCISE

Some studies find a beneficial effect of exercise on the response of RMR during caloric restriction. For example, Nieman et al.[34] examined 21 mildly obese women during a 5-week, 1300 kcal/day diet, with or without exercise. The exercise program occurred five times per week, consisting of 45-min walk/jog sessions at 60% VO_2 max. The two groups lost a similar amount of body weight. The exercise group showed a 6% increase in RMR (kilocalories/day) measured 48 hr postexercise, whereas no significant changes were noted for the nonexercising group. A significant correlation was found between percentage changes in VO_2 max and weekly RMR ($r = 0.56$; $p = 0.01$). The results of this study suggest that the intensity of exercise may play a role in increasing RMR.

Lennon et al.[35] examined 75 obese subjects following 12 weeks of a 1200 to 1800 kca/day diet, with or without exercise training. The exercise training consisted of either self-selected brisk walking or a prescribed jogging program. No significant differences were found in weight loss or body composition changes between the groups. A significant correlation was found between the percentage change in VO_2 max and percentage change in RMR ($r = 0.31$; $p < 0.01$). Furthermore, the improvement in VO_2 max was directly related to the exercise training intensity, suggesting that a threshold of exercise intensity may be necessary to increase RMR. However, since VO_2 max was expressed per kilogram of body weight, the apparent increase in the relative VO_2 max may have been a function of weight loss.

The type of exercise may also affect the response of RMR. For example,

Lemons et al.[22] found no significant differences in weight loss, fat loss, or FFM loss in 60 obese females during an 8-week, 450 kcal/day diet followed by an 8-week, 1500 kcal/day diet, with or without exercise. Exercise consisted of various endurance-type activities (walking/cycling) or weight training. The RMR per kilogram of FFM in the group combining caloric restriction and weight training was restored to 107% of the initial RMR by week 16 despite a large weight loss (>11 kg). The results of this study suggest that weight training may enhance RMR per kilogram of FFM during caloric restriction.

A combination of caloric restriction and exercise has been shown to have no effect on RMR. Hammer et al.[36] examined 26 obese women following an 800 kcal/day diet for 16 weeks, with or without exercise. Exercise consisted of walking/jogging for 5 days per week, progressing from 1.8 to 4.8 km/session at an intensity of ⩾60% HR max. The exercise groups had a greater weight loss than the nonexercise group; however, almost no change in FFM, as estimated by hydrostatic weighing, occurred in either group. No change in RMR, expressed as kilocalories/day or per kilogram of FFM, was observed in either group.

In contrast, some studies find similar reductions in RMR with a combination of caloric restriction and exercise compared to caloric restriction alone. Hill et al.,[12] as described in the previous section, reported that exercise produced a more favorable body composition change than did caloric restriction. However, exercise did not prevent the 20% decline in RMR. These results are consistent with those of Van Dale et al.,[37] who found that caloric restriction in combination with exercise resulted in greater preservation of FFM than caloric restriction; however, the decline in RMR was not prevented. This study investigated 23 obese females following 14 weeks of an 840 kcal/day diet, with or without exercise. Exercise consisted of 4 days per week of aerobics, jogging, and fitness training at an intensity of 60% VO_2 max. The estimated energy expenditure of the exercise was 380–450 kcal/session and corresponded to the extra fat loss in the exercise groups. Significant reductions in absolute RMR and per kilogram of FFM were found after 5 weeks. Although the exercise groups had a slight increase in RMR from weeks 5 to 14 compared to a continued decline in the nonexercisers, the differences were not significant.

Henson et al.,[38] using a crossover design, examined seven obese females during 9 weeks of an 800 kcal/day diet. During weeks 4–6, subjects engaged in a 5 day per week exercise program consisting of 30 min of cycling at 70% VO_2 max. Subjects lost an average of 9.5 kg. RMR per kilogram of FFM decreased 13% during the initial 3 weeks of caloric restriction only and remained decreased during the diet-plus-exercise period. Thus, exercise does not appear to "boost" RMR after a period of diet restriction.

Other studies found that the combination of exercise and severe caloric restriction may accelerate the decline in RMR compared to caloric restriction alone. Heymsfield et al.[39] investigated the use of a 900 kcal/day diet in 12 obese females over a 5-week period, with or without exercise. Exercise consisted of supervised brisk walking increasing to 5.6 km over the study period. The energy cost of exercise was approximately 345 kcal/day. Total weight loss between groups was similar; however, the exercise group lost more fat (-5.3 ± 1.0 kg vs. -4.4 ± 1.6 kg; $p < 0.001$) and less FFM (-2.2 ± 0.8 kg vs. -2.6 ± 0.6 kg; $p < 0.001$) than the nonexercise group. RMR per kilogram of FFM decreased by 16% in the exercise group compared to 8% in the nonexercise group ($p < 0.025$). The authors suggest that the greater energy deficit of the combined diet and exercise group caused the greater decline in RMR.

Phinney et al.[14] also reported a greater decrease in RMR with exercise combined with severe caloric restriction compared to caloric restriction only. The study protocol was described in the previous section. Results showed that resting oxygen consumption (milliliters/minute) declined in both groups by 10% in the first week of dieting; however, the exercising group showed a further reduction of 17% by the conclusion of the study. Furthermore, the addition of exercise was not shown to increase weight loss or fat loss and did not exert any effect on the change in FFM. This study suggests that during severe caloric restriction, the addition of large quantities of exercise (10 hr/week) introduced over a short training period (4–5 weeks) increases the diet-induced decline in RMR.

POSSIBLE EXPLANATIONS FOR THE INCONSISTENT FINDINGS

Inconsistent changes in both the direction and the magnitude of RMR have been found during a combination of caloric restriction and exercise. Table 7–2 presents a summary of the studies reviewed. These discrepant results reflect short-term adaptations in RMR and may be a function of the differences among studies in the following areas:

1. *Magnitude of caloric restriction:* The ability of exercise to have a positive influence on RMR may be lost with severe caloric restriction. Exercise contributes to the negative energy deficit created by caloric restriction, which, in turn, may force the body to adapt by decreasing RMR to a greater extent than with caloric restriction alone.
2. *Changes in VO_2 max:* A significant increase in VO_2 max may be necessary to elicit a positive change in RMR during weight loss. The ability of exercise training to increase VO_2 max is a function of the intensity, duration, and frequency of exercise, as well as the duration of exercise training and the initial fitness level.
3. *Timing of RMR measurement:* It is possible that the elevation in postexercise energy expenditure may be prolonged for several hours. Thus, RMR should be measured at least 24 hr after the last exercise bout to ensure a true resting state.[32]

TABLE 7-2 Comparison of RMR Changes Among Studies

<table>
<tr><th rowspan="2">Study</th><th rowspan="2">Caloric Intake (kcal/day)</th><th rowspan="2">Weeks</th><th colspan="2">Weight Loss (kg)</th><th colspan="2">RMR (% Change)</th></tr>
<tr><th>Diet</th><th>Diet and Exercise</th><th>Diet</th><th>Diet and Exercise</th></tr>
<tr><td>Nieman et al.[34]</td><td>1300</td><td>5</td><td colspan="2">~5.5</td><td>NC</td><td>+6.0</td></tr>
<tr><td>Hammer et al.[36]</td><td>800</td><td>16</td><td colspan="2">5 to 11</td><td>NC</td><td>NC</td></tr>
<tr><td>Hill et al.[12]</td><td>800</td><td>5</td><td colspan="2">~8.1</td><td>−17.3</td><td>−19.1</td></tr>
<tr><td>Phinney et al.[14]</td><td>720</td><td>4–5</td><td colspan="2">~6.7</td><td>−10.0</td><td>−27.0*</td></tr>
<tr><td>Heymsfield et al.[39]</td><td>900</td><td>5</td><td colspan="2">~7.0</td><td>−9.6</td><td>−20.3*</td></tr>
</table>

*Significant difference diet versus diet and exercise. NC, no change.

4. *Spontaneous activity:* Subjects may decrease their activity during nonexercising hours to compensate for the energy expended during the required exercise training. This could result in an energy expenditure similar to that of a caloric restriction–only condition. Use of the doubly labeled water technique to measure total daily energy expenditure in free-living subjects may enable us to study this hypothesis.

METHODOLOGIC CONSIDERATIONS FOR FUTURE STUDIES

The following factors should be taken into consideration in future studies that examine the effect of a combination of exercise and caloric restriction on body composition changes and energy expenditure in the treatment of obesity:

1. Study periods should be long enough to allow physiologic adaptations to exercise to occur and to enable subjects to reach a steady state of exercise training. The American College of Sports Medicine suggests that a minimum of 15 to 20 weeks of exercise training is necessary for structural and functional adaptations to occur. Additionally, initial fitness levels should be taken into consideration, since the magnitude of adaptation is inversely related to the initial fitness level.[8]
2. The level of exercise should be adequately documented. This includes the mode, frequency, intensity, and duration of the exercise sessions. The energy cost of exercise can thus be estimated, allowing comparisons among studies regarding similar energy deficits created by different combinations of exercise and caloric restriction.
3. Accurate measurements of body composition should be employed. Numerous methodologies exist for assessment of body composition, some being more acceptable (hydrostatic weighing, total body water) than others (skinfold measurements, infrared interactance). New advances in the field of body composition will increase the ability of clinicians to accurately assess changes in body composition with weight loss.
4. Accurate measurement of RMR should be employed. Numerous variables affect this measurement. The ideal conditions for measurement of RMR include a postabsorptive state, a minimum of 24 hr postexercise, measurement early in the morning, and values taken after a sufficient adjustment period for the subject.
5. An adequate sample size is required to decrease the incidence of statistical error. A limitation of many studies is their small sample sizes, which decreases the statistical power to observe significant differences among treatment groups.
6. Healthy, nutrient-dense, hypocaloric diets should be utilized to ensure an adequate quality and quantity of macro- and micronutrients. Adequate fluid and electrolyte intake to ensure hydration and a higher quantity of dietary protein is required when caloric intake is below that required to maintain body weight.[18,40]

7. Compliance with both caloric restriction and exercise protocols should be adequately monitored.
8. Differences in fat patterning should be taken into consideration. It has been suggested that body fat distribution characterized as either gluteal-femoral or abdominal influences RMR.[41] Abdominal body fat may also be easier to lose than gluteal-femoral fat.[42]

SUMMARY

To date, the literature examining various combinations of caloric restriction and exercise has been plagued with discrepancies. It appears that some endurance exercise routines may have no additive effects on loss of total body weight, especially with severe caloric restriction. Furthermore, some investigators have found greater loss of fat and greater preservation of FFM in exercise-diet treatments, whereas others have found no added benefit of exercise on body composition changes with substantial weight loss. The discrepant results have been attributed to numerous factors, including nutrient adequacy of the diet; magnitude of caloric restriction; initial body fat status; body fat distribution; genotype; the use of numerous exercise and diet combinations; methodologic differences; measurement error; and the lack of consideration of other confounding variables.

Regardless of the current inadequacies, it appears that the benefits derived from exercise diminish as the severity of the caloric restriction increases, particularly to semistarvation. This is seen in the body's ability to lose weight, spare FFM, and defend RMR. These findings may be a function of the magnitude of the energy deficit. With severe caloric restriction, adding endurance exercise contributes to a negative energy deficit, causing the body to adapt to a greater extent than with caloric restriction alone. Further investigation is needed to determine if an energy or nutrient deficit threshold exists for preservation of FFM and RMR.

Although further investigation of the mechanisms and rationale is needed, a combination of resistance training and caloric restriction may prove to be an optimal way of deriving body composition and RMR benefits during weight loss. Since resistance exercise is a relatively low-energy activity, it would not contribute significantly to the energy deficit created by caloric restriction, and this would overcome the observations of Phinney et al.[14] That is, no greater reduction in RMR would be found with a combination of weight training and caloric restriction compared to caloric restriction alone. Furthermore, weight training may have a greater ability to spare FFM compared to endurance exercise during weight loss and may affect the energy efficiency of the residual FFM, as proposed by Lemons et al.[22]

Further examination of the relationships between endurance exercise, resistance exercise, and caloric restriction is needed to elucidate an optimal combination.

REFERENCES

1. Wing RR, Jeffrey RJ. Outpatient treatment of obesity: A comparison of methodology and results. *Int J Obes* 3:261, 1979.
2. Scientific Affairs Council. Treatment of obesity in adults. *JAMA* 260:2547, 1988.
3. Position of the American Dietetic Association: Very-low-calorie weight loss diets. *J Am Diet Assoc* 90:722, 1990.
4. Fisler JS, Drenick EJ. Starvation and semistarvation diets in the management of obesity. *Ann Rev Nutr* 465, 7:465, 1987.
5. Forbes GB. Body composition: Influence of nutrition, disease, growth, and aging, in Shils ME, Young VR (eds), *Modern Nutrition in Health and Disease,* ed. 7. Philadelphia, Lea & Febinger, 1988, pp. 533–556.
6. Poehlman ET, Tremblay A, Nadeau A, et al. Heredity and changes in hormones and metabolic rates with short-term training. *Am J Physiol* 250:E711, 1986.
7. Stern JS, Lowrey P. Obesity: The role of physical activity, in Brownell KD, Foreyt JP (eds), *Handbook of Eating Disorders: Physiology, Psychology, and Treatment of Obesity, Anorexia, and Bulimia.* New York, Basic Books, 1986, pp. 145–158.
8. American College of Sports Medicine: Position Stand. The recommended quantity and quality of exercise for developing and maintaining cardiorespiratory and muscular fitness in healthy adults. *Med Sci Sports Exerc* 22:265, 1990.
9. Hagan RD, Upton SJ, Wong L, et al. The effects of aerobic conditioning and/or caloric restriction in overweight men and women. *Med Sci Sports Exerc* 18:87, 1986.
10. Hill JO, Schlundt DG, Sbrocco T, et al. Evaluation of an alternating-calorie diet with and without exercise in the treatment of obesity. *Am J Clin Nutr* 50:248, 1989.
11. Pavlou KN, Steffee WP, Lerman RH, et al. Effects of dieting and exercise on lean body mass, oxygen uptake, and strength. *Med Sci Sports Exerc* 17:466, 1985.
12. Hill JO, Sparling PB, Shields TW, et al. Effects of exercise and food restriction on body composition and metabolic rate in obese women. *Am J Clin Nutr* 46:622, 1987.
13. Wishnofsky M. Caloric equivalents of gained or lost weight. *Metabolism* 1:554, 1952.
14. Phinney SD, LaGrange BM, O'Connell, et al. Effects of aerobic exercise on energy expenditure and nitrogen balance during VLCD. *Metabolism* 37:758, 1988.
15. Krotkiewski M, Toss L, Bjorntorp P, et al. The effect of a very-low-calorie diet with and without chronic exercise on thyroid and sex hormones, plasma proteins, oxygen uptake, insulin and c peptide concentrations in obese women. *Int J Obes* 5:287, 1981.

16. Van Dale D, Saris WHM, Schoffelen PFM, et al. Does exercise give an additional effect in weight reduction regimens? *Int J Obes* 11:367, 1987.

17. Ballor DL, Katch VL, Becque MD, et al. Resistance weight training during caloric restriction enhances lean body weight maintenance. *Am J Clin Nutr* 47:19, 1988.

18. Hoffer LJ, Bistrian BR, Young VR, et al. Metabolic effects of very low-calorie weight reduction diets. *J Clin Invest* 73:750, 1984.

19. Bray GA. Exercise and Obesity, in Bouchard C, Shepard RJ, Stephens T, et al. (eds), *Exercise, Fitness, and Health: A Consensus of Current Knowledge*. Champaign, Ill, Human Kinetics Books, 1990, pp. 497–510.

20. Ballor DL, Tommerup LJ, Smith DB, et al. Body composition, muscle and fat pad changes following two levels of dietary restriction and/or exercise training in male rats. *Int J Obes* 14:711, 1990.

21. Wadden TA, Foster GD, Letizia KA, et al. Long-term effects of dieting on resting metabolic rate in obese outpatients. *JAMA* 264:707, 1990.

22. Lemons AD, Kreitzman SN, Coxon A, et al. Selection of appropriate exercise regimes for weight reduction during VLCD and maintenance. *Int J Obes* 13 (Suppl 2): 119, 1989.

23. Donnelly JE, Pronk NP, Jacobsen DJ. Effects of a very low calorie diet and physical training regimens on body composition and resting metabolic rate in obese females. *Am J Clin Nutr* 54:56, 1991.

24. Fleck SJ, Kraemer WJ. Resistance training: Physiological responses and adaptations. *Phys Sports Med* 16:108, 1988.

25. Poehlman ET. A review: Exercise and its influence on resting energy metabolism in man. *Med Sci Sports Exerc* 21:515, 1989.

26. Harris S, Benedict F. *A Biometric of Basal Metabolism in Man*. Pub No. 279. Washington, DC, Carnegie Institution, 1919.

27. Danforth E. The role of thyroid hormones and insulin in the regulation of energy metabolism. *Am J Clin Nutri* 38:1006, 1983.

28. Bray GA, Atkinson RL. Factors affecting basal metabolic rate. *Prog Food Nutr Sci* 2:395, 1977.

29. Ravussin E, Lillioja S, Knowler WC, et al. Reduced rate of energy expenditure as a risk factor for body weight gain. *N Engl J Med* 318:467, 1988.

30. Miller AT, Blyth CS. Lean body mass as a metabolic reference standard. *J Appl Phys* 5:311, 1953.

31. Keys A, Brozek J, Hanschel A, et al. *The Biology of Human Starvation*. Minneapolis, University of Minnesota Press, 1950.

32. Poehlman ET, Melby CL, Goran MI. The impact of exercise and diet restriction on daily energy expenditure. *Sports Med* 11:78, 1991.

33. Poehlman ET, Melby CL, Badylak SF. Resting metabolic rate and postprandial thermogenesis in highly trained and untrained males. *Am J Clin Nutr* 47:793, 1988.

34. Nieman DC, Haig JL, DeGuia ED, et al. Reducing diet and exercise training effects on resting metabolic rates in mildly obese women. *J Sports Med Phys Fitness* 28:79, 1988.

35. Lennon D, Nagle F, Stratman F, et al. Diet and exercise training effects on resting metabolic rate. *Int J Obes* 9:39, 1985.

36. Hammer RL, Barrier CA, Roundy ES, et al. Calorie-restricted low-fat diet and exercise in obese women. *Am J Clin Nutr* 49:77, 1989.

37. Van Dale D, Schoffelen PFM, Ten Hoor F, et al. Effects of addition of exercise to energy restriction on 24-hour energy expenditure, sleeping metabolic rate and daily physical activity. *Eur J Clin Nutr* 43:347, 1989.

38. Henson LC, Poole DC, Donahoe CP, et al. Effects of exercise training on resting energy expenditure during caloric restriction. *Am J Clin Nutr* 46:893, 1987.

39. Heymsfield SB, Casper K, Hearn J, et al. Rate of weight loss during underfeeding: Relation to level of physical activity. *Metabolism* 38:215, 1988.

40. Clark N, Blackburn GL. The theoretical basis of nitrogen balance, in Blackburn GL, Bray GA (eds), *Management of Obesity by Severe Caloric Restriction*. Littleton, PSG Publishing, 1985, pp. 54–62.

41. Weststrate JA, Dekker J, Stoel M, et al. Resting energy expenditure in women: Impact of obesity and body-fat distribution. *Metabolism* 39:11, 1990.

42. Krotkiewski M, Bjorntorp P, Sjostrom L, et al. Impact of obesity on metabolism in men and women: Importance of regional adipose tissue distribution. *J Clin Invest* 72:1150, 1983.

CHAPTER 8

The Psychology of Obesity, Weight Loss, and Weight Regain: Research and Clinical Findings

Gary D. Foster, M.S. and Thomas A. Wadden, Ph.D.

Despite the serious medical conditions associated with obesity[1], an expert panel, composed predominantly of physicians, concluded: "Obesity creates an enormous psychological burden. In terms of suffering, this burden may be the greatest adverse effect of obesity."[2]

The purpose of this chapter is to assess the nature and extent of the psychological burden of obesity from several perspectives. First, we will review the consequences of being overweight in a society preoccupied with thinness. Second, we will outline the role of psychological factors in the etiology of obesity. Third, we will discuss the effects of weight loss and regain on psychological functioning in the obese.

BEING OBESE IN A THIN WORLD

Any psychological burden of obesity is certainly exacerbated by our nation's marked preoccupation with thinness. Thin is definitely "in." One need venture no further than the supermarket checkout line to gain some insight into popular notions of beauty. The covers of *Vogue, Cosmopolitan,* and *Elle,* as well as the advertisements within them, display svelte, tall women. Displays of overweight women are typically limited to tabloids accompanied by an expose revealing how weight gain has ruined their lives or ads describing a new secret for how to lose weight.

Cultural Ideals of Beauty

It is interesting to note that this svelte ideal was not always viewed as desirable. During the Renaissance, for example, the paintings of Rubens portrayed beauty as women with large bellies, thighs and breasts. These women probably represented cultural values of reproduction and prosperity. By today's standards, such figures would be considered extremely obese.

As women sought roles in addition to childbearing, the ideal shape took an extreme turn to the tall, almost anorectic shape of the flapper in the 1920s. Women during this time used restrictive garments and devices to create a body shape devoid of curves. The ideal shifted again in the 1950s to a plumper version of beauty embodied by Jane Russell and Marilyn Monroe. These curvaceous "knockouts" of their time would be considered overweight by today's standards. Our current cultural ideal for women is slightly heavier than the anorectic Twiggy of the 1970s but still retains a long, lean appearance (e.g., Jamie Lee Curtis, Julia Roberts). For a more detailed history of the evolution of cultural ideals of beauty, the reader should consult the works of Bennett and Gurin[3] and Schwartz.[4]

A review of popular magazines over the last century further illustrates the varying ideals of body shape. Using the breast:waist ratio as an indicator of body shape preference, Silverstein et al.[5] reviewed photographs of models in *Vogue* and *Ladies Home Journal* from 1901 to 1980. The ratio ranged from nearly 2.0 in 1910 to 1.1 in 1925 to 1.5 in 1950 to 1.25 by 1981. Support for a more lean cultural ideal is also derived from a study that found Miss America contestants and Playboy centerfolds had become increasingly thin, relative to their peers, between 1960 and 1979.[6] Independent of the evolution of the current ideal, it is clear that an obese, even slightly overweight, individual senses her deviation from the svelte ideal.

Ideal versus Real

As the cultural ideal of beauty has become leaner, our nation has become heavier, with women twice as likely as men to experience a major (approximately 15 kg) weight gain.[7] A personal example of a *Self* magazine writer, Penny Ward Moser, forcefully illustrates the extremity of today's ideal.[8] Moser is 5 ft 7 in. and weighs 124 lb. Using the Barbie doll as one indicator of the cultural ideal, she compared her measurements to those of the doll. Using the hips as a constant, Moser calculated that to achieve the same proportions as Barbie, Moser's bust would have to increase by 12 in., her waist decrease by 10 in., and her height increase by 22 in.!

This discrepancy between ideal and real has created an "insatiable desire for new information programs, devices, books and medicines that will make us healthier, slimmer, fitter and more aesthetically appealing."[9] Dieting has become a way of life for many Americans, who spend an alarming $33 billion per year on diet foods, weight loss programs, diet books, or special reducing agents. Dieting, however, is not the only method of pursuing the ideal body. Plastic surgery procedures increased 63% between 1981 and 1988. Abdominoplasty procedures (tummy tucks) have increased 45% since 1981, and liposuction has increased 81% since 1984.[9]

As Brownell[9] has suggested, the two assumptions underlying the quest for the aesthetic ideal are dubious. First, the body is not infinitely malleable by diet and exercise. There are clearly biological limits to body shape and weight, including genetics,[10–12] resting metabolic rate,[13,14] and fat cell number.[15,16] Second, the perceived benefits of an ideal weight may be more illusory than real.[17] Achieving an ideal weight does not guarantee improved relationships, better jobs, or more friends. These benefits may occur, but they are not governed exclusively by weight. In addition, as reviewed later in this chapter, there is no evidence that persons of average weight are any more happy or any less disturbed than those who are overweight.[18]

Increased Pressure on Women

Although the societal pressure to be thin and fit is extreme in the 1990s, it is particularly intense for women. Despite the advances of the women's movement, there is still considerably more pressure for women to be attractive (i.e., thin) than for men. A study by Silverstein et al.[5] illustrated marked gender differences in messages conveyed by the mass media. The authors performed a content analysis of articles and advertisements that dealt with body shape, dieting, food, cooking, and drinking that appeared in eight magazines in which at least 75% of the readership was male (*Field and Stream, Playboy, Popular Mechanics,* and *Sports Illustrated*) or female (*Family Circle, Ladies Home Journal, Redbook,* and *Women's Day*). The ratio of ads and articles for diet foods in women's compared to men's magazines was 63:1, that for ads or articles about body shape was 8:1, and that for total number of food ads was 79:1. Interestingly, ads or articles about alcoholic beverages appeared 33 times more frequently in men's magazines. The message that women receive from the popular press and Madison Avenue is a contradictory, if not impossible, one: Stay in shape and be thin while eating all of the delicious foods you want. This contradictory message is represented on almost every cover of popular women's magazines. One recent cover included one article on how to make "devastatingly delicious brownies" and another on "10 ways to keep your tummy trim."

TABLE 8–1 Degree of Worry About Typical Concerns of Female High School Students (N = 453)

Variable	Mean Score
Looks	7.74[a]
Figure	7.11[b]
Relationships with the opposite sex	7.03[b,c]
Weight	6.77[b,c]
Popularity with the opposite sex	6.55[c]
The future	5.92[d]
Money	5.86[d,e]
Complexion	5.82[d,e]
Grades	5.75[d,e]
Family	5.39[e,f]
Popularity with the same sex	4.95[f,g]
Parents	4.90[f,g]
Health	4.83[g]
Nuclear war	3.60[h]
Sports	3.54[h]

Means sharing a common superscript are not significantly different. 1, none at all; 5, moderate amount; 10, extreme amount.

Source: Adapted from Ref. 19 with permission.

The gender differences in the concerns about weight and figure seem to be internalized by adolescence. We surveyed 453 girls and 355 boys in the 10th grade to assess how much they worried about weight in relation to a variety of other issues.[19] Girls worried most about their looks, figure, relationships with the opposite sex, weight, and popularity with the opposite sex, in that order (Table 8–1). Boys worried most about money, looks, popularity with the opposite sex, relationships with the opposite sex, and the future, in that order. Boys rated weight as 13th among 15 concerns (Table 8–2). These findings suggest that financial success may hold the same prominent position for adolescent boys that weight and figure do for girls.

Gender differences are also evident among college students' perception of desirable and current weight. Using silhouettes to assess current and ideal weight, Fallon and Rozin[20] found that females rated their current weight as heavier than ideal, while males considered their current weight as ideal.

Increased Dieting

This increased pressure has resulted in an increased prevalence of dieting among women. Despite a similar prevalence of obesity among men and women, as many as 24% of men compared to 40% of women are trying to lose weight

TABLE 8–2 Degree of Worry About Typical Concerns of Male High School Students (N = 355)

Variable	Mean Score
Money	6.57[a]
Looks	6.45[a]
Popularity with the opposite sex	6.41[a]
Relationships with the opposite sex	6.28[a]
The future	5.64[b]
Physique	5.15[b,c]
Grades	5.06[b,c,d]
Sports	4.98[c,d]
Complexion	4.82[c,d]
Family	4.74[c,d]
Health	4.60[c,d]
Parents	4.46[d,e]
Weight	3.92[e]
Popularity with the same sex	3.87[e]
Nuclear war	2.46[f]

Means sharing a common superscript are not significantly different. 1, none at all; 5, moderate amount; 10, extreme amount.

Source: Adapted from Ref. 19 with permission.

at any given time.[21] The rate of dieting among adolescent females has doubled over the past 20 years and now approaches 60–70%.[22,23] Women exceed men by a ratio of 4:1 in commercial weight loss programs.[24] The irony of this increased societal pressure for women to lose weight is that the medical consequences of overweight are more significant for men. Recent research indicates that body fat carried below the waist (most common in women) is associated with far fewer medical consequences than fat carried above the waist (most common in men).[25] Thus, minimal pressure is exerted on obese men to lose weight despite the clear medical need for them to do so. In general, men—not women—should reduce excess weight.

Discrimination Against the Obese

It would be expected that an overweight person in a society preoccupied with thinness would suffer discrimination. Regrettably, there are plenty of examples. The most disturbing studies about the stigma of overweight reveal that weight alone can elicit a host of negative attributes and characterizations. Children as young as 6 years of age label silhouettes of obese youngsters as "lazy, stupid, cheats, lies, and ugly." Even more troublesome is that these judgments are made by obese youngsters as well.[26] College students rate obese persons as less intelligent, hard-working, and successful than nonobese persons.[27] In another study, students were asked to rate various categories of persons for their suitability as a marriage partner. Embezzlers, cocaine users, shoplifters, and blind persons were all rated as more suitable spouses than obese individuals.[28] Sadly, health care professionals share this negative view of the overweight. Physicians consider their obese patients to be weak-willed, ugly, and awkward.[29]

Discrimination is also found in schools and in the workplace. The obese are less likely to be accepted into high-ranking colleges despite equivalent high school grades, academic qualifications, and application rates.[30] Even landlords are less likely to rent to overweight persons.[31] Obese persons are less likely to be considered good employees.[32,33] A survey revealed that only 9% of executives who earned $25,000 to $50,000 were more than 10 lb overweight, whereas 39% of those earnings $10,000 to $20,000 were similarly overweight. The authors calculated that each pound of fat could cost an executive $1000 per year.[34]

In addition to these formal studies, there is informal discrimination against the obese that is harder to measure but still evident. For example, both of us have been asked questions such as "How can you work with fat people all day? Doesn't it feel futile?" Incredibly, it is assumed that overweight persons are so different, so unappealing, that it would be unpleasant to work with them. Jokes about overweight individuals are still fair game for sure laughs by comedians. One need only tune in David Letterman or Jay Leno to hear jokes underscoring erroneous stereotypes of the overweight as sloppy, lazy, gluttonous, or unable to perform or enjoy sex. Television sitcoms regularly reinforce these stereotypes. A "My Turn" column in *Newsweek* exemplifies society's contempt for the obese: "This information [about genetic determinants of obesity] should be withheld from the fat multitudes because the obese will latch onto any excuse for failing to lose weight. . . . Face it Chubbo, when was the last time you were force-fed?"[35]

PSYCHOPATHOLOGY AND OBESITY

Obese persons might well be expected to show higher levels of depression and other psychological disturbances in view of the prejudice and discrimination to which they are subjected. It would seem almost impossible to maintain a positive self-image in a society such as ours, which scorns the overweight. Investigations of this topic, however, have yielded some surprising findings.

Population Studies

Adults. Population studies have generally failed to find significant differences in psychological function (as measured by self-report inventories) between obese and non-obese persons.[18] Moore and colleagues,[36] in a study of 1660 people in midtown Manhattan, found that obese individuals scored significantly higher than nonobese persons on three of nine measures of psychological functioning—immaturity, suspiciousness, and rigidity. Differences between groups on these measures were so small, however, as to be judged clinically insignificant. Small differences were similarly observed in a study by Stewart and Brook[37] of 5817 persons. In this investigation, however, obese individuals were found to be significantly less depressed and anxious than were their nonobese counterparts.

Results of these American studies are supported by findings from two British studies. Crisp and McGuiness[38] found that obese Britons reported significantly less anxiety and depression than did their nonobese counterparts, findings strikingly similar to those of Stewart and Brook. Silverstone[39] also found no evidence of increased psychopathology in the obese "even when any possible influence of age and social class had been controlled for." Five additional European studies confirm the impression that there are few significant differences in psychological functioning among obese and nonobese persons in the general population.[40–44]

Children. Findings for children parallel those for adults. Our research team has conducted four studies of children and adolescents, which revealed no significant differences between obese and nonobese youngsters in self-esteem and measures of dysphoria.[19,23,45,46] Sallade[47] similarly reported that obese and nonobese children did not differ significantly on measures of personality function. Obese children were found to have slightly lower self-esteem, but their scores fell well within normal limits.

Clinical Studies

In contrast to population investigations, studies of markedly overweight persons seeking treatment for their obesity have suggested that psychological disturbance is common in the obese. Numerous studies have assessed psychopathology using the Minnesota Multiphasic Personality Inventory (MMPI).[48] Ten such investigations found at least mild elevations in depression, as defined by a T score of 60 (one standard deviation above the mean).[49–58] Mild to moderate elevations have also been observed on scales measuring hypochondriasis, hysteria, and impulsivity (i.e., psychopathic deviancy). We have observed similar findings in patients whom we have treated with very-low-calorie diet and behavior therapy.[59] Thus, there is no question that a significant minority of persons presenting for treatment will report significant psychological distress, which may require treatment by psychotherapy and/or pharmacotherapy (as discussed later).

From an academic standpoint, it is important to note that some investigators may have overestimated the contribution of psychopathology to the development of obesity as a result of failing to study appropriate control groups. This is a critical omission because individuals seeking clinical care, regardless of their specific disorder, often report increased dysphoria and other psychological disturbance. This fact is revealed by Swenson and colleagues'[60] analysis of the MMPIs of 18,328 women treated for general medical and surgical procedures at the Mayo Clinic. Mean scores for this sample on the hypochondriasis, depression, and hysteria scales were 61, 60, and 62, respectively—the criterion for psychopathology in the studies of obese patients. Moreover, approximately 15% of patients in the Mayo Clinic study had a T score of 70 on each of these scales, which is two standard deviations above the mean and is indicative of clinically significant psychopathology.

These findings suggest that although some obese individuals may display mild to moderate psychological distress, the psychological functioning of obese patients as a group does not differ significantly from that of other clinic patients. Carefully controlled studies using either the MMPI[58,61] or other measures of psychological status support this view.[62,63]

Psychological Disturbance Specific to Obesity

Findings of generally normal psychological functioning in overweight individuals are a tribute to the obese, given the prejudice and discrimination that they endure. Despite these positive findings, we believe that obesity is likely to be associated with a number of weight-specific problems that may adversely affect quality of life, even if they are not severe enough to result in clinically significant complications. Moreover, most psychological inventories do not assess weight-related difficulties, which means that such problems would go undetected if they did exist.

This belief is supported by findings of two studies of adolescent girls that we conducted.[19,23] In neither study did obese girls score significantly higher in dysphoria (anxiety and/or depression) than did their nonobese classmates. The obese girls, however, reported significantly greater dissatisfaction with and worry about their weight and figure than did the nonobese girls. While such dissatisfaction and worry may not reach clinically significant levels of depression, it is still likely to adversely affect an individual's quality of life. Klesges[64] has reported comparable findings in obese college students.

Similarly, the feelings of guilt and shame that many obese individuals report concerning their inability to control their weight[65] are likely to reduce self-esteem in some areas of functioning, even if not sufficiently to affect global self-esteem. Perhaps the greatest benefit of group treatment for obesity is that it allows patients to share such feelings and to realize that they are not alone with them.

Body image disparagement. Although dissatisfaction with weight and figure are currently so common in adolescent females as to approach a "normative discontent,"[66] these problems are likely to be most severe in the obese. Many obese individuals feel that their bodies are ugly and despicable, and that others view them with hostility and contempt. As Stunkard and Mendelson[67] have written, "it makes no difference whether the person be also talented, wealthy, or intelligent; his weight is his only concern, and he sees the whole world in terms of his weight."

This disorder is most likely to be observed in young upper-middle-class Caucasian women, in whom the prevalence of obesity is very low (i.e., 5%) and thus, the sanctions against it are quite high. Within this population, the disturbance is most severe in women who have been obese since childhood, who have a generalized neurotic disturbance, and whose parents chided them for their weight problem. The disturbance appears to result from an internalization of parental and peer criticism and persists in the absence of continued derogation. Adolescence appears to be the period of greatest risk for development of the disorder.[68,69]

Weight-specific psychological complications of obesity, including body image disparagement, are likely to be far less severe, and perhaps completely absent, in persons from lower socioeconomic status. This is because obesity is common in the lower class[1] and thus may be more readily accepted. There may also be racial differences in preferred body type that affect psychological responses. African-Americans and other minorities do not appear to value thinness to the same extent as Caucasians,[70,71] a finding that may explain the low prevalence of eating disorders in minority populations.[72]

PSYCHOGENIC EXPLANATIONS OF OBESITY

The majority of the population and clinical studies described above were not conducted to assess the psychological consequences of prejudice and discrimination against the obese. Instead, many sought to assess the contribution of psychopathology to the development of obesity.

Psychoanalytic Perspective

In the 1950s, at the height of its influence, psychoanalytic theory held that obesity was a presentation of a basic personality problem.[73] As one analyst noted, "It is a particular way of handling one's difficulties in human relationships, and, even more, one's poor relationship with one's self. . . . Excessive eating becomes a form of acting out unconscious conflicts which can find no other solution or expression."[74] While early theorists frequently discussed the obese individual's "oral" conflicts, later investigators conceptualized overeating as a means of coping with depression and other negative feelings.[75,76]

There are few research data to support the psychoanalytic view of obesity, and those that have been offered are subject to multiple interpretations. For example, the fact that obese individuals in some studies scored lower in depression and anxiety than nonobese persons has been offered as evidence that overeating represents a defense against these emotions. If this hypothesis were correct, we would expect obese individuals to become depressed or anxious when they dieted. As discussed later, however, obese individuals usually show improvement in psychological functioning with dieting and weight loss.[77] Moreover, when obese individuals do overeat in response to emotional distress, they may do so primarily because negative emotions disrupt their normal ability to control their food intake, as suggested by proponents of restraint theory.[78]

Obese personality type. Consistent with the psychoanalytic view, some investigators proposed that there was an obese personality type. According to this view, obese individuals may appear jolly and carefree in social interactions, but they suffer from feelings of inferiority, are very passive-dependent, and have a deep need to be loved.[79] Although some obese individuals certainly display these characteristics, so do some nonobese persons.[80] Moreover, efforts to identify an obese personality type have yielded the opposite finding; there is remarkable heterogeneity of personality types among obese individuals, as revealed by the results of investigations that used a statistical method known as *cluster analysis*.[81–83] In each sample of subjects studied, as few as 3 and as many as 10 personality subtypes were identified; about one-third of the subjects did not fit any of the subtypes. There could not be a stronger demonstration of the heterogeneity of personality functioning in obese individuals.

Behavioral Perspective

In sharp contrast to the psychoanalytic view, behavior therapists writing in the 1960s and 1970s argued that obesity was a learned disorder in which inappropriate eating habits (including overeating) resulted from and were amenable to principles of conditioning. Stuart's[84] landmark report of the highly successful behavioral treatment of eight clients led to hundreds of studies of this approach and to its widespread use in commercial and hospital-based programs.

There is little research evidence, however, to support the behavioral view of obesity. Laboratory studies generally have failed to find consistent differences in the eating habits of obese and nonobese persons.[85] In addition, the vast majority of studies that compared the daily caloric intake in the two groups, as determined from self-reports, failed to find significant differences.[86,87]

More recent studies, using the technique of doubly labeled water, have found that most obese individuals do have higher caloric requirements (and thus higher caloric intakes for weight maintenance) than their nonobese counterparts.[88,89] The higher energy intake is usually equal to that required to maintain the extra fat-free mass in obese individuals. Even when it is shown, however, that obese individuals consume more food than the nonobese, behavioral theory does not necessarily provide satisfactory explanations of this finding. Thus, to conclude that an individual eats more because he or she is positively reinforced to do so does not identify the physiologic or other mechanisms that make this individual more susceptible to hunger signals, the palatability of food, or other factors that may determine food intake.[90] Moreover, behavioral and psychoanalytic explanations may be very similar in some cases. A behaviorist, for example, might argue that some individuals are negatively reinforced to overeat because it reduces emotional distress. (*Negative reinforcement* refers to the increase in a behavior that reduces or terminates an aversive condition.) Such an argument is very similar to the psychoanalytic view that overeating is a defense against negative emotions.

Externality hypothesis. A very popular theory in the 1970s explained overeating in the obese in terms of their increased sensitivity to external cues, including times, places, sights, and smells associated with food.[91] Eating in the obese was thought to be influenced by these external factors to a far greater degree than it was in average-weight individuals, in whom eating was thought to be regulated primarily by internal signals such as gastric motility. Subsequent research, however, failed to show consistent differences in externality between obese and nonobese individuals.[92,93]

PROBLEMS WITH RESEARCH ON PSYCHOLOGICAL FACTORS

Two factors may have prevented investigators from isolating the possible effects of psychological factors on the development of obesity: the heterogeneous nature of this disorder and the failure to conduct longitudinal studies. We will briefly review each of these factors.

Heterogeneity of Obesity

Research during the past two decades has shown that obesity is a very heterogeneous disorder that may result from a variety of factors.[17] Thus, obese persons may differ in the age of onset of this disorder,[94] the presence of hyperplastic versus hypertrophic obesity,[16] and the principal areas in which fat is stored (i.e., upper- vs. lower-body obesity).[25] Moreover, obesity may result from decreased physical activity, overconsumption of food, a low resting metabolic rate, and genetic factors.[73,95]

Efforts to assess the contribution of psychological factors to obesity might prove more successful if investigators controlled for the effects of the physiologic factors cited. This would require studying relatively "pure" subtypes of obese individuals. Thus, for example, the influence of psychological and environmental factors could be studied in identical twins reared apart. Holding genetic factors constant would permit a clearer assessment of the influence of environmental variables. In the absence of such designs, the possible effects of psychosocial factors may well be masked by more powerful physiologic variables.

Longitudinal Investigations

The other major shortcoming in this area is that the effects of psychological variables are usually investigated after subjects have become obese. Thus, investigators administer psychological inventories to obese and nonobese subjects, and when greater psychopathology is discovered in the obese, it is frequently interpreted as a factor contributing to the weight difficulty. As noted above, however, this method is unable to differentiate between factors that may be a consequence rather than a cause of obesity. Thus, prejudice and discrimination may be responsible for the depression observed in some persons, rather than depression causing obesity.

To solve this problem, longitudinal studies are needed in which subjects are assessed on a variety of psychosocial dimensions before the onset of their obesity. One such study was recently completed in a group of 132 obese and nonobese children, 3 to 5 years of age, who were followed annually for 3 years.[96] Initial body fat was the best predictor of increases in fat over this period. Only one of the psychosocial variables studied, physical self-esteem was consistently related to the development of obesity but only during the first 2 years. It accounted for less than 5% of the variance in changes in body fat. It should be noted that variables including general self-esteem and maternal and parental regard were not associated with changes in body fat.

Additional studies of this nature are needed in which subjects are examined for longer periods of time. In particular, children should be studied through adolescence, a time at which the prevalence of obesity increases markedly. Only by conducting such studies can investigators determine the true contribution of psychological factors to obesity.

BINGE EATING IN THE OBESE

Recent findings concerning binge eating in obese individuals underscore the need for longitudinal studies of psychosocial variables. Several research teams have reported in the past decade that approximately 20–30% of the patients who enter weight loss programs experience problems with binge eating, consuming large amounts of food in a short period of time.[97–100] Unlike persons with bulimia nervosa, who compensate for their binging by vomiting or using laxatives, obese binge eaters do not purge. Purging or other compensatory behaviors may assist persons with bulimia nervosa to maintain a relatively normal body weight, while the absence of such compensation may contribute to weight gain in obese binge eaters. Thus, research is needed to illuminate the relationship between binge eating and obesity. It is possible that patients initially become obese in the absence of binge eating. They may start to binge in response to efforts to lose weight that are often associated with severe dietary deprivation.[101] Studies have shown that the vast majority of persons with bulimia nervosa report that their first binge occurred while they were dieting.[102]

Regardless of the etiology of binge eating, there are important psychological differences between obese bingers and nonbingers.[80] Binge eaters report greater psychological distress than do nonbingers on standard measures of psychopathology and have a higher lifetime prevalence of psychiatric illness, particularly affective disorders.[103–106] They also report greater dietary disinhibition than do nonbingers[99,105] and lower self-efficacy with regard to dieting.[97,105] Binge eating may also be associated with an increased risk of greater attrition[105], although this is not a consistent finding.[107–109]

Obese binge eaters, like persons with bulimia nervosa, are likely to display significant cognitive distortions related to food and eating.[65] They frequently have lists of "good" and "bad" foods, the latter of which they try to avoid while dieting. When bingers overeat or consume some of their "bad" foods, they often become emotionally upset and harangue themselves with statements such as "You're pathetic. You have no self-control. I can't believe how you've blown your diet." This self-derogation frequently leads to greater emotional distress and further overeating.

Patients tend to overestimate greatly the extent of their dietary transgressions. Cognitive therapy is used with such individuals to help them identify their distorted self-statements and to replace them with more rational thoughts. This approach has been used successfully with persons with bulimia nervosa and has been tried with encouraging results in obese binge eaters.[110]

EFFECTS OF DIETING AND WEIGHT LOSS

Given the high prevalence of dieting, especially among the obese, it is important to assess the psychological sequelae of dieting and weight loss. Studies examining the psychological effects of dieting have yielded contradictory results. Stunkard and Rush[111] reviewed seven studies published between 1951 and 1973, all of which reported adverse emotional reactions associated with dieting. Wing et al.,[112] by contrast, reviewed 10 studies published between 1969 and 1983 that reported that dieting was associated with either improvements or no worsening in mood. The most obvious difference between these two groups of studies was the use of behavior therapy in the latter ones. This has led some invcstigators[109] to attribute the lack of adverse emotional reactions to behavior therapy. There are, however, other methodologic differences between the two groups of studies that may better explain their divergent findings.[77,113]

When mood was assessed by objective psychometric instruments (e.g., Beck Depression Inventory,[114] State-Trait Anxiety Inventory[115]) there was no change in mood or improvement. Open-ended assessment, typically by psychiatric interview, consistently revealed adverse mood changes. This phenomenon was especially evident in one study that used both methods in the same sample of patients.[113] Objective tests showed improvements in mood, while open-ended methods yielded some indication of untoward changes.

The frequency of assessment also affected the outcome. Smoller et al.[77] found that all 11 studies that assessed mood only at pre- and posttreatment reported benign changes. Of the 13 that assessed mood more frequently throughout treatment, 46% reported benign changes while 54% reported adverse changes. It may be that more frequent assessment measures the effects of dieting, while pre- to posttesting assesses the effects of weight loss. Intermittent assessments are more likely to reveal the transient stresses associated with restricting caloric intake below usual levels and attempting to adopt a more active lifestyle. Pre- to postmeasurements are more likely to reflect the emotions associated with a retrospective look at successful weight loss rather than the temporary setbacks (e.g., less than expected weight loss, life stressors that affect adherence) most dieters encounter during the course of treatment.

The relationship between weight loss and mood is more complicated. Of those studies in which mean weight losses exceeded 20 lb (9 kg), 46% reported adverse consequences. When weight losses averaged 20 lb (9 kg) or less, no studies reported adverse effects. It is important to note that the relationship between weight loss and mood does not appear to be linear and that the large weight losses associated with surgical procedures are associated with surprisingly few symptoms.[116] Treatment setting (inpatient versus outpatient), length of treatment, and attrition do not seem to be related to psychological outcome.[77]

EFFECTS OF WEIGHT REGAIN

Much less is known about the emotional consequences of weight regain. This is an important issue to investigate given the high prevalence of relapse among dieters[117,118] and the frequency of repeated cycles of weight loss and regain.[119] The few studies conducted suggest that weight regain is universally associated with adverse emotional reactions. Brownell and Stunkard[120] showed that depression decreased in patients as they lost weight during 6 months of treatment. Depression levels returned towards baseline, however, as patients regained weight during a 1-year follow-up period. Scores did not fall into the clinically significant

TABLE 8–3 Effects of Weight Regain on Physical and Psychological Status in 36 Females at 3-year follow-up evaluation

Variable	Mean Score
Satisfaction with appearance	6.39
Self-esteem	5.97
Self-confidence	5.95
General level of happiness	5.66
Physical health	5.61
Recreational activities	5.36
Job performance	5.21
Social activities	5.18
Outlook on the future	5.17
Relationship with spouse/partner	5.03
Sex life	4.97
Relationship with family members	4.61

1, very positive effect; 4, no effect; 5, slightly negative effect; 6, moderately negative effect; 7, very negative effect.

Source: From Ref. 121, p. 927, with permission.

range of depression at baseline or follow-up, but these data suggest that dysphoria is positively correlated with weight gain.

The only other study of the psychological effects of weight regain (to our knowledge) was conducted as part of a 3-year follow-up evaluation of patients treated with a very-low-calorie diet (VLCD), behavior therapy, and a combination of the two.[121] Patients in the VLCD-alone and behavior therapy conditions showed significant reductions in depression scores at the end of treatment and at the 1-year follow-up. At the 3-year follow-up, at which time patients had regained a majority of their weight loss, scores increased so that they were no longer significantly different from baseline. Patients in the VLCD-alone condition showed no significant changes in depression at any time during treatment or follow-up. The effect of weight regain on physical and psychological health was assessed in 36 patients across all conditions. Patients were asked to rate the effect of weight regain on a variety of variables listed in Table 8–3. Weight regain had the most negative effect on satisfaction with appearance, self-esteem, self-confidence, happiness, and physical health.

CLINICAL IMPRESSIONS

Research on psychosocial factors associated with the etiology and treatment of obesity lags behind our clinical knowledge in many instances. In this section, we briefly summarize our principal clinical impressions of the relationship between obesity and psychological status.

Personality and Psychopathology

We have found that personality style is as diverse in the obese as it is in persons of average weight. Thus, in any group of 10 patients receiving treatment, we usually observe several who are outgoing, socially skilled, and productive group members. They participate constructively in the meeting and help to care for other group members. One or two additional individuals are likely to be somewhat shy and reserved but can contribute appropriately to the group when asked to do so.

Each group is also likely to contain one or two individuals with a personality disorder. Persons with borderline personality disorder frequently are popular among group members during the early stages of treatment. They may disclose intimate thoughts and feelings about themselves and develop engaging relationships with group members. Over time, however, they are likely to flood the group with reports of their troubled personal relationships and difficulties in coping with life's challenges. In addition, they frequently are emotionally volatile in group situations and may develop intense positive or negative feelings toward staff and other group participants.

Persons with a passive-aggressive personality style never become this emotionally involved with the staff or group members. They are, however, likely to drain the group's energy by their constant complaints that they are not "getting anything out of treatment" and that none of the suggestions offered by group members are helpful. Such persons were first identified in traditional group psychotherapy and have been referred to as *help-rejecting complainers*.

Interpretation. As indicated, we normally find a wide range of personality styles among our overweight patients, as well as a wide range of mental health. The great majority of individuals fall into the normal range of psychological functioning, but clearly there are exceptions.

In the case of personality disorders, it is tempting to speculate that the patient's obesity is dynamically related to the personality dysfunction. Thus, the borderline patient may eat to ease feelings of profound emptiness or binge in response to overwhelming impulses that may also be associated with drug abuse, sexual promiscuity, and self-mutiliation. The passive-aggressive individual may overeat as an expression of anger and defiance, and the resulting obesity may silently communicate the message "Don't try to get too close to me." Obesity in persons with low self-esteem may simply be an outward expression of their negative feelings toward themselves.

More research is clearly needed on the relationship between obesity and personality dysfunction. At present, in the absence of definitive data, we think that the relationship between obesity and psychopathology may well be coincidental. The psychiatric complications and personality disorders described above are also found in individuals of average weight. Thus, these complications may occur independent of weight status. Regardless of the etiologic relationship, it is important that persons with personality disorders and other psychopathology receive the care that they require, which is above and beyond that needed to manage their obesity. In many cases, such individuals should be referred for adjunctive therapy.

Life Stressors

We are increasingly impressed by the effects of untoward life events on patients' psychosocial functioning and on their ability to control their weight. During a 1-year treatment program, it is not unusual for at least one group member to have a death in the family and another to experience significant work-related or financial problems. Such occurrences are likely to be associated with anxiety, depression, and other adverse emotions, as they are in persons of average weight. In obese individuals, such experiences also are frequently associated with weight gain, as patients lose control of their customary efforts to manage their weight.

Practitioners should be prepared to support patients during such difficult times. In some instances, a couple of brief meetings (10 to 15 min) are sufficient to help the individual cope with the difficulties. In cases in which the patient's dysphoria does not remit within a few weeks, the practitioner should consider a referral for individual psychotherapy. Supportive therapy may be more appropriate than psychodynamic treatment in such instances.

Weight Loss and Dieting

Our clinical experience is consistent with research findings of both positive and negative emotional responses to weight reduction. In terms of benefits, patients gain a sense of mastery over a chronic problem, which increases their self-efficacy. They are justifiably proud of their weight losses and their ability to engage in health-promoting behaviors (such as being more assertive about food choices, increasing their activity level, and requesting and obtaining social support). Many patients enjoy a sense of well-being as their medical conditions improve. Decreases in blood lipids, glucose, blood pressure, and the medications for obesity-related conditions improve patients' moods. Positive reinforcement in the form of praise from friends and family also results in improvements in mood.

Concomitant with these extremely positive emotions, some patients experience occasional annoyance and sometimes distress. One of the most common problems associated with weight loss is the increased attention patients receive. Such attention and praise are especially difficult for shy patients who are not accustomed to receiving compliments. Often this attention takes the form of asking questions about the diet and heaping praise on the patient. One patient remarked, "I wish I could just go out and not have to talk about my diet all night." We have found it useful to role-play such situations with patients in group sessions in order to increase their social skills and their comfort in receiving compliments and directing the conversation to other topics.

Any type of increased attention after weight loss is a double-edged sword. On the one hand, it is nice to be recognized for a difficult accomplishment (i.e., weight loss). On the other, some patients resent the praise (i.e., "Why are they so nice to me now that I've lost weight? I'm still the same person I was 40 pounds ago").

Attention from the opposite sex can be particularly disconcerting for some patients, especially those who have a history of sexual or physical abuse.[122] Weight loss may bring with it a sense of increased vulnerability. We have seen this anxiety heightened in patients who approach a weight at which they were victimized. One patient with a history of sexual abuse reported that she no longer felt safe walking in areas where she had previously walked for months. She concluded, "I guess my weight made me feel safe. I didn't think any man would want to attack me. Now that I am looking better, I'm more scared for my safety."

Stuart and Jacobson reviewed the delicate balance between weight, sex, and marriage[123] and found that weight loss may expose certain functions of obesity. For example, some patients reported using weight to deter sexual attention from a spouse. Losing weight increases the likelihood of this unwanted event. Some patients also have reported using weight to deter themselves from extramarital affairs. Their increased weight decreases the number of potential extramarital partners. Losing weight opens up the possibility of flirting and engaging in affairs. Independent of marriage, losing weight certainly heightens any fears of intimacy that patients may possess.

Another potential adverse emotional consequence associated with weight loss is the stress and anxiety associated with redefining roles in the family or the workplace. A patient, for example, may decide not to serve three dinners each night as various members of the family come home. It may be appropriate for some patients to change their household duties to avoid high-risk eating situations (e.g., cleaning up after dinner, food shopping). This requires negotiation among family members, and the change may be unsettling for all. It is not uncommon to hear family members ask, "When can we go back to the way things used to be?"

Social as well as professional roles may also change as a result of weight loss. Coworkers or friends who were formerly buddies may now approach thinner patients as prospective dates. Some patients report that resisting such romantic overtures may dramatically alter a friendship. As patients become more assertive, they may not be as well liked in work or social settings. Those interested in the emotional responses to weight loss and dieting should consult the eloquent and moving description of these experiences provided by Jasper.[124]

It is important to note that these adverse reactions do not happen in all or even a majority of patients. They do happen frequently enough, however, that practitioners should be alert for their occurrence and intervene promptly. Before treatment, practitioners should ask about previous weight loss efforts to determine any history of adverse emotional reactions to weight loss and/or dieting to assess the likelihood of similar untoward occurrences. Role-playing and assertiveness training may be adequate for some patients, while others may require psychotherapy. One indication of the need for intervention is weight gain or weight stabilization during a period in which weight loss is expected. A small minority of patients may be too anxious to proceed with weight loss and return, consciously or unconsciously, to a more comfortable weight. The cost of further weight loss may not be comparable to the benefits. Although there are no data to support this contention, we believe that the adverse emotional consequences of weight loss (especially when unexpected) may be the primary reason for weight regain in a select minority of patients.

Weight Regain

Our clinical experience suggests that there are no unequivocally positive effects of weight regain. As patients begin to regain weight, they become frustrated. They express feelings of disbelief and powerlessness: "I can't believe that I regained 5 pounds in 2 weeks. It took me over 1 month to lose 5 pounds. Why even bother? It's no use." Some may respond by denial with comments such as "Three pounds is no problem. I can take it off, I've just lost 30." This denial typically just delays the frustration.

Patients also experience anger as weight is regained. The anger may be directed at the treatment providers, but almost always it is turned inward. "How can I let this happen to me? I've worked so hard, and now I am blowing it." We find it helpful clinically to acknowledge these emotions as a natural and expected part of long-term weight control. It is normal to be upset by weight gain. It triggers fears of being out of control and returning to a heavier weight. We encourage patients to focus on reversing small weight gains before they become larger. We do this by helping patients develop specific strategies to reverse the gain and contingency plans if weight loss is not accomplished (Wadden & Foster, 1992).[65] Unfortunately, the emotions associated with weight regain (i.e., shame, anger, and depression) are not conducive to enacting these plans. Thus, we strongly encourage patients to attend sessions, especially when they are having difficulty.

A FINAL NOTE

As this review has indicated, the psychological burden of obesity can be great and is exacerbated by a society preoccupied with thinness. In many cases, overweight patients have been ridiculed, scorned, and rejected, not only by passing strangers but also by family and friends.[125] Each time patients lose weight and regain it, their self-respect erodes and feelings of shame and inadequacy increase. The very prospect of undertaking another weight loss effort may be frightening to patients, since it may represent another potential failure.

Unfortunately, health care providers, like the public at large, harbor a host of negative stereotypes toward the obese that are likely to be aroused when patients fail to lose weight.[126] Patients are likely to have encountered health care providers who have accused them of not trying hard enough or lacking self-discipline. Blaming patients for their condition only adds to the pain of obesity. In some cases, patients will have followed treatment protocols rigidly without losing weight. In other cases, life stressors may have affected their ability to adhere. In neither case, however, can practitioners afford to blame patients for lack of progress.

Practitioners should examine any negative feelings they experience toward patients, for these are often the same feelings experienced by the patient: impotence, frustration, anger, and sadness. In many cases, the greatest service that the practitioner can provide is to allow patients to verbalize their feelings of anger, sadness, or disappointment and to respond empathically. In all cases, overweight persons should be treated with the greatest respect and compassion. Particularly with persons who are unable to lose weight, the goal of treatment is to help them recover their lost self-esteem and to realize that they can live a rich and fulfilling life, regardless of their weight.

REFERENCES

1. Van Itallie TB. Health implications of overweight and obesity in the United States. *Ann Intern Med* 103:983, 1985.
2. National Institutes of Health Consensus Development Panel. Health implications of obesity. *Ann Intern Med* 103:1073, 1985.
3. Bennett W, Gurin J. *The Dieter's Dilemma*. New York, Basic Books.
4. Schwartz H. *Never Satisfied: A Cultural History of Diets, Fantasies and Fat*. New York, Free Press, 1986.
5. Silverstein B, Perdue L, Peterson, et al. The role of mass media in promoting a thin standard of attractiveness for women. *Sex Roles* 14:519, 1986.

6. Garner DM, Garfinkel PE, Schwartz D, et al. Cultural expectation of thinness in women. *Psychol Rep* 47:483, 1980.
7. Williamson DF, Kahn HS, Remington PL, et al. The 10-year incidence of overweight and major weight gain in US adults. *Arch Intern Med* 150:665, 1990.
8. Moser PW. Double vision: Why do we never match up to our mind's ideal? *Self Magazine,* January, pp. 51–52, 1989.
9. Brownell KD. Dieting and the search for the perfect body: Where physiology and culture collide. *Behav Ther* 22:1, 1991.
10. Stunkard AJ, Sorensen TIA, Hanis C, et al. An adoption study of human obesity. *N Engl J Med* 314:193, 1986.
11. Stunkard AJ, Harris JR, Pedersen NL, et al. The body mass index of twins who have been reared apart. *N. Engl J Med* 322:1483, 1990.
12. Bouchard C. Heredity and the path to overweight and obesity. *Med Sci Sports Exerc* 23:285, 1991.
13. Foster GD, Wadden TA, Mullen JL, et al. Resting energy expenditure, body composition and excess weight in the obese. *Metabolism* 37:467, 1988.
14. Garrow JS, Durrant ML, Mann S, et al. Factors determining weight loss in obese patients in a metabolic ward. *Int J Obes* 2:441, 1978.
15. Krotiewski M, Sjosttrom L, Bjorntorp P. Adipose tissue cellularity in relation to prognosis for weight reduction. *Int J Obes* 1:395, 1977.
16. Bjorntorp P. Fat cells and obesity, in Brownell KB, Foreyt JP (eds), *Handbook of Eating Disorders*. New York, Basic Books, 1986, pp. 88–98.
17. Brownell KD, Wadden TA. The heterogeneity of obesity: Fitting treatments to individuals. *Behav Ther* 22:153, 1991.
18. Wadden TA, Stunkard AJ. The psychological and social complications of obesity. *Ann Intern Med* 103:1062, 1985.
19. Wadden TA, Brown G, Foster GD, et al. Salience of weight related worries in adolescent males and females. *Int J Eating Dis* 10:407, 1991.
20. Fallon AE, Rozin P. Sex differences in perceptions of desirable body shape. *J Abnorm Psychol* 94:102, 1985.
21. NIH Technology Assessment Conference Panel. Methods for voluntary weight loss and control. Ann Intern Med 119:764, 1993.
22. Rosen JC, Gross J. Prevalence of weight reducing and weight gaining in adolescent girls and boys. *Health Psychol* 6:131, 1987.
23. Wadden TA, Foster GD, Stunkard AJ, et al. Dissatisfaction with weight and figure in obese girls: Discontent but not depression. *Int J Obes* 13:89, 1989.
24. Wadden TA, Foster GD, Letizia KA, et al. A multi-center evaluation of a proprietary weight reduction program for the treatment of marked obesity. *Arch Int Med* 152:961, 1992.
25. Sjostrom L. Impact of body weight, body composition and adipose tissue distribution on morbidity and mortality, in Stunkard AJ, Wadden TA (eds), *Obesity: Theory and Therapy*. New York, Raven Press, 1993, pp. 13–42.

26. Staffieri JR. A study of social stereotype of body image in children. *J Pers Soc Psychol* 7:101, 1967.
27. Harris MB, Harris RJ, Bochner S. Fat, four-eyed and female: Stereotypes of obesity, glasses and gender. *J Appl Soc Psychol* 12:503, 1982.
28. Venes AM, Krupka LR, Gerard RJ. Overweight/obese patients: An overview. *Practitioner* 226:1102, 1982.
29. Maddox GL, Liederman V. Overweight as a social disability with medical implications. *J Med Educ* 44:214, 1969.
30. Canning H, Mayer J. Obesity: Its possible effects on college admissions. *N Engl J Med* 275:1172, 1966.
31. Karris L. Prejudice against obese renters. *J Social Psychol* 101:159, 1977.
32. Larkin JC, Pines HA. No fat persons need apply. *Soc Work Occup* 6:312, 1979.
33. Roe DA, Eickwort KR. Relationships between obesity and associated health factors with unemployment among low-income women. *J Am Med Wom Assoc* 31:193, 1976.
34. Fat execs get slimmer paychecks. *Industry Week* 180:21, 1974.
35. Hecht K. Oh, come on fatties. *Newsweek,* September 3, 1990, p 8.
36. Moore ME, Stunkard AJ, Srole L. Obesity, social class and mental illness. *JAMA* 181:962, 1962.
37. Stewart AL, Brook RH. Effects of being overweight. *Am J Pub Health* 73:171, 1983.
38. Crisp AH, McGuiness B. Jolly fat: Relation between obesity and psychoneurosis in general population. *Br Med J* 3:7, 1976.
39. Silverstone JT. Psychosocial aspects of obesity. *Proc R Soc Med* 61:371, 1968.
40. Floderus B. Psycho-social factors in relation to coronary heart disease and associated risk factors. *Nord Hyg Tidskr* Suppl 6:1974.
41. Hallstrom T, Noppa H. Obesity in women in relation to mental illness, social factors and personality traits. *J Psychosom Res* 25:75, 1981.
42. Hallberg L, Hogdahl A-M, Nilsson L, et al. Fetma hos kvinnor: Sociala data, symtom och fynd. *Lakartidn* 63:621, 1966.
43. Kittel F, Rustin RM, Dramaix M, et al. Psychosocio-biological correlates of moderate overweight in an industrial population. *J Psychosom Res* 22:145, 1978.
44. Larsson B. Obesity: A population study of men, with special reference to the development and consequences for the health. Dissertation Gotab, Kungalv, Sweden, University of Goteborg, 1978.
45. Kaplan KK, Wadden TA. Childhood obesity and self-esteem. *J Pediatr* 109:367, 1986.
46. Wadden TA, Foster GD, Brownell KD, et al. Self-concept in obese and normal weight children. *J Consult Clin Psychol* 52:1104, 1984.
47. Sallade J. A comparison of the psychological adjustment of obese vs. nonobese children. *J Psychosom Res* 17:89, 1973.

48. Hathaway SR, McKinnley JC. *Minnesota Multiphasic Personality Inventory*. Minneapolis, University of Minnesota, 1982.

49. Johnson SF, Swenson, WM, Gastineau CF. Personality characteristics in obesity: Relation of MMPI profile and age of onset of obesity to success in weight reduction. *Am J Clin Nutr* 29:626, 1976.

50. Kollar EJ, Atkinson RM, Albin DL. The effectiveness of fasting in the treatment of superobesity. *Psychosomatics* 10:125, 1968.

51. Lauer JB, Wampler RS, Lantz JB, et al. Psychosocial aspects of extremely obese women joining a diet group. *Int J Obes* 3:153, 1979.

52. Leon GR, Eckert ED, Teed D, et al. Changes in body image and other psychological factors after intestinal bypass surgery for massive obesity. *J. Behav Med* 2:39, 1979.

53. McCall RJ. MMPI factors that differentiate remediably from irremediably obese women. *J Commun Psychol* 1:34, 1973.

54. Pomerantz AS, Greenberg S, Blackburn GL. MMPI profiles of obese men and women. *Psychol Rep* 41:731, 1977.

55. Rosen LW, Aniskiewicz AS. Psychosocial functioning of two groups of morbidly obese patients. *Int J Obes* 7:53, 1983.

56. Solow C, Silberfarb PM, Swift K. Psychosocial effects of intestinal bypass surgery for severe obesity. *N Engl J Med* 290:300, 1974.

57. Svanum S, Lantz JB, Lauer JB, et al. Correspondence of the MMPI and the MMPI–168 with intestinal bypass surgery patients. *J Clin Psychol* 37:137, 1981.

58. Webb WW, Phares R, Abram HS, et al. Jejunoileal bypass procedures in morbid obesity: Preoperative psychological findings. *J Clin Psychol* 32:82, 1976.

59. Wadden TA, Stunkard AJ, Brownell KD, et al. Treatment of obesity by behavior therapy and very-low-calorie diet: a pilot investigation. *J Consult Clin Psychol* 52:692, 1984.

60. Swenson WM, Pearson JS, Osborne D. *An MMPI Source Book*. Minneapolis, University of Minnesota Press, 1973.

61. Crumpton E, Wine DB, Goot H. MMPI profiles of obese men and six other diagnostic categories. *Psychol Rep* 19:1110, 1966.

62. Holland J, Masling J, Copley D. Mental illness in lower class normal, obese and hyperobese women. *Psychosom Med* 32:351, 1970.

63. Mendelson N, Weinberg N, Stunkard AJ. Obesity in men: A clinical study of twenty-five cases. *Ann Intern Med* 54:660, 1961.

64. Klesges RC. Personality and obesity: Global versus specific measures? *Behav Assess* 6:347, 1984.

65. Wadden TA, Foster GD. Behavioral assessment and treatment of markedly obese patients, in Wadden TA, Van Itallie TB (eds), *Treatment of the Seriously Obese Patient*. New York, Guilford Press, pp. 290–330.

66. Rodin J, Silberstein L, Streigel-Moore R. Women and weight: A normative discontent, in Soneregger TB (ed), *Psychology and Gender. Nebraska Symposium on Motivation*. Lincoln, Lincoln University of Nebraska Press, 1988, pp. 257–307.

67. Stunkard AJ, Mendelson M. Disturbances in body image of some obese persons. *J. Am Diet Assoc* 38:328, 1961.
68. Stunkard AJ, Mendelson M. Obesity and the body image: I. Characteristics of disturbances in the body image of some obese persons. *Am J Psychiatry* 123:1296, 1967.
69. Stunkard AJ, Burt V. Obesity and the body image: II. Age at onset of disturbances in the body image. *Am J Psychiatry* 123:1443, 1967.
70. Wadden TA, Stunkard AJ, Rich L, et al. Obesity in black adolescent girls: A controlled clinical trial of treatment by diet, behavior modification, and parental support. *Pediatrics* 85:345, 1990.
71. Stern MP, Pugh JA, Gaskill SP, et al. Knowledge, attitudes, and behavior related to obesity and dieting in Mexican Americans and Anglos: The San Antonio heart study. *Am J Epidemiol* 115:917, 1982.
72. Andersen AE, Hay A. Racial and socioeconomic influences in anorexia nervosa and bulimia. *Int J Eating Dis* 4:479, 1985.
73. Stunkard AJ. Some perspectives on human obesity: its causes. *Bull NY Acad Med* 64:902, 1988.
74. Becker BJ. The obese patients in psychoanalysis. *Am J Psychother* 14:322, 1960.
75. Garetz FK. Socio-psychological factors in overeating and dieting with comments on popular reducing methods. *Practitioner* 210:671, 1973.
76. Kornhaber A. The stuffing syndrome. *Psychosomatics* 11:580, 1970.
77. Smoller JW, Wadden TA, Stunkard AJ. Dieting and depression: A critical review. *J Psychosom Res* 31:429, 1987.
78. Stunkard AJ, WAdden TA. Restrained eating and human obesity. *Nutr Rev* 48:78, 1990.
79. McReynolds WT. Toward a psychology of obesity: Review of research on the role of personality and level of adjustments. *Int J Eating Dis* 2:37, 1982.
80. O'Neil PM, Jarrell MP. Psychological aspects of obesity and dieting, in Wadden TA, Van Itallie TB (eds), *Treatment of the Seriously Obese Patient*. New York, Guilford, pp. 252–71.
81. Barrash, J, Rodriguez EM, Scott DH, et al. The utility of MMPI subtypes for the prediction of weight loss after bariatric surgery. *Int J Obes* 11:115, 1987.
82. Blankenmeyer BC, Smylie KD, Price PC, et al. A replicated 5 cluster MMPI typology of morbidly obese female candidates for gastric surgery. *Int J Obes* 14:235, 1990.
83. Duckro PN, Leavitt JN, Beal DG, et al. Psychological status among female candidates for surgical treatment. *Int J Obes* 7:477, 1983.
84. Stuart RB. Behavioral control of overeating. *Behav Res Ther* 5:357, 1967.
85. Stunkard AJ. Obesity, in Bellack AS, Hersen M, Kazdin AE (eds), *International Handbook of Behavior Modification and Therapy*. New York, Plenum Press, 1982, pp 535–573.
86. Garrow J. *Energy Balance and Obesity in Man*. New York, Elsevier, 1974.

87. Wooley SC, Wooley OW, Dyrenforth SR. Theoretical practical and social issues in behavioral treatment of obesity. *J Appl Behav Analysis* 12:3, 1979.
88. Bandini LG, Schoeller DA, Cyr HN, et al. Validity of reported energy intake in obese and nonobese adolescents. *Am J Clin Nutr* 52:421, 1990.
89. Schoeller DA. Measurement of energy expenditure in free-living humans by using doubly labeled water. *J Nutr* 118:1278, 1988.
90. Rodin J, Schank D, Striegel-Moore R. Psychological features of obesity. *Med Clin North Am* 73:47, 1989.
91. Schachter S. Some extraordinary facts about obese humans and rats. *Am Psychol* 26:129, 1971.
92. Rodin J. The externality theory today, in Stunkard AJ (ed), *Obesity*. Philadelphia, WB Saunders, 1980, pp 226–239.
93. Rodin J. The current status of the internal-external obesity hypothesis: What went wrong? *Am Psychol* 36:361, 1981.
94. Price RA, Stunkard AJ, Ness R, et al. Childhood onset (age $<$ 10) obesity has high familial risk. *Int J Obes* 14:85, 1990.
95. Wadden TA, Bell ST. Obesity, in Bellack AS, Hersen M, Kazdin AE (eds), *International Handbook of Behavior Modification and Therapy*. New York, Plenum Press, 1990, pp 449–473.
96. Klesges RC, Haddock CK, Klesges LM et al. Relationship between psychosocial functioning and body fat in preschool children: A longitudinal investigation. *J Consult Clin Psychol* 60:793, 1992.
97. Gormally J, Black S, Daston S. The assessment of binge eating severity among obese persons. *Addict Behav* 7:47, 1982.
98. Marcus MD. Binge eating in obesity, in Fairburn CG, Wilson GT (eds), *Binge Eating: Nature, Assessment and Treatment*. NY, Guilford Press, pp. 77–96.
99. Marcus MD, Wing RR, Lamparski DM. Binge eating and dietary restraint in obese patients. *Addict Behav* 10:163, 1985.
100. Spitzer RL, Yanovski S, Wadden TA, Walsh BT, et al. Binge eating disorder: Its further validation in a multisite study. *Int J Eating Dis*. 13:137, 1993.
101. Polivy J, Herman CP. Dieting and binging: A causal analysis. *Am Psychol* 40:193, 1985.
102. Striegel-Moore R, Silberstein L, Rodin J. Toward an understanding of risk factors for bulimia. *Am Psychol* 41:246, 1986.
103. Hudson JI, Pope HG, Wurtman J, et al. Bulimia in obese individuals. Relationship to normal-weight bulimia. *J Nerv Ment Dis* 176:144, 1988.
104. Kolotkin RL, Revis ES, Kirkley BG, et al. Binge eating in obesity: Associated MMPI characteristics. *J Consult Clin Psychol* 55:872, 1987.
105. Marcus MD, Wing RR, Hopkins J. Obese bing eaters: Affect, cognitions, and response to behavioral weight control. *J Consult Clin Psychol* 56:433, 1988.
106. Marcus MD, Wing RR, Ewing L, et al. Psychiatric disorders among obese binge eaters. *Int J Eating Dis* 9:69, 1990.

107. Telch CF, Agras WS. The effects of a very low calorie diet on bing eating. *Beh Ther* 24:177, 1993.

108. Wadden TA, Foster GO, Letizia KA. Response of obese binge eaters to behavior therapy combined with a very low calorie diet. *J Consult Clin Psychol* 60:808, 1992.

109. Wadden TA, Foster GO, Letizia KA. One-year behavioral treatment of obesity: Comparison of moderate and severe restriction and the effects of weight maintenance therapy. *J Consult Clin Psychol* 1994, in press.

110. Telch CF, Agras WS, Rossiter E, et al. Group cognitive-behavioral treatment for the non-purging bulimic: An initial evaluation. *J Consult Clin Psychol* 58:629, 1990.

111. Stunkard AJ, Rush J. Dieting and depression reexamined: A critical review of untoward responses during weight reduction for obesity. *Ann Intern Med* 81:526, 1974.

112. Wing RR, Epstein LH, Marcus MD, et al. Mood changes in behavioral weight loss programs. *J Psychosom Res* 28:189, 1984.

113. Wadden TA, Stunkard AJ, Smoller JW. Dieting and depression: A methodological study. *J Consult Clin Psychol* 54:869, 1986.

114. Beck AT, Ward CH, Mendelson M, et al. An inventory for measuring depression. *Arch Gen Psychiatry* 4:561, 1961.

115. Spielberger CD, Gorsuch RL, Lushene R. *The State-Trait Anxiety Inventory*. Palo Alto, Calif, Consulting Psychologists Press, 1983.

116. Stunkard AJ, Wadden TA. Psychological aspects of severe obesity. *Am J Clin Nutr* 55:524, 1992.

117. Wadden TA, Sternberg JA, Letizia KA, et al. Treatment of obesity by very low calorie diet, behavior therapy and their combination: A five year prospective. *Int J Obes* 13:39, 1989.

118. Kramer FM, Jeffery RW, Forster JL, et al. Long-term follow-up of behavioral treatment for obesity: Patterns of weight regain among men and women. *Int J Obes* 13:123, 1989.

119. Wadden TA, Bartlett SJ, Letizia KA, et al. Relationship of dieting history to resting metabolic rate, body composition, eating behavior and subsequent weight loss. *Am J Clin Nutr*. 56:203, 1992.

120. Brownell KD, Stunkard AJ. Couples training, pharmacotherapy, and behavior therapy in the treatment of obesity. *Arch Gen Psychiatry* 38:1233, 1981.

121. Wadden TA, Stunkard AJ, Liebschutz J. Three-year follow-up of the treatment of obesity by very low calorie diet, behavior therapy and their combination. *J Consult Clin Psychol* 56:925, 1988.

122. Felitti VJ. Long-term medical consequences of incest, rape and molestation. *South Med J* 84:328, 1991.

123. Stuart RB, Jacobson B. *Weight, Sex and Marriage*. New York, WW Norton, 1987.

124. Jasper J. The challenge of weight control: A personal view, in Wadden TA, Van Itallie, TB (eds), *Treatment of the Seriously Obese Patient*. New York, Guilford Press, pp. 411–436.

125. Coleman JA. Discrimination at large. *Newsweek* August 2, 1993, p. 9.

126. Frank A. Futility and Avoidance: Medical professionals in the treatment of obesity. *JAMA* 269:2132, 1993.

Long-Term Health Effects Associated with Significant Weight Loss: A Study of the Dose–Response Effect

CHAPTER 9

Beatrice S. Kanders, Ed.D., M.P.H., R.D., Francis J. Peterson, Ph.D., Philip T. Lavin, Ph.D., Dawn E. Norton, B.S., Nawfal W. Istfan, M.D., Ph.D., and George L. Blackburn, M.D., Ph.D.

INTRODUCTION

Obesity is associated with an increased risk of several diseases, including diabetes, hypertension, stroke, cardiovascular disease, gallstones, and certain types of cancer.[1–5] The health benefits of weight loss are well known and have been

Acknowledgments

The authors gratefully acknowledge the editorial assistance of Michelle Kienholz, as well as suggestions and comments of Dr. Thomas Wadden. The authors also wish to acknowledge the contributions of the following Optifast Clinics and clinic personnel: S. Baumann, Central Ohio Nutrition, Columbus, OH; R. Brandeis, Northwest Clinical Nutrition Center, Seattle, WA; M. Carrillo, Kaiser Permanente, San Diego, CA; J. DeMarco, Mt. Sinai Hospital, Minneapolis, MN; C. Dufour, 7th Ward General Hospital, Hammond, LA; S. Flood, University of Rochester Medical Center, Rochester, NY; B. Gapinski, Waukesha Memorial Hospital, Waukesha, WI; R. Harrisman, University of Arkansas Metabolic Management Clinic, Little Rock, AR; E. Kinsey, Weight Management Center, Charleston, SC; D. Miller, Normandy Osteopathic Hospital South, St. Louis, MO; F. Normann, Fountain Valley Hospital, Fountain Valley, CA; C. Owsiany, Baylor University Medical Center, Dallas, TX; T. Schmidt, Yorba Linda Medical Center Clinic, Inc., Yorba Linda, CA; K. Sweeney, York Hospital Nutrition & Weight Management Center, York, PA; and E. Tekula, University Community Hospital, Tamarac, FL.

This study was supported by grants from Sandoz Nutrition Company (Minneapolis, MN) and from the Center for Nutritional Research Charitable Trust Fund (Boston, MA).

reviewed elsewhere.[6–10] However, few studies have evaluated the amount of weight loss needed to achieve a significant improvement in health status. Is there a dose–response relationship for weight loss in the improvement in such weight-related diseases as diabetes or hypertension, or is there a certain percentage of weight loss beyond which no additional health benefit it achieved? The long-term effects of sustained weight loss on health outcome also remain undocumented.

This chapter will address each of these issues through analysis of the 18-month medical outcome data of 783 individuals who participated in a medically supervised very-low-calorie diet (VLCD) as part of a multidisciplinary obesity treatment program. In designing this study, the primary goal was to evaluate and compare the effects of both short-term weight loss and long-term follow-up on health outcome in a prospectively defined obese population. Specific attention was paid to diabetes and hypertension, as these chronic diseases are most frequently associated with obesity.[11] Secondary objectives were to characterize this sample of VLCD patients; to determine the duration of treatment and the degree of weight loss for these patients; and, finally, to monitor the impact of weight loss as a medical intervention, as evidenced by changes in health, medication usage, and medical conditions.

METHODS

Study Design

In the spring of 1986, the names of 50 Optifast clinics in the United States were solicited from Sandoz Nutrition Company (Minneapolis, Minn). Of these clinics, at least 2 from each of six geographic zones were asked to assist in the investigation; a total of 15 clinics agreed to participate.

Charts for 100 consecutive obese patients[12] were reviewed at each clinic, and standardized forms were completed by trained data monitors. All patients were to have begun treatment prior to December 31, 1985; one clinic had treated only 29 subjects prior to this date. Eligibility was based on the completion of at least 3 weeks of active weight loss. Patients were excluded from study entry if they had previously participated in the same VLCD program.

Fourteen of the 15 clinics participated in a follow-up telephone survey, and patients from these clinics were contacted to obtain data approximately 18 months after enrolling in the VLCD program. At least three attempts were made to contact each patient.

Treatment

The patients were treated with a liquid formula VLCD[13,14] that provided a minimum of 70 g/day of protein, as well as essential vitamins and minerals.

Patients were screened by a dietitian, a nurse, and/or a physician prior to enrolling. The initial medical evaluation included a medical history, a physical examination, the calculation of body mass index (BMI), an electrocardiogram (ECG), and comprehensive blood tests; psychological assessments were also performed if necessary.[15] No patient was admitted to the program if a VLCD was contraindicated for either medical or psychological reasons.

While consuming the VLCD, patients were monitored weekly by a dietitian, a nurse, and/or a physician; laboratory tests and ECGs were performed as necessary. All patients underwent biweekly and, later, monthly laboratory analysis. Information on nutrition, exercise, and behavior modification was presented at weekly group sessions led by a trained health professional.[16] Mild physical activity, such as brisk walking, was strongly encouraged.

The active weight loss (AWL) phase was defined as the period in which patients consumed two-thirds or more of their daily calories as the liquid formula. Patients were permitted to remain in AWL for up to 20 weeks, and one-third of the clinics permitted patients to use the VLCD beyond 20 weeks. The physician determined which formula to prescribe (420 vs. 800 kcal) based on each patient's sex, degree of obesity, level of physical activity, existing medical conditions, and rate of weight loss.

Following AWL, patients entered a 3- to 5-week period of refeeding during which self-prepared meals were gradually reintroduced as patients were weaned off the liquid formula diet. Weekly physician visits and group behavior therapy continued. Patients decided whether to participate in active maintenance (AM), which began at the conclusion of the refeeding phase. During AM, patients consumed less than one-third of their calories as the liquid formula. While no standard maintenance program existed across the sites, each clinic encouraged patients to attend maintenance groups.

The liquid formula was discontinued at the end of AM, and patients were instructed to comply with a new calorie-controlled diet based on the U.S. Dietary Guidelines[17] adjusted to sustain their new body weight. Nutrition education focused on reducing dietary fat and controlling the quantity and quality of all calories consumed. Moderate aerobic exercise was encouraged, and physician visits and behavior therapy continued according to each patient's willingness to attend.

Data Collection

Clinical data were abstracted from patient charts. Data monitors were trained to abstract charts and to conduct the follow-up telephone survey according to a procedure manual presented at a 2-day training session. Clinic representatives practiced filling out actual data collection forms using fictitious charts. Forms were reviewed at the training session by experienced clinical data monitors. Data on body weight, medical status (medication use, number of physician visits), and use of the liquid formula recorded in patient charts during AWL and AM were abstracted.

Follow-up data were obtained through a structured telephone interview conducted by trained interviewers 18 ± 2 months after patients started the VLCD program. Data were collected on weight, dieting experience, and medical status. The presence of diabetes and hypertension was based on a diagnosis by the primary care physician, as documented in the patient's chart. Patients with both diabetes and hypertension were counted separately in each disease category.

Medical outcome was classified according to the following definitions used by data monitors: (1) no medical intervention, (2) medical visit but no medication, (3) medical visit and medication, (4) hospitalization, and (5) life-threatening. Information was collected on all medication use, including over-the-counter drugs, aspirin, and nonsteroidal anti-inflammatory drugs.

Statistical Analysis

In the presentation of the data, means and standard deviations are used unless otherwise indicated. The sample size chosen permitted 95% confidence intervals with a width of less than 5% for population proportions and of less than 20% of the standard deviation for percentage weight loss within major sex-diet subgroups. It was also sufficiently large to detect a positive relationship between percentage weight loss and improvement in medical condition (2% slope for the regression line) with 90% power according to a one-sided test of significance with 5% type I error.

The effects of baseline BMI and sex were evaluated by the use of multivariate regression analyses for AWL duration and AWL percentage weight loss. The percentage weight loss regression was run first with AWL duration excluded and then included as a covariate. The prevalence of diabetes mellitus and hypertension was determined at baseline and at 18 months and compared using McNemar's paired comparison test (two-sided). The relationship between percentage weight loss and percentage with medical problem improved was determined by using a Kruskal-Wallis exact test.

RESULTS

Baseline Characteristics

The mean age, sex, weight, percentage above ideal body weight,[18] and BMI of the 1429 patients at program entry are shown in Table 9–1. At study entry, 154 patients had an initial diagnosis of diabetes, 421 had hypertension, and 100 had both diseases.

TABLE 9–1 Baseline Characteristics of the Study Population

Variable	Males	Females	Combined
Number	356	1073	1429
Age (years)	43.6 ± 10.3	42.0 ± 11.3	42.4 ± 11.1
Percent above ideal body weight[a]	67.9 ± 32.2	65.2 ± 30.3	65.8 ± 30.8
BMI (kg/m^2)	39.1 ± 7.5	36.1 ± 6.7	36.9 ± 7.0
Diabetes (*n*)	47	107	154
Hypertension (*n*)	135	286	421

[a]Based on 1959 Metropolitan Life Insurance tables.[18]

Duration on Program

Males and females remained in AWL for 17 ± 11 and 19 ± 11 weeks, respectively. Of the original 1429 patients enrolled, 700 participated in both AWL and AM. Females stayed in the program for an average of 27 ± 18 weeks, males for an average of 26 ± 18 weeks. Among males and females, a higher initial degree of obesity was associated with significantly longer participation in active treatment ($p < 0.0001$).

Change in Weight

During AWL, males lost 1.7 ± 0.7 kg/week (3.7 ± 1.6 lb/week) or 1.4 ± 0.6 % of initial body weight per week. Females lost 1.0 ± 0.5 kg/week (2.2 ± 1.0 lb/week) or 1.1 ± 0.5% of initial body weight per week. The total percentage weight loss during AWL was 20 ± 9% among males (28.9 kg) and 19 ± 9% among females (19.0 kg). BMI decreased 8.0 ± 4.6 kg/m^2 in males and 6.9 ± 4.1 kg/m^2 females.

Body weights at the end of maintenance were available for 655 of the 700 patients who began AM. During AM, males regained 2.1% of initial body weight (0.54 kg/m^2) and females regained 2.6% (0.67 kg/m^2). Compared with males who did not enter AM, male participants had lower initial body weights (164% vs. 172% ideal body weight) and lost more weight during AWL (23.0% vs. 16.4%); female participants also lost more weight during AWL (23.2% vs. 14.4%) but had higher body weights at study entry (170% vs. 166% ideal body weight).

Change in Health Status

Clinically significant health benefits were observed for patients with diabetes and hypertension (Table 9–2). Of the 154 patients initially diagnosed with diabetes, 88 showed significant improvement ($p < 0.0001$) at the end of AWL, as did 230 of the 421 patients initially diagnosed with hypertension ($p < 0.0001$).

TABLE 9–2 Relationship Between Percentage Weight Loss and Improvement in Diabetes and Hypertension at the End of AWL

Outcome	0–9% Weight Loss	10–19% Weight Loss	≥20% Weight Loss
Diabetes (*n*)	32	54	61
Improved (*n*)[a]	13*	26*	46*
Improved (%)	42	48	75
95% confidence intervals (%)	25, 61	35, 61	62, 83
Hypertension (*n*)	74	147	181
Improved (*n*)[b]	26**	67**	128**
Improved (%)	35	46	71
95% confidence intervals (%)	25, 47	38, 54	63, 77

[a] Three patients with diabetes at baseline for whom AWL weight data were missing also showed improvement.

[b] Nine patients with hypertension at baseline for whom AWL weight data were missing also showed improvement.

*$p = 0.0003$.

**$p = 0.0001$.

During the 1100 person-years reviewed throughout AWL and AM, there were no new diagnoses of diabetes and only three new diagnoses of hypertension.

Significant reductions were noted in the use of insulin and hypoglycemic agents among diabetic patients. Half of the patients using insulin and half of those using other diabetic agents at study entry discontinued their use by the end of AWL. Six of the eight patients who discontinued insulin had lost ⩾20% of body weight, as had three of seven patients who discontinued other diabetic agents (Table 9–3). During AWL, only one patient started using insulin and only seven patients started using other diabetic agents.

Approximately 40% of hypertensive medications were discontinued. Eighty-one patients were taken off their baseline hypertension medication, and six patients stopped using diuretics. Again, greater weight loss was associated with a higher likelihood of discontinuing medication: 46 of the 81 patients who discontinued hypertensive medication lost ⩾20% of body weight, as did 1 of the 6 patients who discontinued diuretics; only 7 and 11 patients began using these drugs, respectively, during AWL.

Eighteen-Month Follow-Up

Of the 1339 patients from 14 clinics contacted, 783 patients took part in a structured telephone interview 18 months after study entry. The most frequent reasons for nonparticipation included relocation and unwillingness to participate. Telephone survey participants and nonparticipants had comparable baseline weights. Male participants lost more weight (21.1% vs. 18.8%) than did nonparticipants during AWL; females participants also lost more weight (19.8% vs. 16.9%) than did nonparticipants. More survey participants continued in AM (56% vs. 39%). Survey participants had a slightly higher incidence of diabetes (13% vs. 10%) and hypertension (34% vs. 28%) at study entry.

Among survey participants, 349 females and 113 males participated in maintenance, while 299 females and 60 males did not. Females and males who participated in AM had lost 14.5% and 15.6% of initial body weight, respectively, at 18 months. In contrast, survey participants who did not enter AM had lost only 8.8% and 10.2%, respectively.

At 18 months, 69 patients had diabetes and 228 had hypertension, including those with improved, the same, or worse disease, as well as 5 patients who developed diabetes and 24 patients who developed hypertension during follow-up. Preexisting conditions were improved in 42 of the diabetic patients and in 108 of the hypertensive patients during follow-up.

Relationship Between Weight Change and Health Outcome

Percentage weight loss from baseline was significantly related to improvement in diabetes ($p < 0.0003$) and hypertension ($p < 0.0001$) at 18 months (Table

TABLE 9–3 Relationship Between Percentage Weight Loss and Change in Medication Use at the End of AWL

Outcome	0–9% Weight Loss	10–19% Weight Loss	≥20% Weight Loss	Unknown
	DIABETES			
Insulin at baseline (*n*)	5	5	6	
Discontinued insulin during AWL (*n*)	1	1	6	
Started insulin during AWL (*n*)				1
Other diabetic agents at baseline (*n*)[a]	4	5	3	
Discontinued other diabetic agents during AWL (*n*)	3	1	3	
Started other diabetic agents during AWL (*n*)				7
	HYPERTENSION			
Hypertensive medication at baseline (*n*)[b]	35	76	84	
Discontinued hypertensive medication during AWL (*n*)	5	30	46	
Started hypertensive medication during AWL (*n*)				7
Diuretics at baseline (*n*)	16	14	10	
Discontinued diuretics during AWL (*n*)	5	0	1	
Started diuretics during AWL (*n*)				11

[a]Two patients who used other diabetic agents at baseline for whom AWL weight data were missing continued to use these medications during AWL.

[b]Of eight patients who used hypertensive medications at baseline for whom AWL weight data were missing, one discontinued use and seven continued to use these medications during AWL.

9–4). Improvements in diabetes and hypertension corresponded directly to the degree of weight loss from baseline. As shown in Table 4–5, weight change (including weight gain) during follow-up was not significantly related to health outcome at 18 months for either diabetes ($p = 0.16$) or hypertension ($p = 0.27$).

Mean percentage weight loss from baseline to 18 months was 18% for patients whose diabetes improved, 7% for those with the same diabetes, and 3% for those with worsened diabetes. Mean percentage weight loss from baseline to 18 months was 19% for patients whose hypertension improved and 10% for those in whom hypertension was the same or worse.

Few patients developed health complications by the time of follow-up and those who did lost the least amount of body weight during AWL. Among patients who lost ≥ 20% of initial body weight, only 2 developed diabetes and only 6 developed hypertension; among those who lost 10–19% of body weight 2 developed diabetes and 10 developed hypertension; among those losing < 10%, 1 developed diabetes and 6 developed hypertension. Five patients developed hypertension for whom weight data were not available. The likelihood of developing diabetes increased from 2% for patients losing 20% or more of initial body weight to 6% for those losing < 20% of initial body weight.

Intercurrent Health Events

No life-threatening events were documented, and only 49 intercurrent health events were reported that required hospitalization: 29 during AWL, 12 during AM, and 8 during follow-up. Nine of the 49 hospitalizations were related to symptomatic gallbladder disease or gallstones, and an additional 6 patients suffered gallbladder attacks (4 during AWL, 2 during AM) that were managed by physician visits and medication. Patients with symptomatic gallstones were significantly heavier at baseline (119.5 kg vs. 103.6 kg, $p = 0.01$); had higher baseline BMIs (43 kg/m^2 vs. 37 kg/m^2, $p = 0.0015$); remained in AWL longer (197 weeks vs. 130 weeks, $p = 0.001$); and had greater percentage weight loss (26.5% vs. 18.9%, $p = 0.001$) than did patients who did not develop symptomatic gallstones. The remaining 40 intercurrent health events requiring hospitalization varied widely, including knee surgery, ovarian cyst, parathyroid tumor, hip replacement, and fractured arm due to an automobile accident.

DISCUSSION

In 1429 obese adults from 15 geographically diverse clinics, we identified clinically and statistically significant improvements in health, as demonstrated by a reduction in active medical problems and in medication use. Improvements in health outcome were associated in a dose–response manner with a reduction in

TABLE 9–4 Relationship Between Percentage Weight Change and Improvement in Diabetes and Hypertension at 18-Month Follow-Up

Outcome	≥1% Weight Gain	0–9% Weight Loss	10–19% Weight Loss	≥20% Weight Loss
Diabetes (*n*)	22	40	18	23
Improved (*n*)[a]	4*	12*	10*	16*
Improved (%)	18	30	55	70
95% confidence intervals (%)	6, 42	15, 50	28, 79	46, 84
Hypertension (*n*)	44	84	71	76
Improved (*n*)[b]	10*	18*	36*	44*
Improved (%)	23	21	51	58
95% confidence intervals (%)	11, 42	13, 33	39, 62	46, 69

[a]Among the 42 patients with improvement in diabetes, 31 discontinued medication use and 1 reduced medication use at 18 months.

[b]Among the 108 patients with improvement in hypertension, 61 discontinued medication use and 7 reduced medication use at 18 months.

*$p = 0.0001$.

TABLE 9–5 Relationship Between Percentage Weight Change and Improvement in Diabetes and Hypertension from the End of AWL to 18-Month Follow-Up

Outcome	≥5% Weight Gain	0–5% Weight Gain	≥1% Weight Loss
Diabetes (*n*)	69	18	16
Improved (*n*)	25	9	8
Same (*n*)	38	8	6
Worse (*n*)	6	1	2
Hypertension (*n*)	166	63	46
Improved (*n*)	61	31	16
Same (*n*)	68	21	19
Worse (*n*)	37	11	11

excess body weight during a multidisciplinary obesity treatment program. Among the 154 diabetic patients and the 421 hypertensive patients who were studied, improvements were noted in 57% of the diabetic patients and in 54% of the hypertensive patients by the end of active weight loss. These changes were sustained throughout the subsequent maintenance phase, and at the 18-month follow-up, the incidence and severity of diabetes and hypertension remained clinically and statistically improved despite a regain of approximately one-third of the initial weight loss.

Improvement in the clinical status of diabetes and hypertension correlated with weight reduction during AWL. Among diabetic patients who lost ⩾20% of their initial body weight, 75% had a significant improvement in their disease, while 48% of the diabetic patients with 10–19% weight loss and 42% of the diabetic patients with <10% weight loss had a significant improvement in their disease. Similar results were noted for the hypertensive patients, with significant improvement in disease occurring among 71% of patients with ⩾20% weight loss; among 46% of patients experiencing 10–19% weight loss; and among 35% with <10% weight loss. Weight gain during maintenance and follow-up did not significantly alter disease status at 18 months. Instead, weight reduction during AWL and the net weight change from study entry to the 18-month follow-up remained the most potent predictors of change in health at 18 months.

Weight loss in this population was comparable to that reported[14,19,20] for other obese patients undergoing multidisciplinary treatment of obesity with a VLCD: Mean losses were 29 kg for males and 19 kg for females over 17 and 19 weeks of active weight loss, respectively. However, despite a 20% reduction in body weight, these patients would still be classified as overweight by standard height-weight charts.[18] These results, as well as those from other recent reports,[3,10,21] suggest that ideal body weight need not be obtained to improve health outcome.

The 18-month follow-up data were obtained by a structured telephone interview. While self-report data are used in many aspects of health assessment, self-reported weight may be subject to inaccuracy and bias.[22] Palta et al.[23] found that weight was underestimated by 1.6% among men and by 3.1% among women. However, a recent survey found that the most obese patients were more likely to underreport their weight loss and that less obese patients were more likely to overstate their change in body weight (Consumer Research Corporation of America, Minneapolis, Minn.; Sandoz Nutrition Company, Minneapolis, Minn.; unpublished data, 1992). Given the large sample size of the present study, some patients probably did underreport body weight. Assuming underreported weight, the overall trends noted would be conservative in that a possibly smaller magnitude of weight loss would be sufficient to achieve significant long-term improvement in health outcome.

The fact that only 59% of the original sample were available for follow-up study may also be of some concern. Other studies that have collected long-term follow-up weight data on participants by telephone or through the mail have reported similar (60%) or lower (35%) response rates.[15,24]

Despite the well-known relationship body weight and health, few studies have documented the long-term effect of weight loss on chronic disease status. Among type II diabetic patients, Wing et al.[3] have reported that a combination of caloric restriction, exercise, and behavior modification produced a 6.9-kg weight loss, as well as significant improvements in glycosylated hemoglobin values, during active weight loss and at 1 year. More recently, Wing et al.[25] demonstrated that glycemic control was significantly improved 1 year after treatment in patients consuming a formula diet compared with those on a standard balanced deficient diet (1200 kcal/day).

Recently, Weinsier et al.[26] examined the relationship between change in body weight and change in comorbidities of obesity over a 4-year study period. Subjects consumed an 800 kcal/day diet during active treatment and lost an average of 13 kg. After an average of 4 years of follow-up, they regained 11 kg. Both weight loss and weight rebound were associated with changes in mean arterial pressure, fasting triglycerides, and high density lipoprotein-cholesterol, and changes in these risk factors were in direct proportion to the change in body weight.

Finally, prescribing the same VLCD program given in the present study, Kirschner et al.[27] reported the acute effects of mean weight losses of 30.0 kg nd 21.5 kg in men and women, respectively. Among patients with hypertension, 83% experienced normal blood pressures following weight loss; among patients with diabetes, 100% discontinued oral hypoglycemics, 87% discontinued insulin completely, and another 10% reduced their insulin dose. All patients with baseline hypertriglyceridemia or hypercholesterolemia demonstrated either normalized or improved serum levels.

The economic importance of the present study is readily apparent. In 1986,

$1.5 billion and $11.3 billion in health care costs were directly attributable to obesity among Americans with hypertension and non-insulin-dependent diabetes mellitus (NIDDM), respectively.[28] A 1985 National Institutes of Health Consensus Conference Statement concluded that the primary dietary treatment for NIDDM should be weight loss through caloric restriction.[29] More recently, weight loss (4.5 kg) was shown to lower blood pressure as well as low-dose drug therapy.[30] Available results from the Trials of Hypertension Prevention have shown a relationship between weight loss and blood pressure: For every 1 kg lost, diastolic and systolic blood pressures decrease by 0.33 and 0.43 mm Hg, respectively.[31] Compared with the hypothetical control group who would have been left to their usual diet (18% protein, 38% fat, 44% carbohydrate) and who would therefore have gained weight[32] and increased their risk of disease, our patients demonstrated significantly lower morbidity and mortality.

SUMMARY AND CONCLUSION

This study of a medically supervised, multidisciplinary VLCD program has shown a dose–response relationship between percentage weight loss and health outcome. Greater weight loss in this significantly obese population resulted in better control of diabetes and hypertension. Improvements in health status remained evident in many patients 1 year after treatment, even among those who had regained weight. Additional long-term studies are needed to examine the relationship between weight loss and the control of chronic disease, including diabetes and hypertension, to help health professionals set appropriate weight loss goals for obese patients.

REFERENCES

1. PI-Sunyer FX. Health implications of obesity. *Am J Clin Nutr* 53 (Suppl 6):1595S, 1991.
2. The Hypertension Prevention Trial. Three-year effects of dietary changes on blood pressure. Hypertension Prevention Trial Research Group. *Arch Intern Med* 150:153, 1990.
3. Wing RR, Koeske R, Epstein LH, et al. Long-term effects of modest weight loss in type II diabetic patients. *Arch Intern Med* 147:1749, 1987.
4. Ashley FW, Kannel WB. Relation of weight change to change in atherosclerotic traits: The Framingham Study. *J Chronic Dis* 27:103, 1974.
5. Manson JE, Colditz GA, Stamper MJ. A prospective study of obesity and risk of coronary heart disease in women. *N Engl J Med* 332:882, 1990.

6. Committee on Diet and Health, National Research Council. *Diet and Health: Implications for Reducing Chronic Disease Risk.* Washington, DC, National Academy Press, 1989.
7. National Institutes of Health Consensus Development Panel on the Health Implications of Obesity. National Institutes of Health Consensus Development Conference Statement. *Ann Intern Med* 103:1073, 1985.
8. NIH Technology Assessment Conference Panel. Methods for voluntary weight loss and control. *Ann Intern Med* 116:942, 1992.
9. Kanders BS, Blackburn GL. Reducing primary risk factors by therapeutic weight loss, in Wadden TA, Van Itallie TB (eds), *Treatment of the Seriously Obese Patient.* New York, Guilford Press, 1992, pp. 213–230.
10. Simopoulos AP, Van Itallie TB. Body weight, health, and longevity. *Ann Intern Med* 100:285, 1984.
11. Reaven GM. Banting lecture: Role of insulin resistance in human disease. *Diabetes* 37:1595, 1988.
12. Trulson M, Walsh ED, Caso EK. A study of obese patients in a nutrition clinic. *J Am Diet Assoc* 23:941, 1947.
13. Vertes V, Genuth SM, Hazelton IM. Supplemented fasting as a large scale outpatient program. *JAMA* 238:2151, 1977.
14. Wadden TA, Foster GD, Letizia KA, et al. A multicenter evaluation of a proprietary weight reduction program for the treatment of marked obesity. *Arch Intern Med* 152:961, 1992.
15. Kirshner MA, Schneider G, Ertel N, et al. Supplemented starvation: A successful method for control of major obesity. *J Med Soc* 76:175, 1979.
16. *Optifast Programs Manual.* Minneapolis, Clinical Products Division, Sandoz Nutrition Corporation, and Cleveland, Ohio, Mt Sinai Medical Center, 1985.
17. US Dept of Agriculture and US Dept of Health and Human Services, *Nutrition and Your Health: Dietary Guidelines for Americans,* ed 2. Home and Garden Bulletin No 233. Washington, DC, US Government Printing Office, 1980.
18. Metropolitan Life Insurance Company. New weight standards for men and women. *Stat Bull* 40:1, 1959.
19. Wadden TA, Stunkard AJ, Brownell KD. Very-low-calorie-diets: Their efficacy, safety, and future. *Ann Intern Med* 99:675, 1983.
20. National Task Force on the Prevention and Treatment of Obesity. Very low-calorie diets. *JAMA* 270:967, 1993.
21. Goldberg DJ. Beneficial health effects of modest weight loss. *Int J Obes* 16:397, 1992.
22. Pirie P, Jacobs D, Jeffery R, et al. Distortion in self-reported height and weight data. *Research* 78:601, 1981.
23. Palta M, Prineas RJ, Berman R, et al. Comparison of self-reported and measured height and weight. *Am J Epidemiol* 115:223, 1982.

24. Lavery MA, Loewy JW, Kapadia AS, et al. Long-term follow-up of weight status of subjects in a behavioral weight control program. *J Am Diet Assoc* 89:1259, 1989.
25. Wing RR, Marcus MD, Salata R, et al. Effects of a very-low-calorie diet on long-term glycemic control in obese type II diabetic subjects. *Arch Intern Med* 151:1334, 1991.
26. Weinsier RL, Hensrud DD, Darnell BE, et al. Effect of weight loss maintenance/rebound on recurrence of co-morbidities (abstract). Workshop on Prevention of Obesity: Populations at Risk, Etiologic Factors and Intervention Strategies. Baltimore, National Institute of Diabetes and Digestive and Kidney Diseases, NIH. 1993, p. 98.
27. Kirschner MA, Schneider G, Ertel NH, et al. An eight-year experience with a very-low-calorie formula diet for control of major obesity. *Int J Obes*. 12:69, 1988.
28. Colditz GA. The economic costs of obesity. *Am J Clin Nutr* 55:503S, 1992.
29. National Institutes of Health Consensus Development Conference Statement. *Diet and Exercise in Noninsulin-dependent Diabetes Mellitus*. 6(8), 1986.
30. Wassertheil-Smoller S, Blaufox MD, Oberman AS, et al. The trial of antihypertensive intervention and management (TAIM) study. *Arch Intern Med* 152:131, 1992.
31. Stevens VJ, Corrigan SA, Obarzanck E, et al. Weight loss intervention in phase I of the trials of hypertension prevention. *Arch Intern Med* 153:849, 1993.
32. Williamson DF, Kahn HS, Remington PL, et al. The 10-year incidence of overweight and major weight gain in US adults. *Arch Intern Med* 150:665, 1990.

TREATMENT OF OBESITY

PART II

Popular Diets and Use of Moderate Caloric Restriction for the Treatment of Obesity

CHAPTER 10

Ann M. Coulston, M.S., R.D. and
Cheryl L. Rock, Ph.D., R.D.

INTRODUCTION

Obesity has been identified as a major public health problem in the United States. Among clinicians, attempts to manage the obese patient are often perceived as frustrating and futile.[1] The National Health Examination Survey estimates the incidence of obesity at about 25% of the U.S. population.[2] At the same time, results from national polls estimate that 50% of women are following a weight reduction diet at least twice per year. News media reports suggest that $9.4 billion per year is currently spent on weight reduction products and programs in the United States. This amount increases to $33 billion when consumer consumption of low-calorie food products, diet drinks, and artificial sweeteners is included.[3]

Since the 1950s, scientific study of the nature and treatment of obesity has proceeded with increasing fervor, yet a truly effective treatment or cure remains to be discovered.[4] Despite recent public health attention to the problem of obesity, the increased availability of reduced-calorie food products, and numerous take-weight-off-fast schemes, indications of success in controlling the problem are not readily apparent. If obesity were classified as a disease, its cure rate compared with those of other disabling diseases would be among the lowest.

Concern about the problem of obesity is more than cosmetic. Excess body weight is associated with an increased incidence of several chronic medical conditions, including non-insulin-dependent diabetes mellitus, hypertension, cardiovascular disease, and some types of cancer.[5–8] Research findings show improvement in the metabolic abnormalities associated with these chronic conditions when body weight is even modestly reduced.[9] Unfortunately, weight regain and various complications associated with treatments for obesity, whether from health care providers or from community-based entrepreneurs, may also result in adverse physiologic and psychological consequences.

BASIC CONSIDERATIONS

The dilemma facing the medical community is how to correct the overweight condition and reverse the symptoms caused either by obesity itself or by an associated chronic disease. Several treatment strategies have been introduced over the past quarter century, yet a few basic considerations are central.

First, calories do count. This has been demonstrated repeatedly during the past century. If a popular diet program promotes weight reduction beyond a short-term weight loss caused by diuresis, caloric intake relative to expenditure has been reduced. Recent evidence suggests that obesity is due to excess fat (vs. carbohydrate) calories in the diet.[10,11] The primary effect of reducing dietary fat intake is that decreased total caloric intake will result.[10–12] Popular diets that focus on diet manipulation to lower fat rather than calories ultimately arrive at diet prescriptions for an average intake of less than 1200 kcal/day.[13]

Second, standards such as the recommended dietary allowances (RDAs), which are often used to evaluate the nutritional adequacy of diet regimens, are based on the usual mix of foods obtained from the U.S. food supply and on adequate caloric intake.[14] Use of these standards for assessing the adequacy of popular and reduced-calorie diets is not always appropriate. For example, mineral balance is greatly affected by modifying any dietary component that influences bioavailability, so RDAs for mineral levels may not be the ideal standard for evaluating the nutritional risk of a popular diet composed of an unusual mix of foods. As another example, protein requirements expressed per kilogram of body weight are increased when caloric intake is reduced.

Unfortunately, it may be unreasonable to assume that obese individuals are likely to avoid a popular diet on the basis of risk of nutrient deficiencies or failure to meet simple criteria such as inclusion of the Food Guide Pyramid. For most patients, the pain of obesity today far exceeds that of any imaginable nutritional deficiency, so that the ill-advised diet may be attempted despite professional opinion against it.[15]

Also, diet patterns associated with successful short-term weight loss may, in fact, be diet patterns or behaviors strongly inversely related to long-term weight maintenance or overall health. As examples, take-weight-off-fast schemes are typically low in carbohydrate, and the positive feedback provided by weight loss during a short-term fast may actually reinforce the use of such an approach.[13,16] Patients often have difficulty evaluating popular diets on the basis of long-term success but instead focus only on short-term results. Table 10–1 lists characteristics and examples of types of popular diets.

FASTING

Total fasting or complete avoidance of calorie-containing foods, with the regular administration of fluids and electrolytes, is a technique for promoting rapid weight loss that has been used for many years. Drenick and associates investigated this treatment approach carefully, demonstrating a 1.0 kg/day weight loss in males for the first week, which then decreases to approximately 0.5 kg/day by 1 month of fasting.[17] Fasting is associated with a number of adverse medical risks and produces discomfort for most patients, so it is rarely practiced for more than a few days except under close medical supervision.[18] An adverse medical outcome of total fasting is the lost of significant amounts of lean body mass. Also, a majority of patients who have fasted to reduce body weight return to their prefasting weight within 1 to 2 years of completing the treatment. Starvation or total fasting is no longer an accepted approach to weight reduction within the medical community; however, semistarvation diets remain widely used.

VERY-LOW CALORIE DIETS

Currently, obese individuals in industrialized nations around the world are spending hundreds of millions of dollars per year on formulas and very-low calorie diets (VLCDs).[19] It has been estimated that in 1990, 20 million Americans spent over $1 billion on liquid diet programs and over-the-counter liquid diet products.

The definition of a VLCD has been traced to a 1979 report from an Expert Panel of the Life Sciences Research Office of the Federation of American Societies for Experimental Biology, which declared that diets containing less than 800 kcal/day were VLCDs.[19] The modern use of such regimens was conceived in the 1970s. This treatment strategy was based on the use of diets composed predominantly of protein to promote rapid weight loss without the loss of visceral and skeletal protein stores.[20]

TABLE 10–1 Popular Diets for Weight Control

Diet Type	Characteristics	Examples*
Very low calorie	Less than 800 kcal/day Increased risk of metabolic complications Require medical supervision	Health Management Resources (HMR) Diet Medifast Optifast Diet
Low carbohydrate	Less than 100 g carbohydrate per day Promotes diuresis	Atkin's Diet Scarsdale Diet Stillman's Diet Woman Doctor's Diet
Very low fat	Less than 20% kcal from fat Limited bioavailability of nutrients Low satiety and limited food choices	Macrobiotic Diet McDougall Diet Pritikin Diet Rice Diet
Moderate caloric restriction	Usually 1000–1800 kcal/day Nutritionally balanced Sound scientific rationale	Calloway Diet LEARN Program Diet Weight Watchers Diet
Novelty approaches	Promote unusual food combinations or eating patterns Unscientific rationale	Fit for Life Diet Berger's Immune Diet Beverly Hills Diet Rotation Diet
Packaged Food or formula approaches	Require prepackaged foods or product beverages Usually 1000–1400 kcal/day Limited nutritional counseling	Bahamian Diet Jenny Craig Diet Nutri/System Diet UltraSlimfast Diet

*This list does not include all currently available weight reduction programs.

Source: Adapted from Ref. 16.

The popularity of these VLCDs, originally composed primarily of hydrolyzed proteins, attracted private industry as well as medical interest. Attention in the lay press and popular diet books resulted in the widespread use of a VLCD formula diet composed of hydrolyzed collagen as a protein source, which was distributed without medical supervision. During the peak of this product's popularity, several deaths in obese but otherwise healthy users of various formula VLCDs prompted the Centers for Disease Control (CDC) to investigate their safety.[21] Users of both high-quality and low-quality protein formula products were among the victims, although many reviewers attribute the sudden deaths that occurred solely to the use of low-quality protein-based products.

Currently, the most widely known VLCDs are provided by medical practices and hospitals. Three examples are Optifast, Health Management Resources (HMR), and Medifast, with similar programs and reliance on a formula product. High-protein liquid drinks are prescribed for use periodically throughout the day to achieve a caloric level of 400–800 kcal/day, depending on the program and specific recommendations for the individual client. An obese woman of moderate height might be prescribed the liquid diet at the 400 kcal/day level, while a tall, obese male might consume the diet at the 800 kcal/day level. This product-based diet is prescribed for approximately 12 weeks, which can result in a loss of total body weight ranging from 1.0 to 4.5 kg/week.

During the refeeding phase, the client is reintroduced to food. Meals consisting primarily of lean meats, vegetable salads, and cooked vegetables replace the liquid formula drinks. Finally, the maintenance phase consists of further instruction and practice in eating at a calorie level designed to maintain the newly achieved body weight. For many severely obese patients, this level may not be at their desirable body weight. After several months, they may repeat the VLCD and refeeding phases in an effort to lose an additional 10–20 kg.

There are some differences among these programs, and diet protocols change as companies compete for market share. Generally, Optifast limits the initial VLCD phase to 12 weeks, while HMR permits use of the VLCD until the client's weight goal is met. Medifast has a protocol that permits the inclusion of some food items from the very beginning of enrollment in the program. Some of these programs include dietitians, psychologists, and exercise physiologists, along with a physician, in an effort to improve long-term success rates. Other programs are delivered solely by the physician provider.

Whatever the protocol used, and despite more than 20 years of use, long-term weight loss as a result of VLCDs has not been shown to occur in a majority of patients. One surprising figure is that only about 50% of obese patients who enroll in one of these popular VLCD programs actually complete the program. Even with the inclusion of behavior therapy and nutritional counseling as key components of the program, 88% of enrollees are reported to regain body weight within 18 months of follow-up.[22]

Due to the potential medical risks associated with rapid weight loss, the VLCD popular diet plans that attract obese patients should be provided only under medical supervision.[23] Also, providers should be well trained in the management of complications associated with starvation, and appropriate medical monitoring is necessary.[24] Variants on fasting and semistarvation diets designed for weight reduction are likely to continue to be among the popular diets.

MODERATE CALORIC RESTRICTION

Diets classified as moderate caloric restriction provide an energy intake that is below maintenance requirements but greater than 800 kcal/day, typically promoting an average weight loss of 1% of body weight per week. Compared with more extreme restrictions, these regimens are rarely associated with consequences such as altered metabolism of nutrients or a marked reduction in resting energy expenditure as long as dietary carbohydrate is sufficient. However, whether scientifically sound or questionable, many of these diets utilize similar marketing techniques or other means of enticing the consumer.

One such technique is the use of a marketing gimmick, such as informing the dieter of a newly discovered remedy, substance, or concept that will "cure" obesity forever. Use of a famous name or place to give credibility is common. Biochemical or scientific claims, which may be speculative, are another typical approach. Elements such as fixed menus, special foods, eating or exercise rituals, or special conditions for eating are often among the instructions.

Macronutrient Restriction

The restriction of one or more of the calorie-contributing nutrients—carbohydrate, protein, or fat—is a treatment strategy promoted by several popular weight reduction diets. Restriction of carbohydrate-containing foods has historically been predominant in this category, because a decreased intake of carbohydrate-containing foods results in marked diuresis. This is appreciated (and misinterpreted) as successful, rapid weight loss in the early days of the program, even though the weight loss is the result of water loss and not stored fat.[25] These popular diets can lead to physiologic dehydration, and ketosis can develop when daily carbohydrate consumption is less than 100 g. Reintroduction of dietary carbohydrate and normal regulatory physiologic mechanisms have the effect of normalizing body weight in the long term, unless a sustained reduction in caloric intake has occurred.[26]

More recently, with the public health emphasis on reduced-fat diets to decrease the risk of cardiovascular disease, weight reduction diets focusing on very-low-fat dietary patterns have become popular. Reports in the literature have indicated that adiposity positively correlates with the percentage of total calories from dietary fat in the diets of obese men and women.[10] Normal-weight subjects who are prescribed low-fat diets in controlled settings eat fewer calories even when caloric intake is not specifically restricted.[10,11]

A reduction in dietary fat may be an advantageous approach for reducing total calories, although evidence suggests that the crucial issue remains total calories consumed.[12,27] The "metabolic cost" of converting excess calories to stored fat, and different effects on metabolic caloric expenditure, are other mechanisms by which low-fat diets theoretically could promote weight loss, but there is no evidence that altering the content of calorie-containing nutrients has metabolic effects that accelerate or retard the loss of body fat beyond that attributable to the energy deficits.[28]

Most investigators agree that a reduction in dietary fat is advisable for many consumers, but the degree of fat restriction necessary to reduce the cardiovascular disease risk is not nearly as severe as proposed in several popular diets.[29–31] The promotion of realistic, permanent changes and long-term compliance may actually be reduced by prescribing severe restrictions that are difficult for patients with normal lifestyles. Nutritionally, essential fatty acid and micronutrient deficiencies may occur in patients who rigidly follow very-low-fat, high-fiber diets due to effects on bioavailability.[32–34] Also, such diets provide limited amounts of high-biologic-value dietary protein, which is of increased importance when caloric intake is restricted.

Novelty Diets

Another strategy utilized by several popular diet programs is to limit or regulate the consumption of specific foods, using some half-truths to explain this as necessity for weight control. These programs typically establish categories of forbidden foods or rituals for eating. For example, in the Fit For Life diet plan, specific food combination schemes are advised, as well as consuming food only in the raw state. The Beverly Hills Diet is based on a diet consisting primarily of fruit, with a prescription for types of fruits to be consumed at specific times during the program. These popular diets result in a net decrease in total caloric intake compared to caloric expenditure.[13,16] However, depending on the degree of proscription, popular diets that follow this model need to be carefully evaluated to ensure that the consumer is obtaining a diet that meets essential nutrient requirements.

NUTRITIONALLY BALANCED, MODERATE CALORIC RESTRICTION

This category of popular diets is defined on the basis of a reduction in calorie intake achieved by a reduction in all foods consumed, without any prohibitions of specific foods or classes of foods, and without periods of starvation or semistarvation. Caloric intake is restricted to a level that permits weight loss without compromising nutrient adequacy or promoting metabolic aberrations that may be medically hazardous. This type of popular diet has few, if any, medical risks, is the most economical because it is based on usual food intake, and involves learning skills for food selection that, when continued, may help to prevent relapse.

Often, popular diet programs that follow this pattern of caloric restriction are coupled with behavioral strategies (as a component of learning the skills required for making choices) and encouragement to exercise regularly. This combination of treatment strategies—that is, calorie deficit, behavior therapy, and regular exercise—is viewed as the most highly recommended treatment approach for obesity.[16,28]

Ultimately, eating a diet that is moderately restricted in calories and engaging in regular exercise are lifestyle patterns that must be permanently adopted in order to maintain weight loss, even when patients have lost weight via VLCD, surgery, or other interventions. It has been suggested that maintenance of weight loss in any treatment program can be ensured only to the extent that strategies to maintain weight loss are central to the intervention itself.[35] Also, a moderate reduction in caloric intake is rarely associated with severe discomfort and deprivation, so that changes are more likely to become a permanent, healthful pattern even if only modest weight loss, rather than "ideal" weight, is achieved.[36]

Community-Based Diet Programs

Several community-based programs, which involve a variety of diet approaches to promote weight loss, are currently available. Although these programs would appear to be a cost-effective approach to weight loss, evidence suggests that high attrition rates are a major problem.[37–39]

Diet Center, with more than 20 years of experience, offers a weight reduction program that focuses on a prescribed diet plan and micronutrient supplements. Its weight loss plan is claimed to be based on control of blood glucose levels. It involves restricting carbohydrate sources and alcohol and daily consumption of three meals with two snacks.

The Weight Watchers program, developed in 1963, is based on a balanced, calorie-restricted diet and also incorporates aspects of behavior modification and regular exercise. The diet plans consist of choices from food groups, and consumers can select from among several levels of caloric restriction, ranging from 1000 to 1600 kcal/day. Weight Watchers food products sold in supermarkets are not promoted as an important (or even an essential) component of the program.

Two commercial, franchised weight loss programs, Nutri/System and Jenny Craig, rely on diet plans consisting primarily of packaged food products purchased from the centers. Individual counseling (from employees who are not necessarily trained professionals), behavior modification classes, and an exercise plan are also provided. The diets prescribed by both of these programs provide 1000–1700 kcal/day, with reduced levels of fat, cholesterol, and sodium. Maintenance plans may be purchased at an additional fee. The popularity of these packaged food-based diet plans has inspired other for-profit community-based programs to experiment with the feasibility of offering the option of packaged food products that can be purchased from the centers.

Slim-Fast is essentially a packaged food-based weight-loss program, although the primary product is a liquid formula mix that is marketed directly to consumers, who purchase the product at drugstores and supermarkets rather than at special franchise outlets. The products are accompanied by diet instructions, sample menus, and other descriptive material to encourage a caloric deficit.

Overeaters Anonymous (OA) is a self-help, nonprofit organization that does not prescribe a specific diet plan. This 12-step program is modeled after Alcoholics Anonymous, with an emphasis on abstinence from compulsive overeating. Some of the groups also focus on avoiding certain carbohydrate sources, such as products containing sugar and refined flour, and the importance of eating regular meals is stressed.

Take Off Pounds Sensibly (TOPS) is a nonprofit diet organization started in 1948. Members pay low monthly dues and have no specific diet, but each member is advised to have medical supervision. Similar to OA, the primary involvement is regular attendance at meetings that provide social support.

POPULAR DIET EVALUATION

All popular diet programs demonstrate successful weight loss in the early stages when followed as prescribed. However, long-term success in the majority of those who participate appears to elude virtually all weight control programs to date. Because the treatment of obesity remains elusive, many popular diet programs will continue to be promoted.

Criteria to help clinicians and consumers select a weight management program that will have the desired outcome, free of additional health risks, have been proposed.[16,40] The Michigan Department of Public Health has established some regulatory guidelines for programs that are available in that state. These guidelines address screening procedures, levels of care, disclosure to clients, and key aspects of the components of weight loss programs.[41]

In general, when evaluating a popular weight loss program, criteria that should be addressed include the following:

Is the rationale on which the program is based scientifically sound?

Is the diet nutritionally adequate? Is the food plan practical, with obtainable foods, and conducive to the establishment of a lasting eating pattern?

Is the program appropriate for the individual's physical condition or severity of obesity?

Does the program teach strategies for behavior change rather than simply provide descriptions of desired behavior?

Is exercise promoted as a strategy for long-term weight control, and are screening and supervision provided where indicated?

What are the credentials, training, and supervision of individuals providing care and counseling?

What is the cost of the program relative to the quality of intervention?

Are there practical or psychological considerations for the patient that may affect long-term participation?

Weight control programs with the potential for success and minimal risk have the following components: They include diet plans that satisfy all nutrient needs except energy; food choices that meet individual tastes and habits with minimal hunger and fatigue; eating plans that are readily obtainable, socially acceptable, favor the establishment of a changed eating pattern, and are conducive to improvement of overall health; and an emphasis on permanent behavior change and regular exercise.[16,40,41]

REFERENCES

1. National Academy of Sciences. *Diet and Health: Implications for Reducing Chronic Disease Risk*. Washington, DC, National Academy Press, 1989.
2. *Obesity and Overweight Adults in the United States*. Vital and Health Statistics, National Center for Health Statistics, Series II, No. 230, 1983.
3. Bray GA, Gray DS. Obesity: Part II treatment. *West J Med* 149:555, 1988.
4. Wooley SC, Garner DM. Obesity treatment: The high cost of false hope. *J Am Diet Assoc* 91:1248, 1991.
5. Ashley FW, Kannel WB. Relation of weight change to changes in atherogenic traits: The Framingham Study. *J Chronic Dis* 27:103, 1974.
6. Chaing BN, Perlman LV, Epstein FH. Overweight and hypertension: A review. *Circulation* 39:403, 1969.
7. Manson JE, Stampfer JM, Hennekens CH, et al. Body weight and longevity: A reassessment. *JAMA* 257:353, 1987.
8. Lew EA, Garfinkel L. Variations in mortality by weight among 750,000 men and women. *J Cronic Dis* 32:563, 1979.
9. Wing RR, Koeske R, Epstein LH, et al. Long-term effects of modest weight loss in Type II diabetic patients. *Arch Intern Med* 147:1749, 1987.
10. Tremblay A, Plourde G, Despres JP, et al. Impact of dietary fat content and fat oxidation on energy intake in humans. *Am J Clin Nutr* 49:709, 1989.

11. Kendall A, Levitsky DA, Strupp BJ, et al. Weight loss on a low-fat diet: Consequence of the imprecision of the control of food intake in humans. *Am J Clin Nutr* 53:1124, 1991.
12. Hill JO, Peters JC, Reed GW, et al. Nutrient balance in humans: Effects of diet composition. *Am J Clin Nutr* 54:10, 1991.
13. Fisher MC, LaChance PA. Nutrition evaluation of published weight-reducing diets. *J Am Diet Assoc* 85:450, 1985.
14. Subcommittee on the Tenth Edition of the RDAs, Food and Nutrition Board, Commission on Life Sciences, National Research Council. *Recommended Dietary Allowances*. Washington, DC, National Academy Press, 1989.
15. Wadden TA, Stunkard AJ. Social and psychological consequences of obesity. *Ann Intern Med* 103:1062, 1985.
16. Rock CL, Coulston AM. Weight-control approaches: A review by the California Dietetic Association. *J Am Diet Assoc* 88:44, 1988.
17. Drenick EJ, Swendseid ME, Blahd WH, et al. Prolonged starvation as treatment for severe obesity. *JAMA* 187:100, 1964.
18. Fisler JS, Drenick EJ. Starvation and semistarvation diets in the management of obesity. *Annu Rev Nutr* 7:465, 1987.
19. Atkinson RL. Usefulness and limits of VLCD in the treatment of obesity, in Oomura Y, Tarui S, Inoue S, et al. (eds), *Progress in Obesity Research*. London, John Libbey, 1990, pp. 473–480.
20. Bistrian BR, Sherman M. Results of the treatment of obesity with a protein-sparing modified fast. *Int J Obes* 2:143, 1978.
21. Sours HE, Frattali VP, Brand CD, et al. Sudden death associated with very low calorie weight reduction regimens. *Am J Clin Nutr* 34:453, 1981.
22. Kirschner MA, Schneider G, Ertel HN, et al. An eight-year experience with a very-low-calorie formula diet for control of major obesity. *Int J Obes* 12:69, 1988.
23. Position of the American Dietetic Association: Very-low-calorie weight loss diets. *J Am Diet Assoc* 90:722, 1990.
24. Wadden TA, Van Itallie TB, Blackburn GL. Responsible and irresponsible use of very-low-calorie diets in the treatment of obesity. *JAMA* 263:83, 1990.
25. DeHaven J, Sherwin R, Hendler R, et al. Nitrogen and sodium balance and sympathetic nervous system activity in obese subjects treated with a low calorie protein or mixed diet. *N Engl J Med* 302:477, 1980.
26. Affarah HB, Hall WD, Heymsfield SB, et al. High-carbohydrate diet: Antinatriuretic and blood pressure response in normal men. *Am J Clin Nutr* 44:341, 1986.
27. Alford BB, Blankenship AC, Hagen RD. The effects of variations in carbohydrate, protein, and fat content of the diet upon weight loss, blood values, and nutrient intake of adult obese women. *J Am Diet Assoc* 90:534, 1990.
28. Council on Scientific Affairs. Treatment of obesity. *JAMA* 260:2547, 1988.
29. Grundy SM, Nix D, Whelan MF, et al. Comparison of three cholesterol-lowering diets in normolipemic men. *JAMA* 256:2351, 1986.

30. Grundy SM, Florentin L, Nix kD, et al. Comparison of monounsaturated fatty acids and carbohydrates for reducing raised levels of plasma cholesterol in man. *Am J Clin Nutr* 47:965, 1988.
31. Wood PD, Stefanick ML, Williams PT, et al. The effects on plasma lipoproteins of a prudent weight-reducing diet, with or without exercise, in overweight men and women. *N Engl J Med* 325:461, 1990.
32. Wene JD, Connor WE, DenBesten L. The development of essential fatty acid deficiency in healthy men fed fat-free diets intravenously and orally. *J Clin Invest* 56:127, 1975.
33. Dimitrov NV, Meyer C, Ullrey DE, et al. Bioavailability of beta-carotene in humans. *Am J Clin Nutr* 48:298, 1988.
34. Kaiserauer S, Snyder AC, Sleeper M, et al. Nutrition, physiological, and menstrual status of distance runners. *Med Sci Sports Exerc* 21:120, 1989.
35. Wilson GT. Behavior modification and the treatment of obesity, in Stunkard AJ (ed), *Obesity*. Philadelphia, WB Saunders, 1980, p. 325.
36. Position of the American Dietetic Association. Optimal weight as a health promotion strategy. *J Am Diet Assoc* 90:1814, 1990.
37. Grimsmo A, Helgesen G, Borchgrevink C. Short-term and long-term effects of lay groups on weight reduction. *Br Med J* 283:1093, 1981.
38. Garb JR, Stunkard AJ. Effectiveness of a self-help group in obesity control. *Arch Intern Med* 134:716, 1974.
39. Volkmar FR, Stunkard AJ, Woolston J, et al. High attrition rates in commercial weight reduction programs. *Arch Intern Med* 141:426, 1981.
40. Weinsier RL, Wadden TA, Rittenbaugh C, et al. Recommended therapeutic guidelines for professional weight control programs. *Am J Clin Nutr* 40:865, 1984.
41. Michigan Health Council Task Force to Establish Weight Loss Guidelines. *Toward Safe Weight Loss: Recommendations for Adult Weight Loss Programs in Michigan*. Lansing, Michigan Department of Public Health, 1990.

Very-Low-Calorie Diets for the Treatment of Obesity

Beatrice S. Kanders, Ed.D., M.P.H., R.D. and George L. Blackburn, M.D., Ph.D.

Very-low calorie diets (VLCDs) have been used since the 1930s and represent one of the most aggressive nonsurgical treatments of obesity. Popularized and unpopularized in the late 1980s by Oprah Winfrey, an estimated 15 million individuals have undertaken a VLCD.[1] This chapter will review the history, clinical application, expected outcome, and safety of the VLCD.

EARLY USE OF VLCDs

VLCDs have been around for more than six decades. In 1929, Evans and Strang first used diets of conventional foods to produce rapid weight loss.[2] These diets provided approximately 400 kcal/day (50 g protein, 12 g fat, and 12 g carbohydrate). Patients were maintained on this diet as outpatients for up to 8 weeks, losing 9.9 kg, or 1.2 kg/week or less. By today's standards, the diet was deficient in a number of micronutrients. This diet was largely forgotten until the 1950s. Simeon[3] developed a 500-kcal version supplemented with injections of human chorionic gonadotropins; this diet produced mean weight losses of 9 to 14 kg in

6 weeks; however, it was also deficient in certain vitamins and minerals. Five years later, interest arose in the use of complete starvation as a method of treatment for obesity. Complete starvation produced remarkable weight loss (2–3 kg/week) and was relatively easy to administer. However, this diet had high risks of morbidity[4] and mortality.[5,6]

The prototype of the modern VLCD was developed in the 1960s by Bollinger and Apfelbaum. These clinicians were searching for a diet that was as effective as complete starvation but without the side effects. Of particular concern was the large loss of lean body mass that accompanied these diets. Bollinger and Apfelbuam achieved apparent nitrogen balance with a modified fast that contained 40–60 g of protein from egg albumin.[7,8] In 1973, Blackburn et al. used lean meat and egg albumin to spare the loss of body protein,[9,10] calling this regimen the *protein-sparing modified fast* (*PSMF*). They identified the need to supply 1.2–1.5 g of protein per kilogram of ideal body weight to promote nitrogen retention. Later, Genuth et al.[11,12] in the United States and Howard et al.[13,14] in the United Kingdom added limited amounts of carbohydrate (30–45 g/day). They found that the inclusion of limited amounts of carbohydrate maximized protein sparing, promoted the retention of electrolytes, and inhibited hyperuricemia.

In the late 1970s, the Last Chance Diet brought public attention to VLCDs. Modeled after the protein-sparing modified fast, the *liquid protein diet,* as it was called, consisted of low-quality protein from hydrolyzed gelatin and collagen and was not routinely supplemented with vitamins and minerals. According to the Centers for Disease Control, 100,000 persons used the Last Chance Diet as their sole source of nutrition for at least 1 month during 1977.[15,16] By January 1978, 60 deaths related to the consumption of this liquid protein diet had been reported to the Food and Drug Administration, an incidence 40 times greater than that of the normal population.[17] These deaths were attributed to myocardial atrophy and arrhythmia caused by the poor-quality protein, lack of vitamins and minerals, and possibly some other undetermined toxic elements found in the liquid formula diet.[18]

Today, VLCDs are regarded as safe when used responsibly.[19] Debate continues on the optimal mix of macronutrients and on the role of carbohydrate and fat. While differences in formula composition can influence nitrogen retention, consensus exists on the need to use high-quality animal protein. The ideal VLCD should maximize the rate of weight loss from adipose tissue while maintaining normal protein nutrition and overall health.

CLINICAL APPLICATION OF VLCDS

VLCDs provide 400–800 kcal/day, although there is no universally accepted definition. These diets are designed to produce rapid weight loss while preserving lean body tissue. Most VLCDs provide 45–100 g of high-quality protein[19] from milk or egg-based sources. VLCDs contain varying amounts of carbohydrate but, as a rule, less than 100 g carbohydrate. Most VLCDs are typically powdered formulas that are mixed with water and consumed five times daily. The PSMF, the lean-meat alternative to the formula diet, provides for 1.2–1.5 g of protein per kilogram of ideal body weight as lean meat, fish, or fowl each day. Most patients consume between 10–15 oz of lean meat, fish, or fowl each day over three to five meals. Every VLCD is supplemented with micronutrients including sodium, potassium, calcium, and magnesium. At least 64 oz of low-calorie fluids must be consumed daily. These diets must be medically supervised and administered as part of a multidisciplinary program to insure safety and long-term efficacy.[19]

PATIENT SELECTION

Because of the radical nature of VLCDs and because these diets are not without risk, patients should be carefully evaluated prior to treatment. VLCDs should be limited to persons who are at least 30% (18 kg) overweight.[19,20] Individuals with clear health risks related to their obesity who would potentially benefit from weight loss, particularly rapid weight loss (often required for surgery), are the most appropriate candidates; individuals seeking cosmetic weight loss should be educated on the need for permanent lifestyle changes to prevent weight regain and future health problems before being accepted into the program. A list of indications and contraindications for using VLCDs is provided in Table 11–1. Infants, and children under age 13, pregnant or lactating women, older adults, and persons with porphyria and gout should not be placed on a VLCD.[21] Severe caloric restriction is also contraindicated in persons with a history of recent myocardial infarction; cardiac conduction disorder; a history of cerebrovascular, renal, or hepatic disease; cancer; type I diabetes; or significant psychiatric disturbance.[19,22] Individuals with a history of eating disorders (i.e. anorexia, bulemia), alcoholism, or drug abuse should also be excluded from this mode of treatment.[21] Angina, particularly unstable angina, is another contraindication, although some physicians believe that stable angina may be an indication for the use of a VLCD, since symptoms may improve rapidly on initiation of treatment.[23]

Based on our own experience, VLCDs should be considered only after more conventional 1200-kcal diets have been tried and proved unsuccessful. Patients should be informed that they must commit to a minimum of 1 year in active treatment, which includes both the weight loss and maintenance phases. In addition, because the administration of these diets is expensive, the patient should be able to make the necessary financial commitment. The rapid weight loss achieved during a VLCD produces almost immediate cosmetic and physical relief

TABLE 11–1 Indications and Contraindications for Use of VLCDs

INDICATIONS
>130% of ideal body weight (1959 Metropolitan Life Insurance Tables)
Prior experience with conservative (1200 ± 200 kcal/day) treatment programs
Willing to commit to at least 1 year of treatment (weekly/monthly visits)
Willing to commit to making major lifestyle changes
CONTRAINDICATIONS
Pregnancy or lactation
≥65 years of age
≤12 years of age
Active gout or a history of gout
Porphyria
Recent myocardial infarction
Cardiac conduction disorder (e.g., unstable angina or arrythmia)
Cerebrolvascular hepatica disease
Congestive heart disease
Cancer drug therapy causing protein wasting (e.g., steroids)
Protein-wasting disease (e.g., lupus erythematosus, Cushing's disease)
Severe psychiatric disease.
History of addictive and/or eating disorders (e.g., bulemia, anorexia, alcoholism, drug abuse).
POSSIBLE CONTRAINDICATIONS
Type I diabetes
Adolescence (ages 13–18)
History of disordered eating (e.g., binge eating)
Electrolyte abnormality
Stable angina
Systemic disease (e.g., cancer)

and improvement in overall health; this helps to promote good compliance with the treatment program. Individuals who have obesity-related diseases (such as hypertension or type II diabetes) will require close medical supervision during weight loss to adjust the medication dosage and frequency as needed.

TREATMENT OUTCOMES

The standard length of time for the supplemented fast is 12 to 16 weeks.[19,22] Heavier patients have more lean body mass and exhibit better nitrogen balance while dieting than their less obese counterparts.[24,25] These patients, because of their excess body fat, may remain on the fast longer (assuming good compliance and medical clearance). Refeeding, the process of gradual weaning from the supplement (or PSMF) back to whole foods, generally takes 3 to 6 weeks. Women lose 1.5 kg/week and men 2.0 kg/week on a standard VLCD[19] for a total of 23 kg. Patients often lose up to 5 kg during the first week due to the naturesis that accompanies the initial days of the diet.

A weight loss of 1–2 kg/week is recommended during a VCLD.[19,22] Greater weight loss suggests excessive loss of lean tissue, which could result in the depletion of visceral tissue proteins located in the heart. Patients losing more than 2 kg/week should be evaluated for noncompliance with the diet program or increased physical activity. In some patients, caloric levels may need to be increased to slow an excessive rate of weight loss. An acceptable composition of weight loss over time is 75% from fat mass and 25% from fat-free mass.[26]

About half of all patients will drop out before completing the program.[27] Approximately 30% of those who complete the program will maintain their weight loss for at least 18 months, and the average patient will maintain one-half to two-thirds of his or her original weight loss over 18 to 24 months.[28] Participation in a structured maintenance program will promote greater maintenance of weight loss.[29]

Attrition

VLCDs can be associated with high attrition rates; thus, careful patient selection is extremely important. Although published data from commercial programs are extremely limited, dropout rates of 35% (after 18 weeks) and 45% (after 26 weeks) have been reported in a time-limited Optifast Program[28] and dropout rates of 24% (after 12 weeks) and 31% (after 16 weeks) by Health Management Resource.[30] Compared with commercial low-calorie diet programs (50% within 6 weeks, 70% within 12 weeks),[31] it appears that the dropout rate from commercial VLCD programs is considerably lower. Dropout rates are always highest during the first 3 weeks of treatment, ranging from 16% to 25%.[30–33]

University-based research programs report greater retention rates, perhaps due to the more selective choice of the patient population. These programs typically have rigorous screening criteria and entry requirements. Attrition rates for these programs average 10–20%[34–36] over 12 to 18 months of treatment and follow-up, although a dropout rate as low as 4% was reported during 2 years of treatment and follow-up.[37]

INITIAL SCREENING AND TREATMENT

Because severe caloric restriction causes physiologic and pathophysiologic changes in a population already at increased risk for disease, medical monitoring by physicians trained in the proper use of VLCDs is mandatory. The medical monitoring of these patients begins with a complete medical history and physical examination. The medical history should document the age of onset of obesity, changes in body weight over the years, dieting history, and events associated with rapid weight gain or loss. The physician should identify medical complications of obesity, including diabetes, hypertension, cardiovascular disease, gallbladder disease, osteoarthritis, sleep apnea, and gout. A family history is also important, with particular emphasis on the heights and weights of immediate family members, as well as any obesity-related disorders. Patients with a history of eating disorders, drug or alcohol abuse, or disordered eating behavior should be excluded from treatment with a VLCD except in rare circumstances.

The physical examination should be thorough, with attention focused on obesity-related complications or factors that might affect treatment (e.g., osteoarthritis). Laboratory tests should include thyroid function, complete blood count and differential, chemistry panel (obtained after a 12-hr fast), electrolytes, total cholesterol, high density lipoprotein cholesterol, triglycerides, glucose, insulin (for crude assessment of insulin sensitivity), renal and liver function tests, and uric acid. A complete urinalysis is also necessary as is a recent electrocardiogram (ECG), as cardiac arrhythmias can be dangerous during a VLCD.

Patients should be placed on a conventional 1200-kcal diet for a minimum of 2 weeks prior to starting the VLCD. Compliance with this preparatory diet can often predict how the patient will do on the VLCD. Many commercial programs do not follow this practice and enroll patients immediately after medical screening. During the preparatory diet, patients attend weekly visits at which weight, blood pressure, and food and activity records kept by the patient are carefully reviewed by the staff. Any individual who complies with this initial treatment will then move on to the active fasting phase.

Few studies have compared liquid formula to food-based VLCDs, although patients achieve comparable weight loss on either regimen. In our clinic, we have found that certain patients will do better on one or another of these programs. Individuals whose professional or personal life requires frequent dining out can comfortably stay on a PSMF. We would recommend that when screening a patient for participation in a VLCD program, careful consideration be given to which of these diets best fits the patients' lifestyles and personal preference.

MEDICAL MONITORING DURING THE VLCD

Once the patient has begun the VLCD, certain medical information must be routinely obtained by the nurse or physician. Weight, blood pressure, and pulse should be measured weekly. Patients should be asked about any possible side effects. Common complaints include fatigue, dizziness, muscle cramping, headache, gastrointestinal distress, constipation, diarrhea, cold intolerance, hair loss, and dry skin. Most of these symptoms can be treated individually and will stop with cessation of the diet. Patients taking medication for diabetes or hypertension should be monitored carefully, as their regimen will likely need to be adjusted.

In addition to this weekly monitoring, biweekly assessment of electrolytes and other relevant (depending on the patient's initial medical condition) laboratory values and biweekly ECGs should be conducted. If any arrhythmia is noted, the VLCD should be discontinued immediately until the patient has been examined further. Although we recommend that electrolyte and other laboratory values be assessed every other week, some investigators have reported good outcomes with less frequent monitoring.[38] Patients should be seen twice a month by the physician unless otherwise indicated.

Nurses, dietitians, exercise physiologists, and behavior therapists knowledgeable about the psychological and pathophysiologic changes associated with rapid weight loss will provide additional care and monitoring. Nurses collect weekly vital signs and information on side effects; dietitians or nutritionists educate the patient on proper nutrition and healthy diet; and behavior therapists lead group support sessions. The use of well-trained allied health care professionals can make the program more cost effective by limiting the physician's time. Finally, although walking is the exercise of choice for most patients, exercise physiologists may be employed to conduct exercise stress tests and fitness evaluations and to create exercise prescriptions for program participants.

MULTIDISCIPLINARY VLCD TREATMENT

Current treatment programs for obesity include diet, physical activity, and behavior modification. These treatment components are mutually supportive and necessary to promote long-term maintenance of weight loss.[22,39] Without participating in such a multidisciplinary program, clients will probably regain 55–67% of their weight loss during the year following treatment.[29,37]

VLCDs are popular because they are simple to follow, produce rapid weight loss, and are generally not associated with hunger after several days on the program.[22,40] While on the diet, however, patients must be taught to modify their eating and exercise habits and lifestyle behavior.

As shown in Figure 11–1, Wadden and Stunkard[29] have compared obesity treatment that uses VLCD alone, behavior therapy alone, and combined diet and behavior modification in 59 obese women over a 6-month diet phase and a 1-year follow-up phase. Mean weight losses at the end of treatment for the VLCD alone, behavior therapy alone, and combined treatment conditions were 14.1, 14.3, and 19.3 kg, respectively. Weight loss using combined therapy was significantly greater than that achieved using either treatment component alone. One

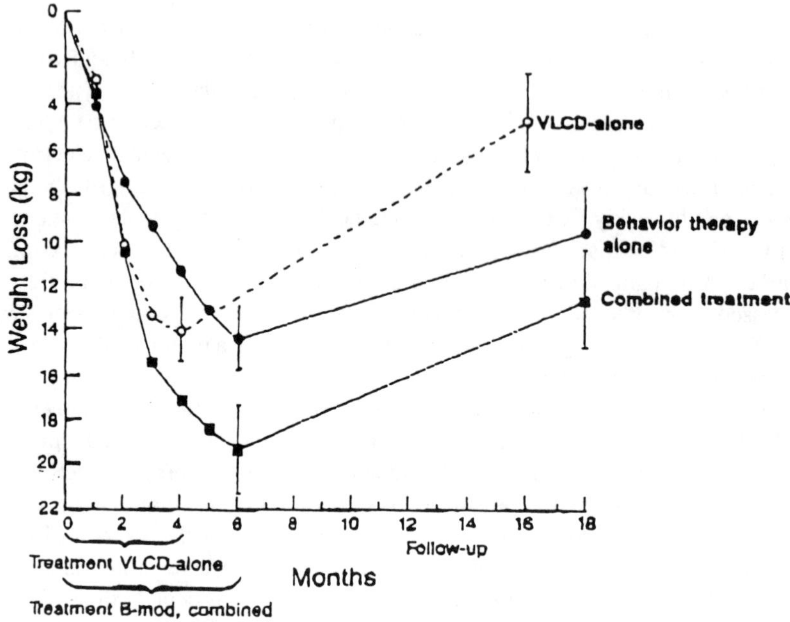

Figure 11–1. Weight changes during treatment and at 12-month follow-up.

(From data in Ref. 29; reprinted with permission)

year following treatment cessation, weight losses were 4.6, 9.8, and 12.5 kg, respectively. Women in the VLCD and combined treatment groups regained two-thirds of their initial weight loss, while women in the behavior change program regained only one-third of their initial weight loss. These data emphasize the importance of including behavior modification therapy in a VLCD program to promote long-term weight control.

The behavior modification component should include self-monitoring, stimulus control, reinforcement, and cognitive restructuring, which are described in detail in Chapter 13. Participants must also be provided with information on diet and nutrition so that they can make informed choices about the foods they will eat as they are weaned from the VLCD and move into maintenance. Finally, while exercise may affect weight loss, only marginally, it appears to be an important determinant of long-term weight maintenance[41,42] and, in conjunction with caloric restriction, may promote favorable changes in body composition.[43,44] In addition, the period of active dieting offers a window of opportunity to teach the exercise skills required to promote long-term weight maintenance. Individuals undertaking VLCDs, however, should be cautioned against excessive endurance exercise during the active weight loss phase. Very strenuous physical activity may depress the metabolic rate during the period of severe caloric restriction rather than raise it.[45] The importance of exercise (both endurance exercise and strength training) in weight control, as well as its practical application, is discussed in detail in Chapters 7 and 12.

NUTRITION PROFILE OF VLCDS

VLCDs differ somewhat in their nutrient composition (Table 11–2) and their subsequent protein-sparing ability and metabolic effects. Calorie level is important in determining nitrogen balance and loss of fat-free mass.[46] When energy intake is low, the body needs more dietary protein for glucogenic amino acids and fuel. Thus, the requirement for protein increases as energy intake decreases. The most important determinant of nitrogen balance, however, appears to be the level of protein intake.[47] Most commercial programs provide 50–90 g of protein daily, and we have reported favorable results when providing 1.2–1.5 g of protein per kilogram of ideal body weight (75 and 55 g/day for men and women, respectively),[48,49] with positive nitrogen balance achieved within 2 weeks of starting the VLCD. It is still unclear what the optimal level of protein intake should be for obese persons undergoing a VLCD; in fact, the optimal level may

TABLE 11–2 Macronutrient Composition and Cost of Selected Formulas VLCDs

Product	Daily Calories	Protein (g)	Carbohydrates (g)	Fat (g)	Weekly Cost ($)*
HMR 500†	520	50	79	1	25.20
70+	520	70	63	1	25.20
800	800	80	97	10	28.70
Medifast 55	435	55	45	4	20.00
70	462	70	37	3	25.00
Plus	848‡	98	60	24	16.00
Optifast 70	420	70	30	2	§
800	800	70	100	13	

*Cost to the doctor for a 1-week supply of packets containing powdered supplement; complete programs involve additional costs.

†Also called Complement 100, 70+, and 800.

‡Formula provides 374 kcal; the remaining calories come from a single 8-oz meal of meat, fish, or fowl plus two cups of salad.

§Packets of Optifast are available only as part of a core 26-week program including a patient manual, weekly classes, physician's visits, and laboratory test. Total cost to the patient averages $2000–$2500.

Modified from the Medical letter on Drugs and Therapeutics 31 (787):22, 1989. Reproduced by permission.

vary among individuals.[50,51] However, it seems prudent to error on the side of providing more rather than less protein and risking protein depletion. A more detailed discussion of the effect of energy restriction on body composition and nitrogen balance, and methods for measuring body composition, is presented in Chapter 3 and elsewhere.[52]

When calories are restricted, dietary carbohydrate may be better than fat in sparing body protein.[53] Adding carbohydrate to the VLCD has also been shown to lessen the decline in metabolic rate, to increase exercise capacity, to improve mood, and to reduce hunger.[22,54–58] Addition of carbohydrates promotes the retention of electrolytes; diminishes the loss of calcium, magnesium, and zinc[59]; reduces ketosis; and inhibits hyperuricemia.[60,61] For these reasons, most commercial products (Table 11–2) today include at least 50 g of carbohydrate.

Although the body has minimal fatty acid requirements, VLCDs may need to include more fat to prevent the formation of gallstones (see Safety on page 207).[62,63] Some reports suggest that consuming at least one meal per day that contains 10 g or more of fat will ensure adequate contraction of the gallbladder.[64] Patients using VLCDs that do not include at least one meal with 10 g or more of fat may therefore be at increased risk for developing gallstones. Commercial formulas currently provide 1–24 g of fat daily, which may make a PSMF (20–40 g/day of fat) a safer choice.

HEALTH BENEFITS

VLCDs have immediate and dramatic effects on the health of obese patients. We have observed significant reductions in glucose and insulin levels after less than 1 week on a VLCD. For individuals with type II diabetes, significant improvements in glycemic control, as measured by fasting blood glucose, the intravenous glucose tolerance test and hemoglobin A_1 testing, are evident at the conclusion of the fast and for up to 1 year after treatment.[35] We have also reported significant improvements in insulin resistance following a VLCD.[65]

Blood pressure also drops dramatically, with the majority of the reduction occurring during the first 3 weeks on the diet.[66] Patients on a VLCD can expect an 8–12% reduction in systolic, and a 9–13% reduction in diastolic blood pressure.[66–68] This reduction in blood pressure is still apparent after 24 months despite weight regain.[66]

Serum total cholesterol, low density lipoprotein (LDL) cholesterol, and triglycerides decrease during VLCD treatment. Total cholesterol decreases approximately 5–15%, with similar or slightly larger decreases occurring in LDL cholesterol.[68] A transient increase in total serum cholesterol may occur after 8 weeks on a VLCD, which will resolve when weight loss ceases.[69] Triglycerides will also decrease 15–50%, depending on the patient's initial level.[68]

Weight loss is generally accompanied by improvements in mood, feeling of well-being, energy level, self-esteem, and quality of life.[29,40,70] These and other psychosocial benefits of weight loss are discussed in greater detail in Chapter 8. A more detailed discussion of the therapeutic benefits of weight loss is presented in Chapter 9 and elsewhere.[71]

SAFETY

VLCDs are associated with a variety of short-term adverse health effects. These include hunger, weakness, fatigue, dizziness, dry skin, constipation or diarrhea, nausea, and cold intolerance. These problems are usually transitory and can be reversed by treating the symptoms or stopping the diet. Constipation can be treated with a bulk laxative and increased fluid intake. Hunger, nausea, and weakness tend to be worse during the first 2 weeks of the program, improving or disappearing later. Dizziness or lightheadedness is treated with increased fluid and sodium intake (usually as bouillon). Diarrhea is treated with an over-the-counter antidiarrhea agent, and dry skin is treated with moisturizers. VLCDs will lower the metabolic rate during the active dieting phase but are not associated with long-term depressions in metabolic rate.[72–74]

Severe caloric restriction is associated with some potentially serious side effects as well. The rate of gallstone formation among patients who undergo rapid weight loss is reported to be 5.8–8.0%.[75,76] In addition, the prevalence of gallstone formation is higher among obese adults, estimated at 28–45% (particularly in morbidly obese adults).[76,77] A linear relationship exists between relative weight and risk of gallstone formation.[77] In our own study,[78] patients who developed gallstones were significantly heavier (body mass index = 43 kg/m^2), remained in active weight loss longer, and lost more weight than did patients who did not develop gallstones. The use of a VLCD may increase the formation of both biliary sludge and cholesterol gallstones, resulting in a higher relative risk for gallstone formation and cholecystectomy.[79] The small caloric load and the restricted fat intake are thought to increase the cholesterol content and sludging of the bile in the gallbladder. In addition, patients appear to be more vulnerable to symptomatic gallstone formation during maintenance.[75,76] A controlled trial demonstrated that the risk of gallstone formation during a VLCD can be significantly reduced by giving patients 1200 mg ursodeoxycholic acid per day.[76] Prophylactic use of ursodeoxycholic acid should thus be considered in appropriate patients treated with VLCDs. In addition, as discussed earlier (Nutrition Profile of VLCDs), patients should consume at least one meal per day that provides 10 g or more of fat.[64]

Plasma uric acid levels also increase transiently at the onset of a VLCD.[80] Although patients with a prior history of gout are at increased risk for exacerbation of symptoms while on a VLCD, precipitation of gout in asymptomatic individuals is uncommon.[81]

MAINTENANCE

In 1991, 5.4% (up from 2.5% in 1989) of the adult U.S. population reported participating in commercial, medically supervised, liquid diet programs.[82] However, very few long-term data are available from such VLCD programs, and most of what is available was collected retrospectively, often including self-reported weights.[30,32] In one published study,[28] of the 55% of men and women who completed a 26-week treatment program, approximately 74% participated in the follow-up evaluation. These patients lost 24.8 kg (24% of their initial body weight) at the end of treatment and regained 9.5 kg over the 13 months following active treatment. The weight loss and weight maintenance reported in this study are comparable to those reported by university-based obesity research programs.[12] Also noteworthy was the significant improvement in health that accompanied the weight loss and that was sustained despite some weight regain at 1 year.

Table 11–3 summarizes randomized clinical trials reported in the literature.[34,35,37,66,83,84] Five of the six studies have follow-up data available 1 to 2 years after treatment, during which time most patients regain 37–52% of their initial weight loss. By 5 years, less than 5% of participants showed significant, lasting weight losses,[34] although one study did report lower body weight at 2 years than at the end of active weight loss.

While initial weight loss using a VLCD is large and impressive, substantial weight is regained by 2 years, and weight maintenance for these patients remains elusive. Clearly, more research is needed to help isolate factors that will promote long-term weight maintenance among reduced obese individuals. For example, several studies have shown that regular contact during the maintenance phase[85,86] will facilitate long-term weight control. Other studies have shown that regular exercise can also promote weight maintenance.[83]

One consequence of a patient's failure to maintain weight loss may be a continued pattern of weight cycling in which body weight fluctuates rapidly and/or in significant amounts. VLCDs produce large, rapid weight losses even in individuals refractory to most treatment attempts and those with morbid obesity. The potential risks of weight cycling should be considered prior to undertaking any weight loss program, particularly a VLCD. Repeated bouts of weight loss and gain have been shown to lower the metabolic rate,[87] to impede efforts to lose weight,[88] to increase adiposity,[89] and to lower self-esteem.[90] However, other studies have shown no adverse effects on metabolic rate,[91,92] body composition,[93] or ability to lose weight[94]; in addition, several studies have indicated that persons

TABLE 11–3 Prospective Randomized Clinical Trials of Obesity Treatment Using VLCDs

Reference	No. of Subjects	Treatment Program and Duration	Initial Body Weight (kg)	Mean Weight Change (kg)	Years of FU from Study Entry (yr)	FU Weight (kg)	Percent Regain
Anderson et al.[37]	50 F, 7 M	VLCD (6 mo)*	120	−22.0	2	−10.0	55
		Gastroplasty + VLCD (9 mo)		−26.1	2	−32.0	0
Sikand et al.[88]	30, F	VLCD + BT (4 mo)	106	−17.5	2	−0.8	95
		VLCD + BT + structured EX (4 mo)		−21.8	2	−9.1	58
DITOH[66]	102 F, 85 M	PSMF + BT (21 wk)	110	−19.1	2.5	−7.1	63
		BT (25 wk)		−13.2	2.5	−5.0	62
Miura et al.[83]	46 F, 24 M	VLCD (up to 2 mo)	148% IBW†	−8.6	2	−4.1	52
		BT (4 mo)		−4.5	2	−6.8	0
		VLCD + BT (up to 2 mo); BT alone (for additional 2 mo)		−10.7	2	−12.8	0
Wadden et al.[34]	76, F	VLCD (8 wk);	106	−13.1	1(5)	−4.7 (+1.0)†	64 (108)
		standard diet (8 wk)		−13.0	1(5)	−6.6 (+2.7)	49 (120)
		BT (6 mo)		−16.8	1(5)	−10.6 (+2.9)	37 (117)
		VLCD + BT (8 wk); BT (8 weeks)					
Wing et al.[35]	26 F, 10 M	VLCD + BT (8 wk);	103	−18.6	1	−8.66	54
		BT additional 3 mos		−10.1	1	−6.8	33
		BT alone (5 mo)					

Note: when not in combination with a VLCD, BT patients are also given a standard 1200 ± 200 kcal/day diet to follow.

M, male; F, female; BT, behavior therapy; PSMF, protein-sparing modified fast; VLCD, very-low-calorie diet; EX, exercise; FU, follow-up.

*Alternating 8-week intervals on VLCD with 2-week intervals on a 900-kcal diet.

† Initial body weight in kg not available

‡ Follow-up data are available at 5 years and are denoted in parentheses.

with a marked history of weight cycling may actually lose more weight than persons with a mild history.[95,96]

So is it better to have lost and gained (weight cycled) than never to have lost at all? While clearly there are putative psychological consequences[97] to weight cycling, at present the effects of weight cycling on dieting and health are unclear. Two recent published epidemiologic studies[98,99] and data from two unpublished prospective studies[100] suggest that weight cycling may have adverse health effects. For this reason, it is wise to screen patients for readiness prior to undergoing a diet. In our clinic, we have patients fill out a questionnaire developed by Dr. Brownell and colleagues to assess diet readiness,[101] keep food and activity records, go on a balanced deficit diet for 3 weeks prior to induction of the VLCD, and come in for weekly clinic visits during this time. Failure to comply with this program or a poor score on the diet readiness questionnaire is an indication that this patient may not be ready to make the necessary commitment to embark on a diet at this time.

CONCLUSION

VLCDs are safe when administered by properly trained medical staff knowledgeable in the physiology and psychology of rapid weight loss. Most patients will lose 18–20 kg in 12–16 weeks on a VLCD. This degree of weight loss can have dramatic effects on the physical and mental health of the patient. In many cases, hypertension, diabetes, and dyslipidemia will be resolved or improved. Rapid weight loss can also improve mood, the feeling of well-being, and self-esteem. Unfortunately, fewer than 5% of individuals who embark on a VLCD will maintain a significant portion of their weight loss for 5 years. Future research must focus on identifying optimal macronutrient composition, promoting better weight maintenance, and reducing potential adverse effects.

REFERENCES

1. Welborn T, Wahlquist ML. Scientific conference on "very low calorie diets." *Med J Aust* 151:457, 1989.
2. Evans FA, Strang JM. A departure from the usual methods of treating obesity. *Am J Med Sci* 177:339, 1929.
3. Simeon AT. The action of chorionic gonadotrophin in the obese. *Lancet* 2:946, 1954.
4. Duncan GG, Duncan TG, Schless GL, et al. Contraindications and therapeutic results of fasting in obese patients, in Brodoff BN (ed), *Adipose Tissue Metabolism*

and Obesity, Vol. 131, New York, Annals of the New York Academy of Sciences, 1965, pp. 632 vol. 131.

5. Spencer I. Death during therapeutic starvation for obesity. *Lancet* 1:914, 1969.
6. Bloom WL. Fasting as an introduction to the treatment of obesity. *Metabolism* 8:214, 1959.
7. Bollinger RE, Lukert BP, Brown RV, et al. Metabolic balance of obese subjects during fasting. *Arch Intern Med* 118:3, 1966.
8. Apfelbaum M, Bostsarron J, Brigant L, et al. La composition du poids diete hydrique. Effets de la supplementation proteique. *Gastroenterol Biol Med* 108:121, 1967.
9. Blackburn GL, Flatt MP, Cloves GH, et al. Protein sparing therapy during periods of starvation with sepsis and trauma. *Ann Surg* 177:588, 1973.
10. Blackburn GL, Flatt JP, Cloves GH, et al. Peripheral intravenous feeding with isotonic amino acid solutions. *Am J Surg* 125:447, 1973.
11. Genuth SM, Castro JH, Vertes V. Weight reduction by supplemented fasting, in Howard AN (ed), *Recent Advances in Obesity Research,* Vol I. London, John Libbey, 1975, pp. 78.
12. Genuth SM, Castro JH, Vertes V. Weight reduction in obesity by outpatient semi-starvation. *JAMA* 230:987, 1974.
13. Howard AN, Grant A, Edwards O, et al. The treatment of obesity with a very-low-calorie liquid-formula diet. An inpatient/outpatient comparison using skimmed milk as the chief protein source. *Int J Obes* 2:321, 1978.
14. Howard AN, McLean Baird I. A long-term evaluation of very low calorie semisynthetic diets: An inpatient/outpatient study with egg albumin as the protein source. *Int J Obes* 1:63, 1978.
15. Gregg MB. Deaths associated with liquid protein diets. *MMWR* 26:383, 1977.
16. Schucker RE, Gunn WJ. *A National Survey of the Use of Protein Products in Conjunction with Weight Reduction Diets Among American Women*. Atlanta, Centers for Disease Control, 1978.
17. Editorial details released on deaths of ten on liquid protein diets. *JAMA* 238:2680, 1977.
18. Howard AN. The historical development of very low calorie diets. *Int J Obes* 13:1, 1989.
19. Wadden TA. Van Itallie TB, Blackburn GL. Responsible and irresponsible use of very-low-calorie diets in the treatment of obesity. *JAMA* 263:83, 1990.
20. Timely statement of the American Dietetic Association: Very low calorie weight loss diets. *J Am Diet Assoc* 89:975, 1989.
21. Dept of Health and Social Security. *Report on Health and Social Subjects No. 31, Use of Very Low Calorie Diets in Obesity*. London, Her Majesty's Stationary Office, 1987.
22. Wadden TA, Stunkard AJ, Brownell KD. Very-low-calorie diets: Their efficacy, safety, and future. *Ann Intern Med* 99:675, 1983.

23. Vertes V. Clinical experience with a very low calorie diet, in Blackburn GL, Bray GA (eds), *Management of Obesity by Severe Caloric Restriction*. Littleton, PSG, 1985, pp. 349–358.
24. Forbes GB. Lean body mass–body fat interrelationships in humans. *Nutr Rev* 45:225, 1987.
25. Forbes GB, Drenick EJ. Loss of body nitrogen on fasting. *Am J Clin Nutr* 32:1570, 1979.
26. Garrow JS. *Treat Obesity Seriously: A Clinical Manual*. New York: Churchill Livingstone, 1981.
27. Glinsmann WH, Hymann GN, Sempos E, et al. Evidence for success of caloric restriction in weight loss and control: Summary of data from industry, in Methods for Voluntary Weight Loss and Control: An NIH Technology Assessment Conference, 1992, Abstracts.
28. Wadden TA, Foster GD, Letizia KA, et al. A multicenter evaluation of a proprietary weight reduction program for the treatment of marked obesity. *Arch Intern Med* 152:961, 1992.
29. Wadden TA, Stunkard AJ. Controlled trial of very-low-calorie diet, behavior therapy, and their combination in the treatment of obesity. *J Consult Clin Psychol* 54:482, 1986.
30. Anderson JS, Hamilton CC, Crown-Weber E, et al. Safety and effectiveness of a multidisciplinary very-low-calorie diet program for selected obese individuals. *J Am Diet Assoc* 91:1582, 1991.
31. Volkmar FR, Stunkard AJ, Woolston J, et al. High attrition rates in commercial weight reduction programs. *Arch Intern Med* 141:426, 1981.
32. Kirschner M, Schneider G, Erter NH, et al. An eight-year experience with a very-low-calorie formula diet for control of major obesity. *Int J Obes* 12:69, 1988.
33. Shapiro H, Weinkove C, Coxon A, et al. Three year hospital experience with control of major obesity by VLCD in medically compromised individuals. *Int J Obes* 13:125, 1989.
34. Wadden TA, Sternberg JA, Letizia KA, et al. Treatment of obesity by very low calorie diet, behavior therapy, and their combination: A five-year perspective. *Int J Obes* 13:39, 1989.
35. Wing RR, Marcus MD, Salata R, et al. Effects of a very-low-calorie diet on long-term glycemic control in obese type 2 diabetic subjects. *Arch Intern Med* 151:1334, 1991.
36. Blackburn GL, Kanders BS, Lavin PT, et al. Dietary Intervention Therapy for Obese Hypertensives (DITOH). *Circulation* 80:II–384, 1989.
37. Anderson T, Backer OG, Stokholm DH et al. Randomized trial of diet and gastroplasty compared with diet alone in morbid obesity. *N Engl J Med* 310:352, 1984.
38. Atkinson RL, Kaiser DL. Nonphysician supervision of a very-low-calorie diet: Results in over 200 cases. *Int J Obes* 5:237, 1981.
39. Council on Scientific Affairs. Treatment of obesity in adults. *JAMA* 260:2547, 1988.

40. Foster GD, Wadden TA, Peterson FJ, et al. A controlled comparison of three very-low-calorie diets: Effects on weight, body composition and symptoms. *Am J Clin Nutr* 55:802, 1992.

41. Van Dale D, Saris WHM, ten Hoor F. Weight maintenance and resting metabolic rate 18–40 months after a diet/exercise treatment. *Int J Obes* 14:347, 1990.

42. Pavlou KN, Krey S, Steffee WP. Exercise as an adjunct to weight loss and maintenance in moderately obese subjects. *Am J Clin Nutr* 49:1115, 1989.

43. Pavlou KN, Steffee WP, Lerman RH, et al. Effects of dieting and exercise on lean body mass, oxygen uptake and strength. *Med Sci Sports Exerc* 17:466, 1985.

44. Wood PD, Stefanick ML, Dreon DM, et al. Changes in plasma lipids and lipoproteins in overweight men during weight loss through dieting as compared with exercise. *N Engl J Med* 319:1173, 1988.

45. Phinney SD, LaGrange BM, O'Connell M, et al. Effects of aerobic exercise on energy expenditure and nitrogen balance during very low calorie dieting. *Metabolism* 37:758, 1988.

46. Rao CN, Naidu A, Rao BS. Influence of varying energy intake on nitrogen balance in men on two levels of protein intake. *Am J Clin Nutr* 28:1116, 1975.

47. Brodoff BN, Hendler R. Very low calorie diets, in Bjorntorp P, Brodoff BN (eds), *Obesity*. Philadelphia, JB Lippincott, 1992, pp. 683–707.

48. Blackburn GL, Bistrian BR, Flatt JP. Role of a protein sparing modified fast in comprehensive weight reduction program, in Howard AN (ed), *Recent Advances in Obesity Research: Proceedings of the First International Congress on Obesity*. London, Newman, 1975, pp. 279.

49. Bistrian BR, Blackburn GL, Stanbury JB. Metabolic aspects of protein sparing modified fast in the dietary management of Prader-Willi obesity. *N Engl J Med* 296:774, 1977.

50. Fisler JS, Drenick EJ, Blumfield DE, et al. Nitrogen economy during very low calorie reducing diets: Quality and quantity of dietary protein. *Am J Clin Nutr* 35:471, 1982.

51. Fisler JS, Kaptein EM, Drenick EJ, et al. Metabolic and hormonal predictors of nitrogen retention in obese men consuming very low calorie diets. *Metabolism* 34:101, 1985.

52. Yang M, Van Itallie TB. Effect of energy restriction on body composition and nitrogen balance in obese individuals, in Wadden TA, Van Itallie TB (eds), *Treatment of the Seriously Obese Patient*. New York, Guilford Press, 1992, pp.

53. Calloway DH, Spector H. Nitrogen balance as related to calories and protein intake in active young men. *Am J Clin Nutr* 2:405, 1954.

54. Apfelbaum M, Fricker J, Igoin-Apfelbaum L. Low- and very-low-calorie diets. *Am J Clin Nutr* 45:1126, 1987.

55. Wadden TA, Stunkard AJ, Brownell KD, et al. A comparison of two very-low-calorie diets: Protein-sparing-modified fast versus protein-formula-liquid diet. *Am J Clin Nutr* 41:533, 1985.

56. Davis PG, Phinney SD. Differential effects of two very low calorie diets on aerobic and anaerobic performance. *Int J Obes* 14:779, 1990.

57. Wadden TA, Mason G, Foster GD, et al. Effects of a very low calorie diet on weight, thyroid hormones and mood. *Int J Obes* 14:249, 1990.

58. Bogardus C, LaGrange BM, Horton ES, et al. Comparison of carbohydrate-containing and carbohydrate-restricted hypocaloric diets in the treatment of obesity. *J Clin Invest* 68:399, 1981.

59. Daive MWJ, Abraham RR, Hewins B, et al. Changes in bone and muscle constituents during dieting for obesity. *Clin Sci* 70:285, 1986.

60. Howard AN, Grant A, Edwards O, et al. The treatment of obesity with a very-low-calorie liquid formula diet: An inpatient/outpatient comparison using skimmed milk as the chief protein source. *Int J Obes* 2:321, 1978.

61. McLean Baird I, Howard AN. A double-blind trial of mazindol using a very low-calorie formula diet. *Int J Obes* 1:271, 1977.

62. Kinwansky S, Chalmers TC. Fat content of very-low-calorie diets and gallstone formation. *JAMA* 40:865, 1992.

63. Sichleri R, Everhart JE, Roth H. A prospective study of hospitalization with gallstone disease among women: Role of dietary factors, fasting period, and dieting. *Am J Pub Health* 81:880, 1991.

64. Gebhard RL, Ansel HJ, Peterson FJ, et al. Gallbladder emptying stimuli in obese and normal weight subjects. *Hepatology* 12:898, 1990.

65. Istfan NW, Plaisted CS, Bistrian BR, et al. Insulin resistance versus insulin secretion in the hypertension of obesity. *Hypertension* 19:385, 1992.

66. Blackburn GL, Kanders BS, Pontes M. et al. Executive summary for the Dietary Intervention Therapy of Obese Hypertension (DITOH). Prepared for the Sixth Data Monitoring and Safety Board Meeting, October 30, 1989.

67. Palgi A, Read L, Greenberg I. et al. Multidisciplinary treatment of obesity with a protein-sparing modified fast: Results in 668 outpatients. *Am J Pub Health* 75:1190, 1985.

68. Anderson JW, Hamilton CC, Brinkman-Kaplan V. Benefits and risks of an intensive very-low-calorie diet program for severe obesity. *Am J Gastroenterol* 87:6, 1992.

69. Phinney SD, Tang AB, Waggoner CR, et al. The transient hypercholesterolemia of major weight loss. *Am J Clin Nutr* 53:1404, 1991.

70. O'Neil PM, Jarrell MP. Psychological aspects of obesity and dieting, in Wadden TA, Van Itallie TB (eds), *Treatment of the Seriously Obese Patient*. New York, Guilford Press, 1992, pp. 252–272.

71. Kanders BS, Blackburn GL. Reducing primary risk factors by therapeutic weight loss, in Wadden TA, Van Itallie TB (eds), *Treatment of the Seriously Obese Patient*. New York, Guilford Press, 1992, pp. 213–230.

72. Foster GD, Wadden TA, Mullen JL, et al. Resting energy expenditure, body composition, and excess weight in the obese. *Metabolism* 37:467, 1988.

73. Foster GD, Wadden TA, Feurer ID, et al. Controlled trial of metabolic effects of a very-low-calorie diet: Short- and long-term effects. *Am J Clin Nutr* 51:167, 1990.

74. Elliot DL, Goldberg L, Kuehl KS, et al. Sustained depression of the resting metabolic rate after massive weight loss. *Am J Clin Nutr* 49:93, 1989.

75. Liddle RA, Goldstein RB, Saxon J. Gallstone formation during weight reduction dieting. *Arch Intern Med* 149:1750, 1989.

76. Broomfield PH, Chopra R, Scheinbaum RC, et al. Effects of ursodeoxycholic acid and aspirin on the formation of lithogenic bile and gallstones during loss of weight. *N Engl J Med* 319:1567, 1988.

77. Bennion LJ, Grundy SM. Effects of obesity and caloric intake on bilary lipid metabolism in man. *J Clin Invest* 56:996, 1975.

78. Kanders BS, Blackburn GL, Lavin P, et al. Weight loss outcome and health benefits associated with the Optifast program in the treatment of obesity. *Int J Obes* 13:S131, 1989.

79. Maclure KM, Hayes KC, Colditz LGA, et al. Weight, diet and risk of symptomatic gallstones in middle-aged women. *N Engl J Med* 321:563, 1989.

80. Kreitzman SN. Clinical experience with a very low calorie diet, in Blackburn GL, Bray GA (eds), *Management of Obesity by Severe Caloric Restriction*. Littleton, MA, PSG, 1985, pp. 359–367.

81. Atkinson RI. Low and very low caloric diets. *Med Clin North Am.* 73:203, 1989.

82. *Dieting and Low-Calorie/Reduced-Fat Products Survey*. Calorie Control Council, Atlanta, Ga., 1991.

83. Miura J, Arai K. Tsukahara S. et al. The long term effectiveness of combined therapy by behavior modification and very low calorie diet: 2 years follow-up. *Int J Obes 13:*73, 1989.

84. Sikand G, Kondo A, Foreyl J, et al. Two year follow-up of patients treated with very low calorie dieting and exercise testing. *J Am Diet Assoc* 88:487, 1988.

85. King AC, Frey-Hewitt B, Dreon D, et al. Diet vs exercise in weight maintenance: The effects of minimal intervention strategies on long-term outcomes in men. *Arch Intern Med* 149:2741, 1989.

86. Perri MG, Shapiro RM, Ludwig WW, et al. Maintenance strategies for the treatment of obesity: An evaluation of relapse prevention training and posttreatment contact by mail and telephone. *J Consult Clin Psychol* 52:480, 1984.

87. Brownell KD, Greenwood MRC, Stellar E, et al. The effects of repeated cycles of weight loss and regain in rats. *Physiol Behav* 38:459, 1986.

88. Blackburn GL, Wilson GT, Kanders BS, et al. Weight cycling: The experience of human dieters. *Am J Clin Nutr* 49:1105, 1989.

89. Reed DR, Contreras RJ, Maggio C, et al. Weight cycling in female rats increases dietary fat selection and adiposity. *Physiol Behav* 42:389, 1988.

90. Wooley SC, Garner DM. Obesity treatment: The high cost of false hope. *J Am Diet Assoc* 91:1248, 1991.

91. Wadden TA, Barlett S, Letizia KA, et al. Relationship of dieting history to resting metabolic rate, body composition, eating behavior, and subsequent weight loss. *Am J Clin Nutr* 56:2035, 1992.
92. Melby CL, Schmidt WD, Corrigan D. Resting metabolic rate in weight-cycling collegiate wrestlers compared with physically active noncycling control subjects. *Am J Clin Nutr* 52:409, 1990.
93. Prentice AM, Jebb SA, Goldberg GR, et al. Effects of weight cycling on body composition. *Am J Clin Nutr* 56:209S, 1992.
94. Wadden TA, Foster GD, Letizia KA, et al. Long-term effects of dieting on resting metabolic rate in obese outpatients. *JAMA* 264:707, 1990.
95. Gonnally J, Rardin D, Black S. Correlates of successful response to a behavioral weight control clinic. *J Counsel Psychol* 27:179, 1980.
96. Bonatol DP, Boland FJ. Predictors of weight loss at the end of treatment and 1-year follow-up for a behavioral weight loss program. *Int J Eat Disorders* 11:573, 1987.
97. Graner DM, Wooley SC. Confronting the failure of behavioral and dietary treatment for obesity. *Clin Psychol Rev* 11:729, 1991.
98. Hamm PB, Shekelle RB, Stamler J. Large fluctuations in body weight during young adulthood and 25-year risk of coronary death in men. *Am J Epidemiol* 129:312, 1989.
99. Lissner L, Odell PM, D'Agostino RB, et al. Variability of body weight and health outcomes in the Framingham population. *N Engl J Med* 324:1839, 1991.
100. Blair SN. Long-term benefits and adverse effects of weight loss: Data from two prospective epidemiological studies, in Program and Abstracts Methods for Voluntary Weight Loss and Control and NIH Technology Assessment Conference, March 1992, pp. 86–93.
101. Brownell KD: Diet Readiness. *Weight Control Digest* 1:1, 1990.

Use of Exercise for Weight Control

CHAPTER 12

Peter Davis, Ph.D.
and Stephen Phinney, M.D., Ph.D.

INTRODUCTION

In the simplest terms, obesity results from an imbalance of caloric intake and caloric output. Although it is well recognized that both the causes of and remedies for obesity are complex and multifactorial, effective weight control can only be achieved through the manipulation of caloric input and output. In this context, increased caloric expenditure by physical activity is a logical approach to either the reduction or maintenance of desired body weight. Because an untrained person can increase caloric expenditure 10-fold over the resting metabolic rate and a well-trained athlete can nearly double this caloric output, moderate physical activity has the potential to contribute to the caloric balance equation when it becomes part of a person's regular schedule.

Not only does physical activity contribute to caloric balance, but it is also well documented that regularly performed physical activity reduces the symptoms and risks of obesity-related co-morbid conditions such as cardiovascular disease, diabetes, pulmonary disorders; and orthopedic conditions.[1] Therefore physical activity has primary benefits in weight control due to its contribution to the caloric balance equation, but it also has secondary benefits due to its positive effect on comorbid conditions.

Although the benefits and results of physical activity appear obvious, the translation of this commonsense rationale into clinical treatment is difficult. It is unfortunately common that the obese individual embarks on a physical activity program, and instead of achieving meaningful results, achieves physical injury or exercise aversion due to either an inappropriate exercise prescription or an overaggressive approach. Not only do obese adults typically have poor cardiovascular fitness levels, but they also usually have limited skills related to sports and physical activity, which further discourages initiation and continuation of appropriate exercise programs. This indicates that exercise needs to be approached from a behavioral change perspective rather than from a purely physiologic point of view. In other words, exercise instruction needs to extend beyond the standard treatment, which teaches the key physiologic outcomes and recommendations for safe and effective exercise, to include an approach that recognizes exercise as a major change in lifestyle. Coaching the patient to increase physical activity thus becomes more a behavioral process than a physiologic one, and standard markers such as heart rate and aerobic capacity should be refocused from indicators of successful outcomes to indicators of a successfully performed behavioral process (i.e., an exercise program).

Another important consideration in the use of exercise for the treatment of obesity is the etiology and mechanism of the disease process itself. Obesity is a chronic, progressive disease, and evidence is beginning to accumulate that strongly suggests a genetic factor in its causation.[2,3] Although exercise is one of the better weapons to counter the accumulation of dietary excesses as adipose tissue, the ability to perform prolonged aerobic exercise may in fact be compromised by the underlying biochemical mechanism that may limit readily oxidizable fuel supplies.[4] In other words, a "Catch 22" situation arises in the sense that the underlying metabolic defect contributing to the development of obesity, resulting in an increase of adipose tissue rather than of carbohydrate stores, may limit the patient's ability to perform the major behavior that can reverse and/or control the disease, that is, physical activity.

In this same context of decreased ability to perform exercise due to poor skills, poor initial aerobic capacity, poor implementation, and the disease process itself, there is also the issue of the method of caloric restriction that is used to reduce excess weight. To be in the best position to maintain a desired body weight with physical activity, the composition of the diet used to achieve weight loss should not leave the patient with limited ability to perform effective exercise. In other words, optimum nutrient intake should be utilized to ensure the best body composition and physical function following weight loss so that patients have the best chance to implement the behaviors that will maintain their desired weight.

The majority of the discussion that follows addresses the issues outlined above as they relate to the treatment of moderate to severe obesity. Various physiologic concerns regarding the use of exercise in the treatment of obesity, such as the combined effects of exercise and caloric restriction on metabolic rate, thermic effect of food, and appetite, are discussed elsewhere in this volume. The effect of exercise as a single mode of intervention in the treatment process will be briefly discussed. Practical solutions to overcome patient resistance to initiating an activity program in terms of the basic approach to exercise instruction will be addressed, as will optimization of the diet composition to enhance the exercise process. The role that exercise plays in the maintenance of weight loss will be discussed. Finally, recommendations for future research in the area of exercise and weight control will be proposed.

EXERCISE ALONE IN THE TREATMENT OF OBESITY

When considering the effect of exercise on weight control, either alone or in concert with other modalities, one must carefully consider several points. One is the wide range of behaviors covered by the definition of *exercise;* another is the variable effect that exercise has on body composition, that is, the fat and lean tissue contained in the various body compartments. To further complicate the issue, one must also consider the effect of exercise alone on body composition during different types or phases of weight control, such as active weight loss by moderate or severe caloric restriction, weight stabilization, or long-term weight maintenance. While this chapter will generally consider exercise to be aerobic and within the guidelines of the American College of Sports Medicine,[5] it should be understood that an exercise program can also be predominantly anaerobic, which may have different results both physiologically and behaviorally.

There is abundant evidence demonstrating that exercise alone is an ineffective method in losing significant weight.[6–9] Wilmore[6] reviewed 55 studies involving exercise as the single modality to achieve weight loss and found that with programs ranging in length from 6 to 104 weeks, the average change in body composition was the loss of a mere 1.6% of body fat. Closer inspection of this review shows that the greatest weight loss by exercise alone was from a program of unknown intensity, 60 min per session, three to five times per week for 15 weeks, during which 20-year-old women lost only 5.7 kg (12.6 lb), or 7% of initial body weight, from 83.4 kg to 77.7 kg.[8] The study employing the heaviest subjects, men weighing 122.4 kg (269 lb), achieved a weight loss of only 3.2 kg (7.1 lb), or 2.6% of initial body weight, which was composed of an increase of 2.6 kg (5.7 lb) of lean weight and a decrease of 3.9% in body fat.[11] The exercise regimen in this study consisted of 9 weeks of aerobic exercise of 60 min duration, five times per week, which for the weight status of the subjects could probably be classified as intense exercise.

More recent studies support these data.[9,12] Meijer[9] studied 15 males and 13 females with a low habitual physical activity level and normal body weight. The subjects completed a 20-week training schedule in preparation to run a half-marathon (13.1 mi or 20 km). Their training schedule was intense, progressing from four running sessions per week of 10–30 min in duration to four sessions per week of 20–60 min in duration and consisting of long-distance running, high-speed running, and interval training. Despite this major effort, body weight did not change, although there were significant changes in body composition, with increases in fat-free mass and decreases in percentage of body fat.

In light of this evidence that exercise alone is generally ineffective in achieving significant weight loss except for the most limited weight loss goals, most recent weight loss programs incorporate a multidisciplinary approach to weight control. The most successful programs utilize a combination of behavior change (exercise and nutrition behavior) and moderate to severe caloric restriction.[13,14] Although these studies did not utilize exercise alone in their treatment, examination of the data provides further information on the contribution of exercise to weight loss. Pavlou et al.[14] showed that there was no significant difference in the rate or amount of weight loss between groups of similar moderate or severe caloric restriction but divided into exercise and nonexercise groups.

Based on the contribution of exercise to both the total amount and rate of weight loss, one might consider the following analogy to describe the role of exercise in moderate to severe weight loss. Exercise is like the fine-tuning control on a television or radio receiver. If persons wish to switch from a high channel to a low channel, they use the channel selector or remote control. However, once they are close to the desired channel, they can use the fine-tune control to lock on to the channel and stay on it during drift. Similarly, if a person wishes to lose large amounts of weight, exercise will not assist to any great extent in getting to the desired weight; but once the desired weight has been achieved, exercise is perhaps the best method to maintain it. Thus exercise functions as a fine-tune controller. The role of exercise in weight maintenance is discussed further in a following section.

EXERCISE AND BODY COMPOSITION

If exercise is not an effective tool for weight loss, then why is so much emphasis placed on a well-designed exercise program during moderate to severe caloric restriction? Apart from the effects of exercise on metabolic rate, thermic effect of food, appetite suppression, or stimulation, and other physiologic variables—

some of which have not been conclusively resolved and remain controversial—the answer appears to lie with the effect of exercise on body composition.

Weltman et al.[15] and Zuti et al.[7] showed a greater percentage of weight loss as fat versus fat-free mass in studies comparing diet-plus-exercise groups to diet-only groups, with the combined-treatment groups achieving a more favorable ratio of body composition change. In the review by Wilmore[6] of weight loss by exercise alone, closer analysis reveals that in the 55 studies reviewed, lean body mass was either preserved or increased in 50 of 54 studies (one paper did not report percentage of body fat or lean body mass). This was achieved by aerobic exercise in 41 studies and by weight training in 13 studies.

This finding is supported by the work of Pavlou et al.,[14] who studied moderately obese men on four different diets, with and without exercise. Since there were no significant differences in weight loss or changes in body composition between the diet groups, they were collapsed into exercise versus nonexercise groups for statistical analysis. The aerobic exercise regimen consisted initially of low-intensity exercise and progressed over the course of the study to moderate to high-intensity exercise involving periods of walking/jogging at 70–85% of maximal aerobic capacity (VO_2 max). Subjects also performed "body weight" calisthenics (i.e., no external weights added to the body weight), such as deep squats, push-ups, sit-ups, and so on. Although, as previously noted, there were no differences in the amount of weight lost between the two groups, there were significant differences in the quality of body mass lost. Body fat was significantly reduced in both the exercise and nonexercise group; however, the reduction in the exercise group (11.2 kg) was significantly greater than that in the nonexercise group (5.9 kg). In terms of lean body mass, there was no change from pre- to posttreatment in the exercise group; however, the nonexercise group showed a significant reduction in lean body mass (3.3 kg). Total weight loss was almost exclusively from body fat stores in the exercise group (95% of weight loss from fat stores, 5% from lean tissue stores) compared to approximately 64% from fat stores and 36% from lean tissue stores in the nonexercise group.

The ability of exercise to contribute to optimal body composition changes is questioned by Van Dale et al.[16] Sixteen obese women were randomly divided into exercise and nonexercise groups. Four times per week, the exercise group participated in 1-hr supervised exercise sessions of aerobic dance, calisthenics, and stretching at an intensity level equivalent to 50–60% of VO_2 max. The diet regimen was a 680-kcal formula diet composed of 76 g carbohydrate, 55 g protein, and 18 g fat for the first 4 weeks of the study. The last 8 weeks of the study used 400 kcal from the formula diet and 800 kcal from free choice of foodstuffs. Subsequent food diary analysis revealed that during the second part of the study, subjects consumed 91 g carbohydrate, 67 g protein, and 20 g fat. In agreement with other studies, there were no differences in weight loss between the exercise and nonexercise groups. However, in contrast to the results of other studies, there were also no differences in the quality of body mass loss. In other words, even though both groups lost significant weight and percentage body fat compared to initial levels, there was no difference between the exercise and nonexercise groups. Similarly, there was no significant difference in the change in fat-free mass between the two groups, with both showing small decreases in fat-free mass throughout the study. It is unclear why the exercise group did not achieve significantly better body composition results, although as the authors point out, a major factor may be that the number of subjects was too small for significant differences to appear. Following a dropout of two subjects in each group, there were only six subjects in each group.

Since resting metabolic rate (RMR) and exercise capacity (VO_2 max) are both highly correlated with lean body mass, it is a major advantage to either maintain or reduce the loss of lean tissue during weight loss. It is logical to assume that by maintaining the highest level of lean tissue and achieving higher levels of exercise capacity, the individual who has exercised during a weight loss program (compared to one who was sedentary during weight loss) is better able to maintain a weight loss. In other words, an individual who exercises during weight loss may be better able to improve the caloric expenditure side of the caloric balance equation. While this in no way ensures long-term weight maintenance, it improves the patient's chances if there have been additional benefits from the other behavioral components of a multidisciplinary weight loss program.

Unfortunately, however, the importance of persistent exercise as a fundamental tool for ensuring the highest-quality weight loss and enhancing the probability of long-term weight maintenance success is often not addressed. This situation will probably remain until there is a shift in the measure of success of a weight loss program (by both clinicians and patients) from achieving maximal weight loss to achieving optimal body composition and function. For this to occur, the standard tool used to measure success, the scale, needs to be either replaced or complemented with clinically appropriate devices that assess body composition and/or performance.

EXERCISE AND WEIGHT MAINTENANCE

As previously mentioned, exercise plays a strong role in achieving optimal weight loss in terms of body composition, and this may make it easier to maintain the desired weight. But what evidence exists to show that exercise is correlated with long-term weight control success? This is a difficult question to answer unequivocally, since effective incorporation of an exercise component into the multidisciplinary treatment approach is a fairly recent development, and long-term statistics are sparse.

In the study by Pavlou et al.[17] of moderately obese men, follow-up 6 and 18 months after completion of their active weight loss phase showed a clear distinction between the exercise and nonexercise groups in regard to their weight status. In this study, male subjects at different levels of caloric restriction were randomized into groups that either did not perform exercise during their active weight loss phase or participated in regular aerobic exercise at 70–85% of VO_2 max. There were no significant changes between prediet weight and follow-up weight at 6 and 18 months for all the exercise groups, regardless of the diet treatment. By contrast, all nonexercise groups regained approximately 60% and 92% of the weight loss at 6 and 18 months of follow-up, respectively.

Similar results were demonstrated in a study by Hakim et al.,[18] who conducted a telephone survey of 122 patients, from an original group of 199 obese patients, 3.5 years after a multidisciplinary, medically supervised weight loss program. Of these 122 patients, 69 (56%) reported regularly performing at least 2.5 hr of aerobic exercise per week, primarily walking. These patients, classified as exercisers, reported a regain of 49% of the weight they had originally lost. Non-exercisers reported a regain of 75% of their original weight loss.

Van Dale[19] confirmed the relationship between exercise and weight maintenance by demonstrating significantly less weight regain in subjects who continued to exercise 18 months after a weight loss regimen compared to subjects who either did not exercise at all or who exercised during active weight loss but then ceased exercising following the weight loss phase.

To determine the amount of exercise necessary to maintain desired weight, Whatley et al.[20] studied 67 moderately obese women who lost a mean of 22 kg (48.5 lb) while performing supervised moderate aerobic exercise for a minimum of 5 weeks. The program included caloric restriction as well as behavioral instruction. At the end of a 32-week follow-up phase, the women were grouped according to how many minutes per week they had exercised during their weight maintenance phase. Eighteen women did not exercise at all during the maintenance phase and regained all the weight they had lost plus an additional 3.2 kg. Twenty-six of the women exercised for less than 100 min and regained all their weight plus an additional 4 kg. Twenty-three women exercised for more than 100 min and not only maintained their weight loss but also lost an additional 1 kg. Unfortunately, this paper does not describe how much less or how much more than 100 min was performed, nor does it quantitate the frequency or intensity of exercise. However, it does suggest that there might be a minimum threshold of exercise necessary to promote long-term weight maintenance. Recent studies link physical activity to a reduction in all-cause mortality and suggest an exercise threshold of approximately 1500–2000 kcal/week, which for moderately fit individuals represents approximately 3–4 hr of exercise per week.[21,22] This is considerably more than the 100 min suggested by Whatley et al.[20] However, the differences could be accounted for by such factors as different intensities, frequencies, modes of exercise, and length of follow-up, as well as the different exercise objectives of the two retrospective studies.

The evidence suggests that since it is relatively easy for poor nutritional and lifestyle choices to override the benefits of exercise, one cannot guarantee that regular physical activity will result in successful long-term weight maintenance. On the other hand, it is safe to assume that physical inactivity will almost certainly result in long-term weight maintenance failure.

INTERACTION OF DIET AND EXERCISE

In research done to date, a major subject has been the role of exercise in improving and/or maintaining both lean body mass and aerobic capacity (as identified by VO_2 max). Since exercise and nutrition are not independent of each other, however, one should also consider the reverse situation: the ability of the diet to allow appropriate exercise to occur. In light of the prevalence of low- and very-low-calorie diets (VLCDs) and the above-stated role that exercise should play in long-term weight management, this section will examine how the composition of the diet used to induce weight loss affects a person's ability to perform exercise, as well as its effect on the preservation of lean tissue.

Obviously, the two macronutrients of major concern are carbohydrate and protein. Carbohydrate is the major choice of fuel for anaerobic exercise (e.g., resistance training), and although it is not the predominant fuel in aerobic exercise, it is the one that ultimately limits endurance time. Protein is required for adequate maintenance of lean body mass.

Is it responsible to assume that adequate levels of exercise can be performed with reduced levels of carbohydrate? Early studies of exercise capacity and carbohydrate restriction employed short periods (14 days or less) of carbohydrate restriction.[23–25] As seen in Table 12–1, studies using longer periods of keto-adaptation resulted in equivalent values for peak aerobic power[26–30] and submaximal endurance[26,27] as long as lean body mass was maintained with adequate protein intake.

The one study of longer keto-adaptation that showed impairment of endurance performance, by Bogardus et al.,[31] may have resulted from the exercise protocol. This study used an intermittent exercise regimen, compared to the continuous regimens used in most other studies, as well as a high intensity level (72% of VO_2 max) for the endurance test.

Taken as a group, the studies shown in Table 12–1 suggest that, given an adequate period for keto-adaptation of 2 weeks or longer, a moderate level of continuous submaximal aerobic exercise is well tolerated.

Although the role of carbohydrate as a fuel during exercise is very important,

TABLE 12–1 Endurance Performance with Carbohydrate Restriction

Reference	Diet			Effect
	Duration	Cho Content	Hypocaloric	
Christenson and Hansen[23]*	7 days	10 g/day	No	Impaired
Bergstrom and Hultman[24]†	14 days	10 g/day	No	Impaired
Phinney et al.[26]	6 weeks	10 g/day	Yes	Same
Bogardus et al.[31]*	6 weeks	10 g/day	Yes	Impaired
Phinney et al.[27]	4 weeks	20 g/day	No	Same
Conlee et al.[28] (rats)	4 weeks	1%	No	Same

CHO, carbohydrate.

*Probably sodium restricted.

† Used intermitent exercise (all other studies employed continuous exercise).

one should not overlook the importance of protein as a determinant of the adequacy of a low-calorie diet or VLCD to support submaximal exercise. Since protein is vital in preserving the functional tissues necessary for exercise, that is, lean body mass, by extension, it is logical that a test of VO_2 max not only provides information on a person's ability to perform exercise but is also a measure of the adequacy of a particular diet in maintaining functional tissue. Thus tests of aerobic capacity, commonly called *graded exercise tests (GXTs),* not only measure fitness but also evaluate the nutritional quality of a low-calorie diet or VLCD. Table 12–2 shows the variability of VLCDs with differing daily protein intake to preserve VO_2 max, which, it should be recalled, is highly correlated with lean body mass. In the VLCDs that were supplemented with daily protein intakes above 1.2 g/kg of ideal body weight (IBW), VO_2 max was preserved[26,29,31]; by contrast, most studies in which daily protein intakes fell below 1.2 g/kg IBW showed a reduction in VO_2 max.[17,32–34] The reduction of aerobic capacity occurred in the lower-protein VLCDs despite the additional carbohydrate provided. These data suggest that VO_2 max, a test of function involving whole body organ systems, may be more sensitive than clinical assessment of body composition or nitrogen balance studies to assess meaningful net change in functional tissue with a major weight loss.

It would appear, therefore, that not only does a well-designed exercise program prepare an individual to maintain the desired weight following major weight loss, but also that the quality and composition of the diet itself increase the ability of the individual to perform the exercise. Therefore the same emphasis must be placed on the nutritional content of the diet and exercise behavior during the active weight loss phase as is placed on these components in the weight maintenance phase if an individual is to succeed in achieving long-term weight control.

TABLE 12–2 VLCD Protein and Preservation of Function

Reference	Exercise	Protein (g/day)	Diet Cho (g/day)	VO_2 max (L/min)	
				Control	VLCD
	Daily Protein ≥1.2 g/kg IBW				
Phinney et al.[26]	No	72	10	2.27	2.45
Bogardus et al.[31]	No	75	75	2.22	2.22
	No	75	10	2.22	1.90
Phinney et al.[29]	No	90	30	1.86	1.97
	Yes	90	30	2.02	2.14
Pavlou et al.[17]	No	90	10	2.80	2.80
	Yes	90	10	2.80	3.40
	Daily Protein ≤1.0 g/kg IBW				
Krotkiewski et al.[32]	No	50	67	1.80	1.70
	Yes	50	67	2.30	2.00*
Gervino[34]	No	56	31	2.26	1.80*
Walberg et al.[33]	Yes	33	94	2.32	2.05*
	Yes	33	44	2.44	2.19*
Pavlou et al.[17]	No	70	30	3.10	2.70*
	Yes	70	30	3.10	3.20

*Significant reduction compared to control.

IMPLEMENTING THE EXERCISE PROCESS

The preceding pages have demonstrated that exercise is both valuable and possible during properly formulated low-calorie diets and VLCDs. However, one of the major dilemmas facing clinicians is how to translate the accumulated scientific knowledge into meaningful information and how to facilitate the process for patients. This is not as simple as teaching a few physiologic concepts, a few relapse prevention strategies, and the standard guidelines for safe and effective physical activity and then giving the command "Go to it!". Even a few strategically placed exercise and/or body composition evaluations are not sufficient to motivate most patients to exercise for the long term. Indeed, despite the valuable research currently being done to assess the role of exercise in the treatment of obesity, the majority of patients who undertake multidisciplinary treatment programs will never initiate or eventually relinquish long-term exercise behaviors. Thus exercise adherence is the biggest problem facing exercise in the treatment of obesity.

For the purposes of this chapter, we now address the fundamental approach to exercise as it relates to obesity treatment. For an in-depth discussion of exercise adherence from a medical and health perspective, including detailed strategies that are used to motivate patients to exercise, the interested reader is directed to the text by Dishman.[35]

Of primary importance is the perspective from which exercise and fitness are viewed. All too often, exercise is defined and evaluated in physiologic terms, focusing on the physiologic products of exercise. These products are the "carrots" used to motivate and encourage patients to exercise. For example, a patient might be told to exercise at a specific intensity, duration, and frequency to produce lowered heart rate, increased VO_2 max, lowered blood pressure, and decreased cholesterol. Using this approach, an endpoint evaluation might measure various products, which would determine whether or not the exercise program had been successful.

While it is true that physical fitness is indeed comprised of many physiologic events and products, exercise is also a behavioral process. It is not enough to teach patients why and how to exercise. They still need to make the psychological commitment to exercise as a positive lifestyle change; and they need to perceive that both the short- and long-term benefits outweigh the risks and effort. In the words of Fox,[36] "Promoting exercise should occur from a process (behavioral) approach rather than from a product (physiological) approach." From this perspective, attempts to achieve a desired behavior (exercise) should be rewarded, rather than focusing on the products of those attempts. All levels of physical activity are valuable because they represent a successful process, even though they may not result in short-term improvements in the products or outcomes of a standard exercise program. This approach not only makes an increase in exercise more achievable for the majority of obese patients (who are generally both unfit and seriously averse to exercise), it also makes exercise more enjoyable and thus more likely to become a repeated behavior.

The process approach does not disregard the importance of physiologic markers and guidelines. Indeed, for high-risk patients, strict exercise guidelines need to be delineated. However, achievement of these markers and guidelines should not be used as the sole standard of success. Thus periodic measurements of physiologic markers can be valuable motivating tools. In addition, rather than using these measurements as successful endpoints, they should be considered indicators of a successful ongoing behavioral process.

Examples of how physiologic outcomes and products of exercise sometimes get in the way of a successful exercise program can be found in some of the recent research involving the complex interrelationship of exercise and obesity. It has been indicated that resistance exercise strategically placed at certain phases of a VLCD might increase lean body mass,[37] that exercise strategically placed at specific times before or after meals might increase the thermic effect of food,[38] and that exercising in a specific way on a specific piece of equipment will maximize caloric expenditure. While much of this research is valuable, and is not being criticized per se, it is a mistake to structure individual exercise programs based on their potential physiologic outcomes if they do not make sense behaviorally. The primary goal of exercise in the treatment of obesity should be to create and validate exercise programs that achieve the greatest behavioral adherence and compliance, followed by the secondary goal of achieving appropriate physiologic change. Until this shift in philosophy occurs, it is doubtful that the poor adherence and compliance data seen in most research and clinical practice will be improved.

A simple strategy to support this approach is relaxation of the standard guidelines of exercise prescription. While upper limits of exercise performance need to be maintained, especially for the high-risk patient, there appears to be no valid reason, using the process approach, for a strict lower limit of exercise performance. In fact, recent studies[39,40] suggest that exercise below the commonly accepted American College of Sports Medicine Guidelines level[5] does result in measurable physiologic changes.

Another strategy that makes sense from a behavioral perspective is monitoring of the recommended or desired activity. This is usually promoted by the practice of keeping diaries or comparing actual performance with predicted goals at routine intervals. This tool is enhanced if the monitoring is provided as feedback to the patient and reinforced by the exercise specialist and/or supervising physician. Self-monitoring alone is not enough. Other strategies are still applicable, of course, but they should be applied with a slightly different objective in mind. The objective is to produce a patient with a behaviorally based, active lifestyle, as opposed to one with a specific physiologic profile.

REFERENCES

1. Harris SS, Casperson CJ, DeFriese GH, et al. Physical activity counseling for healthy adults as a primary preventive intervention in the clinical setting: Report for the US Preventive Services Task Force. *JAMA* 261:3590, 1989.
2. Stunkard AJ, Sorenson TIA, Hanis C, et al. An adoption study of human obesity. *N Engl J Med* 314:193, 1986.
3. Bouchard C, Tremblay A, Despres JP, et al. The response to long-term overfeeding in identical twins. *N Engl J Med* 322:1477, 1990.
4. Phinney SD, Davis PG, Johnson SB, et al. Obesity and weight loss alter serum polyunsaturated lipids in humans. *Am J Clin Nutr* 53:831, 1991.
5. American College of Sports Medicine. *Guidelines for Exercise Testing and Prescription,* ed 3. Philadelphia, Lea & Febiger, 1986.
6. Wilmore JH. Body composition in sport and exercise: Directions for future research. *Med Sci Sports Exerc* 15:21, 1983.
7. Zuti WB, Golding LA. Comparing diet and exercise as weight reduction tools. *Phys Sports Med* 4:49, 1976.

8. Gwinup G. Weight loss without dietary restriction: Efficacy of different forms of aerobic exercise. *Am J Sports Med* 15:275, 1987.
9. Meijer GAL. Physical activity: Implications for human energy metabolism. Ph.D. thesis, University of Limburg at Maastricht, 1990.
10. Oscai LB, Williams BT. Effect of exercise on overweight middle-aged males. *J Am Geriatr Soc* 16:794, et al., 1968.
11. Kolias J, Boileau RA, Barlett HL, et al. Pulmonary function and physical conditioning in lean and obese subjects. *Arch Environ Health* 25:146, 1972.
12. Hill JO, Sparling PB, Shields TW, et al. Effects of exercise and food restriction on body composition and metabolic rate in obese women. *Am J Clin Nutr* 46:622, 1987.
13. Council on Scientific Affairs. Treatment of obesity in adults. *JAMA* 260:2547, 1988.
14. Pavlou KN, Steffee WP, Lerman RH, et al. Effects of dieting and exercise on lean body mass, oxygen uptake, and strength. *Med Sci Sports Exerc* 17:466, 1985.
15. Weltman A, Matter S, Stamford BA. Caloric restriction and/or mild exercise: Effects on serum lipids and body composition. *Am J Clin Nutr* 33:1002, 1980.
16. Van Dale D, Saris WHM, Schofflen PFM, et al. Does exercise give an additional effect in weight reduction regimens? *Int J Obes* 11:367, 1987.
17. Pavlou KN, Krey S, Steffee WP. Exercise as an adjunct to weight loss and maintenance in moderately obese subjects. *Am J Clin Nutr* 49:1115, 1989.
18. Hakim MJ, Holden JH, Darga LL, et al. Effects of exercise on long term weight loss maintenance. *J Cardiopulmonary Rehabil* 9:505, 1989.
19. Van Dale D. Diet and exercise in the treatment of obesity. Ph.D. thesis. University of Limburg at Maastricht, 1989.
20. Whatley J, Istfan N, Blackburn GL. Effect of exercise duration on maintenance of weight loss. *Int J Obes* 10:431A, 1986.
21. Paffenbarger RS Jr, Hyde RT, Wing AL, et al. Physical activity, all-cause mortality, and longevity in college alumni. *N Engl J Med* 314:605, 1986.
22. Blair SN, Kohl HW III, Paffenbarger RS Jr, et al. Physical fitness and all-cause mortality. *JAMA* 262:2395, 1989.
23. Christensen EH, Hansen O. Zur Methodik der respiratorischen Quotient—Bestimmungen in Ruhe und bei Arbeit. *Skand Arch Physiol* 81:137, 1939.
24. Bergstrom J, Hultman E. A study of glycogen metabolism during exercise in man. *Scand J Lab Clin Invest* 19:218, 1967.
25. Pernow B, Saltin B. Availability of muscle substrates and the capacity for prolonged heavy exercise in man. *J Appl Physiol* 31:416, 1971.
26. Phinney SD, Horton ES, Sims EAH, et al. Capacity for moderate exercise in obese subjects after adaptation to a hypocaloric ketogenic diet. *J Clin Invest* 66:1152, 1980.
27. Phinney SD, Bistrian BR, Evans WJ, et al. The human metabolic response to chronic ketosis without caloric restriction: Preservation of submaximal exercise capability with reduced carbohydrate oxidation. *Metabolism* 32:769, 1983.

28. Conlee RK, Hammer RL, Winder WW, et al. Glycogen repletion and exercise endurance in rats adapted to a high fat diet. *Metabolism* 39:289, 1990.
29. Phinney SD, LaGrange BL, O'Connell M, et al. Effects of aerobic exercise on energy expenditure and nitrogen balance during very low calorie dieting. *Metabolism* 37:758, 1988.
30. Davis PG, Phinney SD. Differential effects of two very low calorie diets on physical performance. *Int J Obes* 14:779, 1990.
31. Bogardus C, LaGrange BM, Horton ES, et al. Comparison of carbohydrate-containing and carbohydrate-restricted hypocaloric diets in the treatment of obesity. *J Clin Invest* 68:399, 1981.
32. Krotkiewski M, Toss L, Bjorntorp P, et al. The effect of a very-low-calorie diet with and without chronic exercise on thyroid and sex hormones, plasma proteins, oxygen uptake, insulin and c-peptide concentrations in obese women. *Int J Obes* 5:287, 1981.
33. Walberg JL, Ruiz VK, Tarlton SL, et al. Exercise capacity and urinary nitrogen loss during high and low carbohydrate hypocaloric diets. *Med Sci Sports Exerc* 20:34, 1988.
34. Gervino EV. The effects of a protein sparing modified fast and acute exercise in fibrinolytic activity and lipoprotein patterns in obese women. Ph.D. thesis. Sargent College, Boston University, 1982.
35. Dishman R. *Exercise Adherence: Its Impact on Public Health*. Champaign, Ill, Human Kinetics, 1988.
36. Fox K. Personal communications.
37. Donnelly J, Jacobsen D, Pronk N, et al. Effects of very low calorie diet (VLCD) and exercise on body composition and metabolic rate. *Med Sci Sports Exerc* 21:S32, 1989.
38. Segal KR, Gutin B, Albu J, et al. Thermic effects of food and exercise in lean and obese men of similar lean body mass. *Am J Physiol* 252:E110, 1987.
39. Ballor DL, McCarthy JP, Wilterdink EJ. Exercise intensity does not affect the composition of diet- and exercise-induced body mass loss. *Am J Clin Nutr* 51:142, 1990.
40. DeBusk RF, Stenestrand U, Sheehan M, et al. Training effects of long versus short bouts of exercise in healthy subjects. *Am J Cardiol* 65:1010, 1990.

Behavioral Management of Obesity

CHAPTER 13

Kelly D. Brownell, Ph.D.
and F. Matthew Kramer, Ph.D.

Behavioral programs are among the most widely used approaches for weight loss. There are books and manuals on this approach and the major commercial weight loss centers such as Weight Watchers, Diet Center, and NutriSystem have integrated behavior modification into their programs. Even fad diets and crazy schemes advertised in tabloid newspapers may come with pamphlets or brochures that discuss the importance of behavior change.

There are several reasons for this wide-scale adoption of behavioral techniques and principles. Well over 100 controlled studies testing behavioral approaches have been published, a number far greater than can be claimed for any other approach. This considerable literature is known to researchers, the press, and individuals in policy-making positions, therefore explaining the wide dissemina-

Supported in part by Research Scientist Development Award MH00319 from the National Institute of Mental Health and the Weight Cycling Project of the MacArthur Foundation, both to Dr. Brownell, and by National Research Service Award DK07452 from the National Institute of Diabetes and Digestive and Kidney Diseases to Dr. Kramer.

tion. In addition, behavioral techniques are particularly helpful in efforts aimed at "lifestyle change," a philosophy that has captured the public fancy.

BEHAVIORAL PROGRAMS: A BRIEF DEVELOPMENTAL HISTORY

Early Behavioral Programs

Published results of behavioral programs began to appear in the early 1970s. The researchers involved in these studies found obesity an appealing disorder because it provided an easily quantifiable outcome from which to test theory. Theory was more important than weight loss, so much excitement was generated by studies reporting weight losses of only 5 to 8 lb.

Even though weight losses were small and follow-up periods were brief, there were two important virtues of this era. First, the core procedures of the behavioral program, namely, self-monitoring and stimulus control, were developed and perfected. Second, a generation of researchers in psychology and, to a lesser extent, psychiatry were lured to the study of obesity because of theoretical interests, but subsequently became interested in obesity per se, a phenomenon that has enriched the field.

The Evolution to Modern-Day Programs

Beginning in the late 1970s, researchers studying the treatment of obesity were called on to produce meaningful weight losses in people with significant degrees of obesity. As a consequence, heavier subjects were used, programs became longer, and more techniques were integrated into programs. Programs became more sophisticated with the addition of techniques derived from work on social support, exercise physiology, and cognitive psychology. These are discussed in more detail later.

THE RESULTS OF BEHAVIORAL PROGRAMS

Short-term Results

In the past decade, several major reviews have described the results of behavioral treatment for obesity.[10,13,20,42] Table 13–1 summarizes the basic characteristics and results of earlier and more recent controlled trials of behavior therapy. Early behavioral programs typically lasted for 8 weeks and produced weight losses of about 8 lb. Follow-up of weight maintenance was minimal.

Trials in the late 1970s and early 1980s employed a behavioral "package" that consisted mainly of stimulus control, self-monitoring, and reinforcement

TABLE 13–1 Summary of Data from Controlled Trials of Behavior Therapy Completed Before and During 1974 and During 1978, 1984, and 1986*

	1974	1978	1984	1986
Number of studies included (%)	15	17	15	6
Sample size	53.1	54.0	71.3	93.3
Initial weight (lb)	163.0	194.0	197.0	210.6
Initial per cent overweight	49.4	48.6	48.1	53.4
Length of treatment (weeks)	8.4	10.5	13.2	16.7
Weight loss (lb)	8.5	9.4	15.4	22.0
Loss per week (lb)	1.2	0.9	1.2	1.4
Attrition (%)	11.4	12.9	10.6	20.7
Length of follow-up (weeks)	15.5	30.3	58.4	44.0
Loss at follow-up (lb)	8.9	9.1	9.8	14.5

*All values are means across studies. Studies are those appearing in the *Journal of Consulting and Clinical Psychology*. *Behavior Therapy*. *Behaviour Research and Therapy*, and *Addictive Behaviors*.

Source: Adapted from Ref 13. Reprinted with permission.

techniques. Treatment length increased slightly, to an average of 10 to 12 weeks, and weight losses averaged approximately 11 lb overall (1 lb per week). There also was increased emphasis on long-term follow-up. In the past several years, reports without a follow-up of at least 12 months rarely have been accepted for publication. Certainly, it is important to assess long-term benefits, but the mandate for long follow-up periods may discourage investigators, particularly graduate students and young faculty members with a pressing need to publish, from exploring innovative approaches to treatment.

An important trend apparent in more recent behavioral trials is the marked increase in weight losses, even though most investigators continue to use the basic behavioral package. As examples, average weight losses reported by Craighead and coworkers[17] were 23.9 lb; Jeffery and colleagues.[22] 28.5 lb; Wadden and Stunkard,[39] 31 lb; and Perri and coworkers,[33] 27.4 lb. Referring to Table 13–1, we can see that the average program now is producing considerably larger losses than the early trials. In addition, the 20- to 30-lb losses achieved in the better programs represent a meaningful clinical effect, at least for individuals who are mildly to moderately obese.

Reasons for Improved Short-Term Losses

The improved results seen in more recent programs probably are the result of several factors. First, today's programs are more comprehensive and refined. This seems to be reflected in the slightly higher rate of loss per week seen in the later studies. Programs also have grown in length, which would be expected to produce larger losses. It is interesting to note, however, that despite the fact that most persons lose fastest early in treatment, later studies still have been able to improve upon the rate of loss.

As weight losses have increased, so have initial weights. In addition, there was a surprising increase in attrition for studies in 1986. This increase in attrition is difficult to explain, but in regard to increased initial weight, it is gratifying to note that not only has weight loss increased, but the percentage of initial weight lost has improved (from 5.2% in 1974 to 10.5% in 1986).

Long-Term Results

Weight loss during active treatment is of obvious importance, but the more crucial concern is whether obese persons can be helped to achieve long-term weight loss. Now that there is a growing body of data on follow-ups of 1 year and longer, investigators have found that there are several ways to interpret the results.[10,24,41]

One issue pertaining to the interpretation of long-term results is what the standard of comparison should be. Figure 13–1 shows three hypothetical patterns of weight change over time for obese persons receiving no treatment. Pattern A appears to be the normative outcome for the average American,[28] pattern C shows a trend for weight loss over time, and pattern B shows stable weight maintenance.

Using the data reported in Table 13–2, the long-term weight loss pattern for persons in controlled trials of behavior therapy for obesity also is shown in Figure 13–1. If one takes pattern A as the appropriate comparison, then behavioral treatments appear to have provided a net long-term benefit. If we assume that the average obese person loses weight over a 5-year period, as suggested by Garn and colleagues,[21] and if we consider the concept of regression to the mean, then treatment has had little impact over the long term. Finally, if relatively stable maintenance of weight is used as a point of reference (as usually is done), then some impact, albeit modest, is apparent. Until further information is accumulated, we are not in a position to evaluate fully the long-term impact of interventions.

A second concern in interpreting follow-up results revolves around the course of weight change over time. Follow-ups are costly in terms of time and money, even if one is assured of retaining the majority of subjects. Thus, subjects typically are weighed at relatively long intervals (1 year). If two persons show a net gain of 10 lb over the course of 1 or more years, we cannot be sure, for example, if both experienced gradual regain or if one gained steadily while the other lost weight and then regained. As the interval between assessments increases, the chances of interpretive errors also increases. Kramer et al.,[24] for example, found that, 4 years after treatment, nearly 30 per cent of women were at or below their post-treatment weight. But only 5.3% were at or below this weight for the four follow-ups, done at 1, 2, 3, and 4 years after treatment ended. Clearly, the 4-year results alone suggest a more positive conclusion than do the combined findings for 4 years of annual assessment.

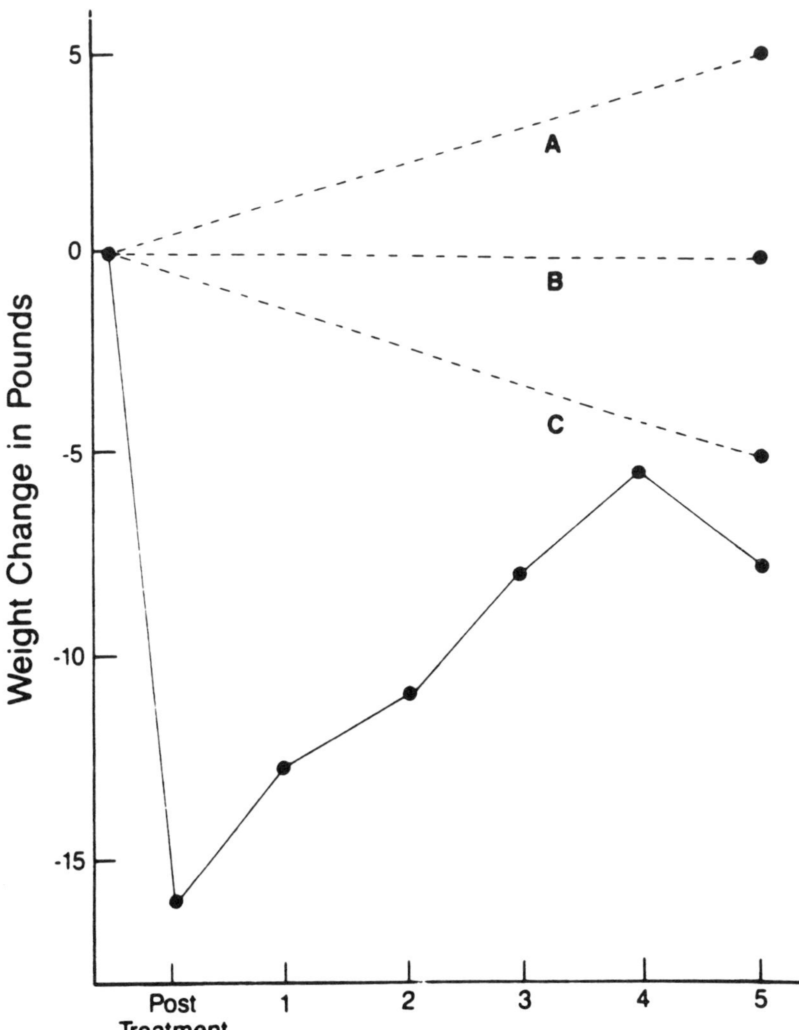

Figure 13–1. Mean weight loss of behavioral programs at posttreatment and at 1, 2, 3, 4, and 5 years of follow-up. Lines A, B, and C represent hypothetical groups of persons receiving no treatment against which to compare the results of behavioral programs. Line A represents the natural history of obese persons receiving no treatment as gradual weight gain. Line B shows stable weight, and line C shows gradual loss.

(From Ref. 10, p. 355. Reprinted with permission)

TABLE 13–2 Net Weight Loss* Over Time in Behavioral Studies with Follow-ups of More than 1 Year

	Posttreatment	1 Year	2 Years	3 Years	4 Years	5 Years
Number of studies (%)	13	8	7	4	4	4
Mean weight loss (lb)	16.0	12.7	11.1	7.95	5.3	7.5

*Averages across studies.

An additional concern in relatively infrequent assessments over a number of years is how to account for the fact that a substantial portion of patients either participate in subsequent treatments or try self-help weight-loss plans. Wadden and associates,[41] for example, found that a net weight loss 3 years after treatment was decreased noticeably if the effects of intervention after the initial treatment were taken into account. The issue is not that our treatments have no long-term impact, but that it is difficult to disentangle the impact of a particular treatment from both later treatments and life events.

As behavioral researchers have placed greater emphasis on maintenance of weight loss, average length of follow-up has increased to about 1 year in studies done in the 1980s. Thus, we have considerable information about change in the first year following treatment. We also are accumulating a database about longer-term outcome.

The results for the first year of follow-ups for behavioral treatment of obesity are encouraging. Reviews such as Wilson and Brownell[42] conclude that weight losses at 1 year typically are similar to those posttreatment and sometimes, slightly better. Even given the fact that some patients suffer substantial regain and that results vary greatly across and within studies, these findings for 1 year lend credence to the value of behavioral interventions.

Table 13–2 shows weight maintenance averaged across studies, with follow-ups of 2 years or more. Consistent with studies with 1 year of follow-up, weight maintenance at 1 and even 2 years posttreatment is, on average, reasonably promising. A clear trend toward regain is present as follow-up continues. The difficulties in interpreting long-term results were discussed earlier. But, even assuming that people who do not enter treatment either gain or maintain their weight, considerable room for improvement still remains.

STATE-OF-THE-ART BEHAVIORAL TREATMENT

Conceptual Model

Behavioral treatment of obesity is grounded in the basic premise of changing daily habits or behaviors in order to achieve the desired goal. The focus is on eating behaviors, attitudes, social support, exercise, nutrition, and other factors related to eating. Contrary to popular belief, behavioral intervention is not merely a matter of applying techniques but is an ongoing process for behavior change. At the center of this model is the evaluation of the antecedents and consequences that influence behavior. Treatment is geared toward modifying the situations that promote eating, eating behavior itself, and the consequences or events that follow eating. Although early programs focused primarily on eating per se, comprehensive programs have broadened considerably to employ general behavioral principles in areas such as nutrition, physical activity, social support, and cognitive psychology (for example, thoughts and feelings) as they relate to weight control.

Components of Behavioral Programs

Behavior therapy for obesity typically is conducted in groups of about 10 patients who meet for 1 to 2 hr a week for 12 to 20 weeks. Many programs offer subsequent booster sessions as well. Some programs also require a financial deposit in order to enhance participation in the program; even a small deposit can have a significant effect on attendance.

Common to both the early behavioral studies and the more comprehensive approaches now in use is a core series of self-monitoring and stimulus-control methods and, frequently, reinforcement techniques. This core formed the basis of most programs until late in the 1970s, when behaviorists began to broaden the scope of their methods. Current programs have incorporated cognitive restructuring approaches, including relapse prevention. There also is an increased emphasis on the role of exercise and social support in the achievement of long-term weight loss. More recently, nutrition also has been given greater consideration. Table 13–3 provides a detailed list of the many specific techniques that may be of value in the treatment of obesity.

Self-Monitoring

Self-monitoring is a standard assessment and treatment component of behavioral interventions. Self-monitoring at the start of treatment is invaluable in assessing the person's eating and exercise behavior. It not only promotes behavior change by increasing awareness of one's behavior but also is a useful index of a person's motivation to put time and energy into the process of change. As treatment progresses, self-monitoring provides a method for evaluating how the person is changing, which techniques are useful, which events or behaviors are especially problematic, and so forth.

Patients typically keep a daily log on which they record what, when, and where they eat as well as the circumstances (that is, who else is there, how they are feeling, what else they are doing). Progress toward meeting one's goals can

TABLE 13–3 Techniques in a Comprehensive Program for Weight Control

LIFESTYLE TECHNIQUES

1. Keep an eating diary
2. Maximize awareness of eating
3. Examine patterns in your eating
4. Prevent automatic eating
5. Identify triggers for eating
6. Weigh yourself regularly
7. Keep a weight graph
8. Use the ABC approach
9. Alter the antecedents to eating
10. Do nothing else while eating
11. Follow an eating schedule
12. Eat in one place
13. Do not clean your plate
14. Put your fork down between bites
15. Pause during the meal
16. Shop on a full stomach
17. Shop from a list
18. Buy foods that require preparation
19. Keep problem foods out of sight
20. Keep healthy foods visible
21. Remove serving dishes from table
22. Leave the table after eating
23. Serve and eat one portion at a time
24. Follow the 5-minute rule
25. Avoid being a food dispenser
26. Use alternatives to eating
27. Use techniques for eating away from home
28. Prepare in advance for special events
29. Plan in advance for high-risk situations
30. Identify your behavior chains
31. Interrupt your behavior chains

EXERCISE TECHNIQUES

32. Keep an exercise diary
33. Understand six benefits of exercise
34. Increase walking
35. Maximize pleasure of walking
36. Increase lifestyle activity

TABLE 13–3 *Continued*

37. Use stairs whenever possible
38. Know the calorie values of exercise
39. Use the pulse test for fitness feedback
40. Choose and use a programmed activity
41. Always warm up and cool down
42. Experiment with jogging
43. Experiment with cycling
44. Experiment with aerobics
45. Counter the exercise-threshold concept

ATTITUDE TECHNIQUES

46. Weigh advantages and disadvantages of dieting
47. Realize complex causes of obesity
48. Distinguish hunger from cravings
49. Confront or ignore cravings
50. Set realistic goals
51. Use the shaping concept for habit change
52. Counter food and weight fantasies
53. Ban perfectionist attitudes
54. Beware of attitude traps
55. Stop dichotomous thinking
56. Counter impossible-dream thinking
57. Focus on behavior rather than weight
58. Banish imperatives from vocabulary
59. Be aware of high-risk situations
60. Distinguish lapse and relapse
61. Outlast urges to eat
62. Cope positively with slips and lapses
63. Use six steps to gain control during lapses
64. Be a forest ranger for urges and lapses

RELATIONSHIP TECHNIQUES

65. Identify and select partner
66. Tell your partner *how* to help
67. Make specific and positive requests of partner
68. Reward your partner
69. Do shopping with your partner
70. Have partner do shopping for you
71. Have partner and family read this manual
72. Exercise with partner
73. Refuse pressures to eat
74. Use pleasurable partner activities

Continued

TABLE 13–3 *Continued*

NUTRITION TECHNIQUES
75. Eat less than 1200 calories per day
76. Be aware of calorie values of foods
77. Know the four food groups
78. Eat a balanced diet
79. Get adequate protein in diet
80. Get adequate carbohydrate in diet
81. Increase complex carbohydrates
82. Limit fat to 30% of total calories
83. Make low-calorie foods appetizing
84. Consume adequate vitamins
85. Take no more than recommended doses of vitamins
86. Increase fiber in diet

Source: Brownell KD. *The LEARN Program for Weight Control.* Dallas: American Health Pub. Co., 1992. Reprinted with permission.

be evaluated by comparing the entries to the daily or weekly goals the patient and group leader have established together. Self-monitoring can be extended to include exercise, nutrition, or social factors as well.

Stimulus Control

Stimulus control methods grew out of observations that obese persons seemed to be particularly responsive to external cues (for example, time of day, setting, sight of food) in their eating behavior.[37] As a result, behaviorists taught clients a variety of ways to reduce their exposure to food and cues associated with eating. Although subsequent research[36] indicates that externality is neither unique to obese persons nor characteristic of all obese persons, the methods that came out of the externality hypothesis remain an integral part of behavioral treatment and, at least for many persons, appear to be of value.[1]

The specific techniques vary from person to person but several methods commonly are employed. First, exposure to food is reduced by keeping food stored out of sight as much as possible, avoiding or reducing the purchase of problematic foods, and reducing food handling and preparation. Second, eating times and places, and activities associated with eating are limited. In other words, eating is limited to few specific times in the day, in only one or two prescribed places, and other activities, such as reading or watching television, are curtailed as much as possible. Third, efforts are made to break habitual or "automatic" eating routines. Instead of automatically making the two pieces of buttered toast for breakfast, for example, one could take out one piece of bread and a small pat of butter, return the remaining bread and butter to their places, and prepare and eat the one slice of bread before making a decision to have a second slice. The idea is to break automatic chains of behavior.

Reinforcement

Reinforcement techniques are used to provide a better balance of positive and negative consequences during weight loss and to provide a bridge to the time when the benefits of weight loss achieve greater potency. The simplest sort of reinforcement is provided though satisfaction that comes from observing (via self-monitoring) desired behavior changes. More powerful reinforcements include self-reinforcement and those provided by family or friends. Although financial rewards may be useful, selecting a highly desirable event as a reinforcement for achieving a specific goal can be helpful. Attending a movie with a friend or buying a new outfit could be used as a reward for meeting one's goal of eating only in certain places and circumstances. Reinforcement helps to maintain the behavior necessary for weight loss and also provides pleasure through something other than eating.

Nutrition

Behavioral programs typically have paid inadequate attention to nutrition. Patients are advised to set a daily calorie goal of approximately 1500 calories for men and 1200 for women, which are adjusted as needed for a given individual. The most vigorous programs, however, also help patients learn more about the constituents of the diet and work toward developing one that not only will be appropriate for weight control but also will increase overall healthfulness. Designing a diet that lowers sodium and fat, for example, is likely to help in weight loss efforts[19] and also to reduce the risks of hypertension, cardiovascular disease, and high cholesterol often associated with obesity. The methods used to control amount of food eaten can be used as profitably to change what is eaten.

Exercise

Just as behavioral methods are helpful in changing eating behavior (energy intake), so too can they be helpful in improving physical activity (energy output). Controversy exists as to whether moderate exercise will decrease appetite and counter the drop in resting energy expenditure induced by dieting. The extra calories used by increased activity, the positive physical and psychological consequences of exercise, and the usefulness of exercise as an alternative behavior to eating, however, all point to the value of including a strong exercise component in the treatment regime.

Patients are taught to increase physical activity in two ways. First, in daily living, people can increase activity by taking stairs rather than elevators or escalators, parking farther from the store, and so on. Second, a programmed exercise component gradually is introduced. For example, the patient may begin by taking a 20-min walk four times a week and, over time, increasing the frequency, length, and pace of walking. As fitness improves, more vigorous activity can be introduced. Starting slowly, avoiding injury, and making the activity as convenient (cost, preparation, and so on) as possible all are important in promoting adherence to the exercise program.

Social Support

For many persons, increasing support and reducing intended or unintended undermining by family members and friends can be an important component for success. Several studies have found that active support by spouses or peers can have positive effects.[9,10] Likewise, offers of food, insistence that the patient prepare high-calorie foods for his or her spouse, and ridicule of the obese person's efforts all can reduce the likelihood of continued behavior change. Patients need to learn, seek support, and deal with social interactions that threaten their efforts.

Cognitive Change

Comprehensive behavioral programs now routinely include components directed toward modifying the attitudes and beliefs that may have an impact on treatment success. Obese persons often hold negative beliefs about themselves and their bodies, as well as about their past and present efforts to attain weight loss. A significant component of their beliefs derives from the omnipresent negative attitudes in Western society about people who are overweight.

Cognitive methods[26] are geared toward modifying those beliefs that are irrational in order to improve the odds of success. A person who sees herself as "a disgusting slob who fails at everything" when she looks in a mirror or overeats at a meal is less likely to continue her efforts than someone who can recognize that success or failure at weight control is only one aspect of her life and that failure at any one point does not make future failure inevitable.

NEW DIRECTIONS FOR MAXIMIZING WEIGHT LOSS

Screening

The effects of a treatment depend on the quality of the program and on the nature of the patients who enter the program. Until recently, attention has been focused almost exclusively on the first factor (improving treatment), and little work has been done on patient selection factors. This is surprising because it is clear that not all patients profit from our intervention.

Important advances are being made in the identification of factors that predict response to treatment.[4] The philosophy underlying this research, however, has been that such identification would permit professionals to devote special attention to individuals with a poor prognosis. There are several possible flaws in this logic.[11] One is the assumption that there is something beyond the treatments now being used that can be offered to such individuals. In the case of clinical programs, the treatment being offered is the most intensive available, so one wonders what the next step would be. In the case of less intensive programs, such as self-help groups, referral to a more intensive program may be useful, but there also are several questionable assumptions in this approach.[11] One assumption is that such persons will succeed if they only can find the correct approach, and another is that the cost of such efforts are justified.

It is possible to take a different perspective on this issue of predicting success.[10,11] If screening criteria could be developed, professionals would be better prepared to (1) match patients to treatments (discussed later), and (2) devote resources to individuals most likely to benefit.

It is a much different philosophy to devote energy and resources to those most likely to succeed than those likely to fail. Screening could be used to target specific programs to those likely to benefit and to spare others the negative consequences of initial weight loss followed by regain. This approach is likely to be more cost effective, which is important for public health reasons.[5]

Screening also might prevent relapse in those who do not have a good prognosis. In a review paper on relapse, Brownell et al.[11] discussed six consequences of relapse: (1) losing and regaining weight can foster feelings of inadequacy; (2) initial weight loss followed by regain may lead to metabolic alterations[8]; (3) failure may convince a patient that the problem is intractable, discouraging him from entering another program later; (4) "negative contagion" can occur in treatment groups, where a person who is not doing well can discourage others who are; (5) the morale of professionals can suffer from failure to help patients; and (6) fewer resources are left for those who might profit.

One way to maximize weight loss from a program is to provide it to those who will respond. This, of course, does raise a number of complex ethical issues and forces us to rely on imperfect screening criteria.[11] We raise the issue here not because screening currently is practical, but because the philosophy of screening may help stimulate more work on screening criteria. In addition, screening may be an effective method for improving the impact of our approaches.

Matching Individuals to Treatments

Many treatments exist for obesity. These include approaches as far-ranging as popular diet books and surgery. There are self-help and commercial groups, exercise programs, and counseling from a variety of professionals. The prevailing logic to comparing these approaches has been to search for the "best." If possible, one would conduct a grand controlled study with millions of subjects assigned randomly to each approach, and from the effort would emerge the victorious program. This mentality of searching for the single treatment of choice has stifled inquiry into approaches that may have some value and has discouraged clinicians from considering a number of possible treatments for any one patient.

As an example, let us say that a controlled trial is undertaken comparing a behavioral approach with a self-help group. In the behavioral program, 60% of the subjects achieve their goal weight loss, whereas only 40% do so in the self-help group. As interesting as the superiority of the behavioral approach might be, we must consider that 40% of those receiving it did not reach goal and that the same percentage did reach goal with the self-help program.

From this perspective, clinicians may serve their patients best by considering the array of treatments available and attempting to match people to those treatments. This is a fruitful area for research because much more needs to be known about the criteria for such matching. Some of the relevant matching criteria might be degree overweight: sex; age; desire for group versus individual treatment; need for a structured diet; need for supervised exercise; cost, frequency, and convenience of meetings; and so forth. Because of the absence of research, we can only speculate about these factors.

We believe this issue is important as we devise ways to maximize weight loss. If individuals find treatments best suited to their personalities and needs, better weight loss is likely to ensue. Both professionals and patients are likely to benefit, and weight losses may be improved over both the short and long term.

Increasing Initial Weight Loss

It is common to hear professionals and dieters alike say that losing weight is easy; keeping it off is the challenge. Certainly, there is much room for improvement in the maintenance of weight loss, but we do not believe the field should be complacent about producing greater initial losses. Even the best behavioral programs produce weight losses of no greater than 30 lb on the average, so increased initial losses would be a great help, especially for individuals with 30 lb or more to lose.

Increasing the initial loss would have several advantages.[10] If we assume that there is a gradual weight gain with most programs once treatment has ended, a substantial initial weight loss would give patients an increased chance of having a clinically meaningful weight loss over the long term. Greater initial losses also provide something substantial to maintain, which should provide more motivation for patients during maintenance phases of programs.

Increasing treatment length. One way to increase weight loss is to increase the length of treatment. As the typical behavioral programs grew in length from 8 to 12 to 16 weeks, the average losses increased from 8 to 11 to 20 lb or more. In a meta-analysis of behavioral programs, Bennett[2] found that program length was one of the best predictors of program success. It is not known how long treatment can be extended without reaching a point of diminishing returns. This is an area where additional research would be helpful, but the existing literature suggests treatment of at least 16 weeks.

Increasing the rate of weight loss. Behavioral programs typically encourage weight losses of 1 to 2 lb per week. More rapid weight loss may be one means of increasing the clinical effectiveness of programs. The most thoroughly tested method of producing large, rapid weight loss is the use of very low calorie diets. These are discussed in detail in this volume and elsewhere.[3,39,40] These can enhance the rate of weight loss, so the major issue remaining is maintenance. Combining aggressive diets with behavior modification may be a fruitful approach in this regard (discussed later).

Tangible incentives. Several investigators have examined the role of financial incentives in enhancing weight loss.[10,22,23,25] Financial contracts have been used in which patients deposit money, which then is refunded in increments based on weight loss. The deposits have been made in a lump sum, by payroll deduction, and by electronic transfer from bank accounts. Controlled studies using this approach show average weight losses about 30% greater than those using the same behavioral program without incentives. Given these positive findings, these procedures deserve further exploration and may be valuable in light of the previous discussion of screening.

Social support. The important ties between social support and susceptibility to and recovery from disease are well documented.[14] This led some obesity researchers to examine the role social support might play in enhancing weight loss. Involving spouses in the treatment process has been examined in a number of studies, but the results do not show a consistently positive effect.[9,12,18] It is our belief that some dieters profit a great deal from the involvement of spouses but, in other relationships, spouse involvement has a negative effect. A research priority is to develop criteria identifying these different types of couples. In the meantime, clinicians should explore with the patient the possibility of involvement of the family, friends, spouses, coworkers, or others who might provide support.

Social support also has been elicited in community settings through weight-loss competitions between groups. This has been done primarily in work-site programs, in which teams of employees compete to reach target weights.[6,7] The initial results of these approaches have been positive, so this method of enhancing motivation can be considered among the possible techniques for increasing weight loss in settings where groups or individuals might enter into competitive programs.

COMBINING TREATMENTS

Behavior therapy offers the greatest hope for maintaining weight losses because of its focus on systematic changes in lifestyle behaviors. It does have limits, however, primarily because it produces weight losses of 30 or fewer pounds on the average. Many patients have more weight than this to lose. This raises the possibility of combining behavioral treatments with other dietary or even surgical approaches, in hope of producing substantial weight losses with the other approaches and maintaining the losses via the behavior modification.

Combining with Very Low Calorie Diets

Much attention has been paid recently to the large and rapid losses produced by aggressive diets. Because this approach now is being used widely, there is great concern about maintaining weight losses. Early reports on these diets suggested rapid regain after the rapid loss, so great hope was held out that behavioral treatments could be used to sustain the losses.

Perhaps the most extensive trial to test this assumption was done by Wadden and Stunkard.[39] Fifty-nine subjects who averaged 89% overweight were assigned to groups receiving either a very low calorie diet alone, behavior therapy alone, or the combination of the diet and behavior therapy. At the end of initial treatment, weight losses were 31 lb for the diet alone, 31.5 lb for behavior therapy alone, and 42.5 lb for the combination.

At a 1-year follow-up, the average weight losses were 10 lb for the diet alone, 21 lb for the behavior therapy alone, and 28.4 lb for the combination. The combined treatment differed significantly from the diet-alone group but not from the behavior therapy alone group. Wadden and Stunkard concluded that

> the results of this study, the first controlled trial of very low calorie diet, confirm the widespread belief that rapid weight loss is followed by almost equally rapid regain. These results also add to the increasing evidence of the effectiveness of behavior therapy. Further research is needed to improve the application of behavior therapy to very low calorie diet.

It is clear from these data that the combination of behavior therapy with aggressive diets is not yet the marriage all had hoped for. It is possible that the regain after cessation of very low caloric diets is inevitable, but we are more hopeful that with further refinement, it will be possible to take advantage of the best of both approaches and to produce greater weight losses that can be sustained subsequently. Currently, however, this is speculation and must await confirmation from controlled trials.

Combining with Pharmacotherapy

The same rationale that led investigators to combine behavior therapy with aggressive diets led to the combination of behavior therapy and drug treatments. As examples, three studies examined the separate and combined effects of fenfluramine and behavior therapy.[12,16,17] In these cases, cessation of the drug led to rapid weight regain, irrespective of whether behavior therapy was used. The combined group in one study[17] did more poorly than the group receiving only behavior therapy, so one could make the interpretation that the drug compromised the effects of behavior therapy.

This literature has not shown the combination of drugs and behavior therapy to be very promising. But only a narrow range of drugs has been tested, and relatively few studies have attempted to combine these approaches. With the advent of drugs that may be more safe and effective than those in the past, more attempts to combine treatments will be in order.

Combining with Surgery

Surgery for obesity would seem to present another opportunity for combining treatments. Some surgery programs include behavioral instruction, but controlled trials using surgery with and without behavior therapy are needed to determine whether this approach's promise can be realized. Because eating patterns and dietary behavior are among the factors the surgical patient must consider, a comprehensive behavioral program may be helpful in the long term.

STRATEGIES FOR MAINTENANCE

Methods for promoting long-term weight loss are of critical importance. Better screening and treatment matching, along with more aggressive means for increasing initial weight loss, will set the stage for an even greater focus on long-term success. Weight loss over the long term thus far has met with limited success; however, recent developments give some reason for optimism about the future.

Although obesity probably is classified most accurately as a chronic rather than an acute problem, most of our interventions have been oriented toward treating it in an acute manner. Some authors are now stressing the importance of taking a long-term viewpoint, however, explicitly recognizing the need for continuing attention in order to achieve continuing success.[10,29]

One major method for improving long-term outcome is greater emphasis on physical activity. Exercise during treatment usually provides some additional benefit, but it is in the long run that incorporating physical activity into the daily routine will provide the maximum benefit. Substantial evidence suggests that better long-term weight loss is found in persons with higher levels of activity.[15,38]

Social support also is an area of great potential for enhancing long-term success. Eating frequently is done with other people, and the way in which the obese person views his or her weight and weight-loss efforts is strongly affected by "significant others." Investigations support the utility of social variables in the form of spouse involvement[9] and competition in the work site.[6] Although much remains to be discovered about tapping the potential of social support, the area deserves attention in our programs.

There has been much interest in recent years in understanding and preventing relapse.[11,27] A failure or slip at some point, which is almost a certainty, often precipitates a predictable sequence of events, involving negative feelings and self-statements, lack of coping ability or skills, and, ultimately, discontinuation of efforts to maintain weight loss. Relapse prevention approaches[27] are aimed at teaching patients skills and changing attitudes so that when lapses do occur, patients are able to cope with them. In addition, as patients learn to identify high-risk situations, they can develop changes in their lifestyle to reduce their exposure to these risky situations.

The work of Perri and colleagues[29,33] exemplifies state-of-the-art treatment combined with the most recent developments in weight loss maintenance. Patients typically are enrolled for a 20-week treatment program. Average weight losses are over 20 lb. As positive as these initial losses are, of greater interest are the variety of maintenance methods these researchers have evaluated.[29–35] This group has examined the impact of posttreatment therapist contact, exercise programs, problem-solving training, relapse prevention, peer support, social influence, and combinations of two or more of these. In addition to evaluating how these methods have affected long-term loss, they also usually evaluated adherence or continued use of the techniques.

This series of studies has found that increasing treatment length and adding an aerobic-exercise component can improve initial weight loss, and during maintenance, exercise may have some additional benefit. Posttreatment therapist contact also proves to be of value, particularly if that contact is aimed at problem solving for specific problems that arise during maintenance. Peer support and social influence approaches were of minimal value as sole maintenance methods but, when combined with other methods such as aerobic exercise, they enhance adherence and weight loss success.

Perri[29,33] concludes that multifaceted strategies are most appropriate. He notes that weight loss is apparent only during active treatment or during posttreatment maintenance and, as a result, he suggests including a tertiary treatment phase in

TABLE 13–4 Possible Methods for Enhancing Long-Term Weight Loss

1. Consider other treatments for our patients.
2. Develop criteria to match patients to treatments.
3. Develop criteria for screening patients to determine if there would be a better time to diet or a better program to join.
4. Increase initial weight losses.
5. Increase the length of treatment.
6. Be more aggressive about attaining goal weight. Consider the "initial treatment phase" as the period necessary to reach goal weight. "Maintenance" should not be considered until there is substantial weight loss to maintain.
7. Increase the emphasis on exercise. Structured, supervised exercise programs need to be tested against current programs in which patients are given only verbal or written advice about exercise.
8. Exploit the social environment as a means to improve long-term adherence. More research is necessary to define the factors in the family, work site, community, and so on that can be used to facilitate weight loss.
9. Financial incentives, which have been effective in producing some of the best losses in behavioral studies, need to be extended for use in the long-term.
10. Combine behavioral programs with other treatments such as commercial and self-help programs, aggressive diets, or surgery.
11. Evaluate the cognitive factors that are included in most programs by consensus, but which have not been studied in detail.
12. Possibly extend stimulus-control methods into the dieter's daily life by considering different mechanisms for food delivery and for supervised exercise.
13. Study the use and timing of relapse prevention methods in more detail.

Source: Ref. 100 Reprinted with permission.

which patients can obtain help as necessary. Table 13–4 describes a variety of methods that can be incorporated into the maintenance phase of treatment. Further work is needed, but Perri's results indicate that well-designed, multifaceted maintenance programs do improve long-term results.

SUMMARY

Much progress has been made in the development of behavioral programs in recent years. As a consequence, the behavioral approach now is integrated into most programs for weight loss.

Because "behavior modification" is practiced so widely, there is a tendency to believe that it consists of little more than a series of techniques or tricks such as record keeping and slowing eating, and that programs do not vary much in how it is employed. This is mistaken. A modern-day, comprehensive program is sophisticated and involves systematic work, not only on eating behavior, but on exercise, attitudes, social relationships, nutrition, and other factors.

The better behavioral programs now are producing weight losses in the range of 25 to 30 lb. The greatest strength of the behavioral approach, however, lies in the maintenance of weight loss. This is an area where exciting developments are occurring. These developments are important, not only to clinicians and programs using behavior modification per se, but to professionals using nearly any approach to weight loss where the maintenance of loss is an issue. The horizon holds much promise for the potential of behavioral approaches, used alone or in combination with other treatments for obesity.

REFERENCES

1. Beneke WM, Paulsen B, McReynolds WT, et al. Long-term results of two behavior modification weight-loss programs using nutritionists as therapists. *Behav Ther* 4:501, 1978.
2. Bennett GA. Behaviour therapy for obesity: A quantitative review of the effects of selected treatment characteristics on outcome. *Behav Ther* 17:554, 1986.
3. Blackburn GL, Lynch ME, Wong SL. The very low calorie diet: A weight-reduction technique, *in* Brownell KD, Foreyt JP (eds), *Handbook of Eating Disorders: Physiology, Psychology, and Treatment of Obesity, Anorexia, and Bulimia*. New York, Basic Books, 1986, pp 198–212.
4. Brownell KD. Behavioral, psychological, and environmental predictors of obesity and success at weight reduction. *Int J Obes* 8:543, 1984.
5. Brownell KD. Public health approaches to obesity and its management. *Annu Rev Public Health* 7:521, 1986.
6. Brownell KD, Cohen RY. Stunkard AJ, et al. Weight-loss competitions at the work site: Impact on weight, morale, and cost-effectiveness. *Am J Public Health* 74:1283, 1984.
7. Brownell KD, Felix, MRJ. Competitions to facilitate health promotion: Review and conceptual analysis. *Am J Health Promotion* Summer 28, 1987.
8. Brownell KD, Greenwood MRC, Stellar E, et al. The effects of repeated cycles of weight loss and regain in rats. *Physiol Behav* 38:459, 1986.
9. Brownell KD, Heckerman CL, Westlake RJ, et al. The effect of couples training and partner cooperativeness in the behavioral treatment of obesity. *Behav Res Ther* 16:323, 1978.
10. Brownell KD, Jeffery RW. Improving long-term weight loss. Pushing the limits of treatment. *Behav Ther* 18:353, 1987.
11. Brownell KD, Marlatt GA, Lichtenstein E, et al. Understanding and preventing relapse. *Am Psychol* 41:765, 1986.

12. Brownell KD, Stunkard AJ. Couples training, pharmacotherapy, and behavior therapy in the treatment of obesity. *Arch Gen Psychiatry* 38:1224, 1981.
13. Brownell KD, Wadden, TA. Behavior therapy for obesity: Modern approaches and better results, in Brownell KD, Foreyt JP (eds), *Handbook of Eating Disorders: Physiology, Psychology, and Treatment of Obesity, Anorexia, and Bulimia*. New York, Basic Books, 1986, pp. 180–197.
14. Cohen S, Syme SL (eds), *Social Support and Health*. New York, Academic Press, 1985.
15. Colvin RH, Olson SB. Winners revisited: 18-month follow-up. *Addict Behav* 9:305, 1984.
16. Craighead LW. Sequencing of behavior therapy and pharmacotherapy for obesity. *J Consult Clin Psychol* 52:190, 1984.
17. Craighead LW, Stunkard AJ, O'Brien RM. Behavior therapy and pharmacotherapy for obesity. *Arch Gen Psychiatry* 38:763, 1981.
18. Dubbert PM, Wilson GT. Goal setting and spouse involvement in the treatment of obesity. *Behav Res Ther* 22:227, 1984.
19. Flatt JP. The difference in the storage capacities for carbohydrate and for fat, and its implication in the regulation of body weight. *Ann NY Acad Sci* 499:104, 1987.
20. Foreyt JP, Goodrick GK, Gotto AM. Limitations of behavioral treatment of obesity: Review and analysis. *J Behav Med* 4:159, 1981.
21. Garn SM, Pilkington JJ, Lavelle M. Relationship between initial fatness level and long-term fatness change, *Ecol Food Nutr* 14:85, 1984.
22. Jeffery RW, Bjornson-Benson WM, Rosenthal BS, et al. Effectiveness of monetary contracts with two repayment schedules on weight reduction in men and women from self-referred and population samples. *Behav Ther* 15:272, 1984.
23. Jeffery RW, Gerber WM, Rosenthal BS, et al. Monetary contracts in weight control: Effectiveness of group and individual contracts of varying size. *J Consult Clin Psychol* 51:242, 1983.
24. Kramer FM, Jeffery RW, Forster JL, et al. Long-term follow-up of behavioral treatment for obesity: Patterns of weight regain among men and women. *Int J Obes*. 13:123–136, 1989.
25. Kramer FM, Jeffery RW, Snell MK, et al. Maintenance of successful weight loss over 1 year: Effects of financial contracts for weight maintenance or participation in skills training. *Behav Ther* 17:295, 1986.
26. Mahoney MJ, Mahoney BK. *Permanent Weight Control: A Total Solution to the Dieter's Dilemma*. New York, WW Norton, 1976.
27. Marlatt GA, Gordon JR (eds). *Relapse Prevention: Maintenance Strategies in Addictive Behavior Change*. New York, Guilford Press, 1985.
28. National Center for Health Statistics. Height and weight of adults ages 18 to 74 years by socioeconomic and geographic variables: United States. Vital and Health Statistics, DHHS Pub No. (PHS) 81–1674. Data from the National Health Survey Series 11, No. 224.

29. Perri MG. Maintenance strategies for the management of obesity, in Johnson WG (ed), *Advances in Eating Disorders,* vol. 1: *Treating and Preventing Obesity*. Greenwich, Conn, JAI Press, 1987, pp. 177–194.

30. Perri MG, McAdoo WG, McAllister DA, et al. Effects of peer support and therapist contact on long-term weight loss. *J Consult Clin Psychol* 55:615, 1987.

31. Perri MG, McAdoo WG, McAllister DA, et al. Enhancing the efficacy of behavior therapy for obesity: Effects of aerobic exercise and a multicomponent maintenance program. *J Consult Clin Psychol* 54:670, 1986.

32. Perri MG, McAdoo WG, Spevak, et al. Effect of a multicomponent maintenance program on long-term weight loss. *J Consult Clin Psychol* 52:480, 1984.

33. Perri MG, McAllister DA, Gange JJ, Jordan RC, McAdoo WG, and Nezu AM. Effects of four maintenance programs on the long-term management of obesity. *J Consult Clin Psychol,* 56:529, 1988.

34. Perri MG, Nezu AM, Patti ET, and McCann KL. Effect of length of treatment on weight loss. *J Consult Clin Psychol*. 57:450, 1989.

35. Perri MG, Shapiro RM, Ludwig WW, et al. Maintenance strategies for the treatment of obesity: An evaluation of relapse prevention training and post-treatment contact by mail and telephone. *J Consult Clin Psychol* 52:404, 1984.

36. Rodin J. The current status of the internal-external obesity hypothesis. *Am Psychol* 36:361, 1981.

37. Schachter S. Rodin J. *Obese Humans and Rats*. Washington, DC, Erlbaum/Wiley, 1974.

38. Stalonas PM, Perri MG, Kerzner AB. Do behavioral treatments of obesity last? A 5-year follow-up investigation. *Addict Behav* 9:175, 1984.

39. Wadden TA, Stunkard AJ. Controlled trial of very low calorie diet, behavior therapy, and their combination in the treatment of obesity. *J Consult Clin Psychol* 54:482, 1986.

40. Wadden TA, Stunkard AJ, Brownell KD. Very low calorie diets: Their efficacy, safety, and future. *Ann Intern Med* 99:675, 1983.

41. Wadden TA, Stunkard AJ, Liebschutz, J. Three-year follow-up of the treatment of obesity by very low calorie diet, behavior therapy, and their combination. *J Consult Clin Psychol,* 56:925, 1988.

42. Wilson GT, Brownell KD. Behavior therapy for obesity: An evaluation of treatment outcome. *Adv Behav Res Ther* 3:49, 1980.

Stress and Weight Maintenance: The Disinhibition Effect and the Micromanagement of Stress

CHAPTER 14

Richard Friedman, Ph.D., Alan Shackelford, M.D., Sarah Reiff, B.A., and Herbert Benson, M.D.

STRESS MANAGEMENT AND WEIGHT MAINTENANCE

The literature on weight loss has shown that stress has a disinhibiting, that is, a facilitating effect on the eating behavior of precisely those individuals likely to be patients in weight loss programs.[1–2,3] Most weight loss programs teach patients behavioral and psychological techniques that are intended to help inhibit inappropriate eating.[4] However, on exposure to situations that are perceived as stressful, individuals who have sought professional help for weight loss are less likely to be able to apply these techniques, thereby allowing disinhibition.[5] Therefore, it is important to address the stress–eating relationship in treatment and to incorporate stress management procedures that prevent disinhibition.

Most behavioral programs that deal with stress and its effects on eating rely

The preparation of this chapter was partially supported by a grant-in-aid from the American Heart Association, Suffolk County, N.Y., and by Sherman/Warburg Fellowships. The authors wish to thank Vivian Stabiner for her assistance.

on patient use of cognitive strategies to prevent inappropriate eating in stressful situations. However, during exposure to stress, previously taught cognitive strategies are likely to be abandoned as anxiety rises and may be least helpful to individuals when they need them most. When confronted with stressful events, patients need a strategy that will allow them to gain quickly and easily the composure necessary to use other behavioral responses. We propose that contingent elicitation of the relaxation response, if it is effectively taught, may be useful as a stress management approach in weight maintenance. In this chapter we will discuss the stress disinhibition effect, the relaxation response, and its use in the micromanagement of stress related to stimulus events likely to trigger inappropriate eating.

The Innate Response to Stress

The physiologic response to stress involves autonomic nervous system activation. More specifically, stress results in increased sympathetic nervous system activity, preparing the individual for physical activity such as fighting or fleeing. This stress response has appropriately been labeled the *fight-or-flight response*.[6] This response involves a dramatic increase in the blood supply to the large muscle groups in the body and an increase in metabolism, heart rate, blood pressure, and respiratory rate. Sympathetic nervous system activation also results in inhibition of gastric motility[7] and promotes the release of sugar into the bloodstream. Hence, on purely physiologic grounds, psychological stress should suppress eating. Indeed, many researchers have pointed out that the physiologic response to stress mimics internal sensations associated with satiety.[8] For many individuals, there is thus a clear inverse relationship between psychological stress and eating.

The Inapt Response to Stress

Despite the physiologic response to stress exhibited by all, two types of individuals appear to increase rather than decrease eating in response to stress: obese individuals and normal-weight dieters.[9] Hence, one important distinction that must be made when discussing the relationship of stress to eating is the response of the dieter/obese individual, occasionally labeled the *restrained eater*, from the response of the nondieter/normal-weight individual, occasionally labeled the *unrestrained eater*.

Unrestrained eaters are individuals who do not deliberately attempt to restrain their food intake. By this, we do not mean to imply that unrestrained eaters do not think about food intake at all or do not actively modulate their eating behavior. They simply do not focus on restraining their food intake or on inhibiting their eating. *Restrained* eaters do focus on inhibition of eating. Examples not related to food may be useful. Behavioral therapists treat individuals who engage in hair twirling, nail biting, or other motoric behavior patterns. Most people occasionally bite their nails or twirl their hair. They are labeled unrestrained. For some however, the behaviors become sufficiently problematic so that clinical intervention is required. The patient is usually taught a series of behavioral and cognitive strategies to reduce the frequency of the problematic behavior and become a successful inhibitor or restrainer. The restrained nail biter or hair twirler is likely to exhibit an increase in the problematic behavior on exposure to stress. This increase in previously restrained behavior is called *disinhibition*. In contrast, the unrestrained nail biter or hair twirler will usually not exhibit an increase in behavior in response to stress. Similarly, unrestrained eaters will usually not increase eating in response to stress; however, restrained eaters will. The most plausible explanation for the relationship between stress and eating in restrained individuals is that stress is a powerful disinhibitor of otherwise inhibited behaviors.

Further discussion of this point requires consideration of a relatively strict behaviorist approach to inhibited behaviors. Inhibited behaviors in general, and restrained eating in particular, presume the existence of a reinforcement contingency. That is, emitting the inhibited behavior will result in acute reinforcement or reward. The long-range consequences of the behavior, however, might be negative. Our behavioral conceptualization is that inappropriate eating is immediately reinforced, although the long-range consequences of the eating are undesirable. A successful weight loss program changes the contingencies so that the patient becomes capable of inhibiting inappropriate eating behaviors associated with immediate reinforcement in order to achieve the delayed reinforcement of the lower body weight. The relative significance of the acute and chronic reinforcement vectors shifts when stress exposure occurs.

A typical example involves alcohol consumption. Problem drinkers who have attempted to curtail their drinking report that they drink because the immediate effects of drinking are reinforced. That is, drinking makes them feel better, that is, less anxious, at the moment, thus reinforcing the drinking behavior. However, problem drinkers also know that the long-range consequences of this reinforcement cycle are very undesirable. Specifically, the increased probability of drinking will have detrimental effects on their physical health, their professional lives, and their social relationships. Hence, the successful inhibitor abstains by employing cognitive strategies that keep the long-range goals more powerful than the immediate gratification. However, in response to stressful, anxiety-provoking situations, the long-range goals can become less relevant and acute anxiety reduction becomes a more salient immediate goal. If the anxiety reduction can be achieved by emitting the previously inhibited behavior, the probability of the occurrence of the inhibited behavior will increase as anxiety rises.

Clinical experiences, literature, and the popular media are filled with examples of this stress disinhibition effect. An experimental report by Higgens and Marlatt[10] provides a typical empirical observation. In this study, several drinkers exhibited a significant increase in alcohol consumption in a laboratory study when exposed to stress. However, some significant variables must be considered before concluding that stress simply increases inappropriate behavior. In particular, the type of stress has recently been shown to be a highly relevant variable.

Type of Stress and Eating

In the Higgens and Marlatt study,[10] the stress that triggered increased drinking was an evaluative ego threat compared to a more fear-inducing stimulus. That is, the drinkers were exposed to a situation in which they felt that others would think poorly of them. The anxiety associated with this ego threat resulted in disinhibition of drinking. When the stress was more fearful, that is, a threat of electric shock, no increase in drinking occurred. Therefore, an important distinction that must be considered in assessing the effects of stress on inhibited behaviors is the type of stress to which the individual is exposed. As for alcohol consumption, recent evidence suggests that stress associated with physical fears reduces eating in unrestrained individuals and that fear does not increase eating in restrained individuals.[11] In contrast, stress associated with ego-threatening circumstances does increase eating in restrained subjects but does not reduce the eating of unrestrained individuals. Thus, the nature of the stressful situation, whether ego or physical threat is involved, as well as dieting status, must be taken into consideration when predicting stress-induced changes in eating behavior.

Self-esteem and Stress-Induced Eating

The complex interactions between the restrained–unrestrained dichotomy and the type of stress exposure is made even more complex by the necessary consideration of dispositional psychological characteristics such as self-esteem. Some recent evidence suggests that restrained eaters with low self-esteem are most likely to exhibit stress-induced increases in eating.

A study by Heartherton et al.[11] clearly describes the relationships discussed above. In their study, 35 restrained and 40 unrestrained female college students were randomly assigned to one of four experimental conditions: shock threat, failure, speech threat, or a control group. All subjects believed that they were participating in a study of perceptual processes that would examine the relationships between perceptual modalities. They were then exposed to one of the four conditions and asked to complete a taste task. During the task, subjects tasted and rated three large bowls of ice cream. They were then encouraged to eat the leftover ice cream. The bowls of ice cream were weighed before and after they were given to the subjects.

In the shock threat condition, subjects were told that they would taste and rate a food, receive an electrical shock, and then be asked to taste and rate the same food again to see if the shock had changed their taste ratings. In the failure condition, subjects were given an unsolvable concept formation problem. Hence, subjects in this group would be unsuccessful and therefore would likely experience an ego threat. The speech threat group was exposed to an anticipated ego threat. These subjects were told that they would be expected to give a 2-min speech in front of five other students, who would grade them on the fluency of their speech and their grammatical style. These subjects were told that they would be given the topic of the speech after they completed a perceptual task. The control group was told that they would compare taste and spatial perceptions, and that after they completed the taste test, they would be given a concept formation task. In the shock threat, speech threat, and control conditions, subjects were given the taste task and then told that the final tasks were canceled, that is, no shocks or speeches would be given. All subjects were given questionnaires to measure anxiety and mood.

The results of group assignment are presented in Figure 14–1.

Figure 14–1. Grams of ice cream eaten as a function of restraint status and experimental condition.

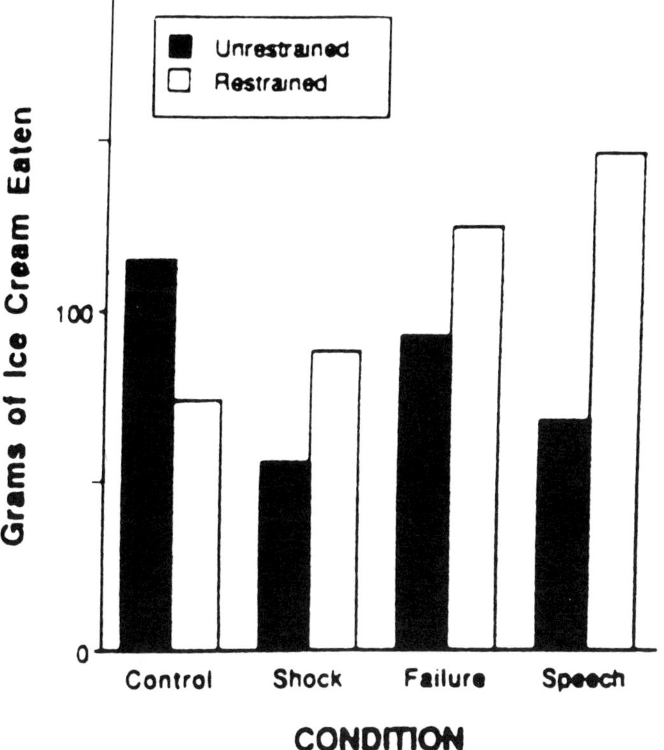

When under stress, the restrained subjects ate more than the unrestrained subjects. Specifically, the restrained subjects in the failure and speech threat conditions ate significantly more than the restrained control subjects. The restrained shock group did not eat significantly more than the restrained control group. In contrast, the unrestrained subjects exposed to the shock condition ate significantly less than the unrestrained control subjects. The unrestrained speech and failure groups both ate non-significantly less than the unrestrained controls.

These results also indicated that self-esteem must be taken into account when determining the effect of stressful events on eating behavior. The data are presented in Table 14–1. As indicated by the authors, "the role of self-esteem was to modify the nature of the restraint-distress interaction such that only the low self-esteem restrained subjects altered their eating in response to the distress conditions; the high self-esteem restrained subjects were unaffected by the distress manipulations" (p. 141). Self-esteem affected the unrestrained eaters in a different respect. The suppressive effect of the shock threat on eating was significant only in subjects with high self-esteem. In addition, the unrestrained subjects with low self-esteem significantly reduced their eating when exposed to the speech threat.

These results, which are representative of the recent literature, suggest that

TABLE 14–1 Grams of Ice Cream Eaten as a Function of Restraint Status, Condition, and Self-Esteem Level

	Restrained		Unrestrained	
Condition	Low Self-Esteem	High Self-Esteem	Low Self-Esteem	High Self-Esteem
Control				
M	53.0	89.8	108. 3	117.9
SE	9.9	8.7	12.4	16.4
n	4	5	3	7
Shock				
M	93.4	84.3	59.8	52.7
SE	13.6	18.0	18.1	9.6
n	4	5	4	6
Failure				
M	156.8	85.0	58.9	107.7
SE	18.4	11.9	17.4	22.5
n	5	4	3	7
Speech				
M	166.2	88.1	36.2	100.2
SE	33.8	50.3	11.7	34.3
n	6	2	5	5

Source: Copyright 1991 by the American Psychological Association. Reprinted with permission.

while stress is not a potent moderator of eating universally, for low self-esteem, restrained eaters (the populations usually seen in clinical weight loss programs), ego-threatening stress may represent a disinhibiting influence resulting in overeating and weight gain. Hence, it is necessary to include stress management as a component of comprehensive weight management.

A Comment on Dieters versus Obese Patients

The distinction between restrained and unrestrained eaters is not the same as the distinction between obese and normal-weight subjects. Dieting is usually associated with restraint, and it is dieting status and not obesity that accounts for the eating response to stress. In clinical practice, the restrained eater is almost always the patient. In research, it is often necessary to distinguish normal-weight, restrained eaters from normal-weight, unrestrained eaters. There are several psychometric instruments that allow this distinction.[12] However, in clinical situations, weight maintenance programs subsequent to clinically induced weight loss will usually involve restrained eaters.

Stress Management Is Not Psychotherapy

The decision to include stress management as a component of weight maintenance programs requires consideration of the appropriate intervention strategy. Often, stress management, especially when ego threats are discussed, is confused with psychotherapy. Once clinicians and patients agree that stress represents a disinhibiting influence and can thereby undermine weight maintenance goals, it is appealing to approach the stress–eating relationship from a psychotherapeutic perspective. Among the goals of psychotherapy is to understand or gain insight into the nature of the stress and to understand why stress may lead to inappropriate eating. These approaches are most often ineffectual and can at times actually be counterproductive. At the crucial moment when the patient is emotionally aroused and about to engage in inappropriate eating, the thought of social support or psychotherapeutically derived insight can and does serve as a rationalization to indulge. Patients report that they feel almost justified in using the behavior, since they have not yet figured out why they behave this way and will at least have something to discuss at a subsequent meeting.

Stress Management Approaches

An alternative behavioral strategy is based on stress management techniques. Rather than concentrating on insight, these techniques are based on conditioning principles that have been successfully used to treat adjunctively a wide variety of clinical disorders.[13] They represent the foundations of the behavioral medicine clinic programs at the New England Deaconess Hospital. They can be easily applied to weight maintenance. The purpose of stress management for weight maintenance is to teach patients to become very sensitive to external and internal stimuli, including ego threats, which are preludes to emotional arousal and are high-risk eating situations. In response to these stimuli, patients are taught to elicit automatically behavioral responses that prevent emotional arousal and reduce the probability of inappropriate eating.

The four basic stress management procedures used in weight maintenance are as follows:

1. Rigorous self-monitoring
   a. Informational value
   b. Therapeutic value
2. Environmental engineering
   a. Manipulating high-risk environments
   b. Manipulating high-risk emotions
3. Relaxation response training
   a. The relaxation response—rationale
   b. The relaxation response—implementation
4. Contingent relaxation
   a. The counterconditioning model
   b. Contingent relaxation response exercises
   c. Long-term goals

Clinical experience indicates that the incorporation of stress management techniques in a comprehensive weight loss program is enthusiastically endorsed by patients. Furthermore, it is relatively simple to use, without a great investment in time or money; practical group application is encouraged and is managed more easily than group psychotherapy. Our clinical experience suggests that it is also an effective long-range therapeutic strategy.

It is important to emphasize at this juncture that we are not suggesting that stress management for weight maintenance is an appropriate intervention strategy *sui generis*. Rather, we are suggesting that this "micromanagement" approach to stress can be effectively embedded in most behavioral treatment plans. For example, Brownell's LEARN program,[14] which we have found to be one of the better behaviorally based weight management programs available, can easily be supplemented by our stress management program.

The LEARN program, like most other behavioral programs, emphasizes self-monitoring and environmental manipulations. In this regard, the program overlaps our stress management approach. In addition, the LEARN program offers wonderful suggestions concerning specific behavioral strategies to help lose weight and keep it off. However, the LEARN program, like most other behavioral packages, does not incorporate specific training in elicitation of the relaxation response and contingent elicitation in response to stressful circumstances. When the concept of stress disinhibition is discussed at all, the recommendation is to engage in a behavior that is incompatible with eating. That is, when the restrained eater is confronted by stress, he or she should react by deciding to do something other than eating. To reiterate a point previously made, at the point of stress exposure, the likelihood of making rational alternative behavioral plans is reduced. The crucial addition to weight maintenance program that we recommend is teaching patients to elicit the relaxation response and to apply it contingently in response to stress. With sufficient practice, the brief reactive relaxation response can become automatic.

Teaching the Relaxation Response

Our approach to self-monitoring and environmental manipulations is essentially the same as described by others. In Chapter 13 of this text, Brownell and Kramer present self-monitoring, stimulus control, lifestyle, and attitude techniques that overlap with our approach and need not be reiterated. We, however, also spend a considerable amount of time on relaxation response training.

The relaxation response is defined as a set of integrated physiologic changes that are elicited when an individual engages in specific thought patterns that involve a repetitive mental focus and the passive ignoring of distracting thoughts. The physiologic modifications that result include decreases in oxygen consumption, heart rate, respiratory rate, and arterial blood lactate and slight increases in skeletal muscle blood flow and in the intensity of slow alpha waves on the electroencephalogram. These changes occur simultaneously and are different from those observed during quiet sitting or sleep. They are consistent with a generalized decrease in sympathetic nervous system tone. Similar physiologic alterations occur during the use of a number of related religious and secular techniques, including progressive muscle relaxation, meditation, autogenetic training, yoga, Zen, and biofeedback.[15]

Two essential components are needed to elicit the relaxation response: (1) mental focusing on a repetitive word, phrase, sound, prayer, or image and (2) the adoption of a passive attitude to intrusive thoughts. Patients are instructed to elicit the relaxation response utilizing a technique that is comfortable for them once or twice daily for 20 min. During group sessions, patients practice the relaxation response together, and considerable time and effort are expended to help patients become familiar with the psychological and physiologic sensations associated with the relaxation response. After several weeks of practice, patients are given exposure to cognitive exercises in which high-risk situations are discussed and then visualized. These discussions are usually included in most behavioral management programs. In our program, however, we ask patients to immediately elicit a "mini" relaxation response for a few seconds as they visualize the stressful stimuli.

At each session, patients are asked to describe situations they have encountered in which they felt stressed or anxious. They are then asked to close their eyes and visualize the situations as vividly as they can. During the visualizations, the patients are repeatedly instructed to elicit the relaxation response when they begin to feel anxious. As the group sessions progress, the specific relationship between stress, anxiety, and eating is addressed and patients are again repeatedly instructed to elicit the relaxation response when anxiety is associated with thoughts of inappropriate eating. After several sessions, it is common for patients to report spontaneous or automatic relaxation response breaks during the week when they are feeling stressed and about to eat. The relaxation response becomes a conditioned response to food-related anxiety.

For those familiar with counterconditioning techniques in behavioral therapy,[16] the procedures we have just described will not be considered innovative. The similarities are deliberate. For the most part, behavioral approaches to weight loss and weight maintenance have relied on operant conditioning principles and cognitive strategies. Classical conditioning procedures have been given relatively little attention. We feel that this balance is appropriate because most of what needs to be accomplished for successful weight loss is achieved by operant conditioning and cognitive restructuring. Again, we refer the reader to Chapter 13 for a detailed description of operant and cognitive conditioning programs. However, given the undesirable aspects of the stress disinhibition effect, behavioral management could be effectively augmented by a classically conditioned response that can be easily integrated into most programs.

CONCLUSION

Preventing the disinhibiting influence of ego-threatening stress is an important therapeutic goal. It would certainly be a formidable task to examine the nature of ego threat in patients whose primary clinical problem is maintaining weight loss. Most patients do not require or desire psychotherapy. According to the literature, time spent gaining insight into the nature of the ego threats or why certain situations are threatening is counterproductive. However, the contingent relaxation response procedures described in this chapter acknowledge the importance of stress in weight maintenance and could offer a simple and feasible approach to the micromanagement of stress.

REFERENCES

1. Herman CP, Polivy J. Anxiety, restraint and eating behavior. *J Abnorm Psychol* 84:666, 1975.

2. Herman CP, Polivy J, Lank C, et al. Anxiety, hunger, and eating behavior. *J Abnorm Psychol* 96:264, 1987.
3. Slochower J, Kaplan SP, Mann L. The effects of life stress and weight on mood and eating. *Appetite* 2:115, 1981.
4. Bennett GA. Behavior therapy for obesity: A quantitative review of the effects of selected treatment characteristics on outcome. *Behav Ther* 17:554, 1986.
5. Ruderman AJ. Dysphoric mood and overeating: A test of restraint theory's disinhibition hypothesis. *J Abnorm Psychol* 94:78, 1985.
6. Cannon WB. *Bodily Changes in Pain, Hunger, Fear and Rage*. New York, Appleton, 1915.
7. Carlson R. *The Control of Hunger in Health and Disease*. Chicago, University of Chicago Press, 1916.
8. Schachter S, Goldman R, Gordon A. Effects of fear, food deprivation, and obesity on eating. *J Pers Soc Psychol* 10:91, 1968.
9. Baucom DH, Aiken PA. Effects of depressed mood on eating among obese and nonobese dieting and nondieting persons. *J Pers Soc Psychol* 41:577, 1981.
10. Higgens RL, Marlatt GA. Effects of anxiety arousal on the consumption of alcohol by alcoholics and social drinkers. *J Consult Clin Psychol* 41:426, 1973.
11. Heatherton TF, Herman CP, Polivy J. Effects of physical threat and ego threat on eating behavior. *J Pers Soc Psychol* 60:138, 1991.
12. Herman CP, Polivy J. Restrained eating, in Stunkard A (ed), *Obesity*. Philadelphia, WB Saunders, 1980, pp. 208–225.
13. Benson H, Stuart E, and the Staff of the Mind/Body Medical Institute. *The Wellness Book: A Comprehensive Guide to Maintaining Health and Treating Stress-related Illnesses*. New York, Crl Publishing Group, 1993.
14. Brownell KD. *The LEARN Program for Weight Control*. Dallas, LEARN Educational Center, 1990.
15. Benson H. *Your Maximum Mind*. New York, Times Books, 1987.
16. Wilson GT, O'Leary KD. *Principles of Behavior Therapy*. Englewood Cliffs, NJ, Prentice-Hall, 1980.

CHAPTER

15 Surgical Treatment of Obesity

Scott A. Shikora, M.D., Peter N. Benotti, M.D., and R. Armour Forse, M.D., Ph.D.

INTRODUCTION

Obesity is generally defined as body weight 20% or more above ideal weight. It is recognized as a major health concern of Western society. The cost in terms of health care dollars and lost production is not insignificant. The National Health and Nutrition Examination Surveys of 1976–80 (NHANES) found that 25% of adult Americans, or about 34 million persons, are obese.[1,2] Of these people, 6 million suffer from morbid obesity (defined as 100% excess body weight or body mass index above 40 kg/m^2).

There is now reasonable unanimity in the medical literature that morbid obesity is associated with serious health hazards and a shortened life span. The multitude of comorbid disease states includes coronary artery disease, diabetes mellitus, hypertension, hepatobiliary disease, endocrine abnormalities, malignancies, degenerative joint disease, cerebrovascular disease, respiratory abnormalities, and sudden death.[3–6] Studies indicate that the relative risks of these conditions have a curvilinear relationship with weight.[3] As weight increases, the prevalence of such illnesses increases disproportionately.[3,7] Van Itallie reports that morbidly obese people have a 3-fold increased likelihood of becoming hypertensive, a 1.5-fold increased likelihood of developing hypercholesterolemia, and a 2.9-fold increased propensity for diabetes.[1] The well-publicized Framingham Heart Study designated obesity as an independent risk factor for cardiovascular disease.[8]

Morbid obesity has also been shown to shorten the life span. Drenick et al. reported a 12-fold excess mortality in morbidly obese males in the 25–34 age group and a 6-fold excess in the 35–44 age group compared to that of men in the general population.[9] Furthermore, Kral found that the mortality rate is double for the morbidly obese compared to the nonobese.[7]

No less significant are the psychosocial aspects of obesity. Poor body image, low self-esteem, depression, and overall poor quality of life have been described.[10]

Although there is much controversy in the medical literature concerning the most effective therapy for obesity, there is unanimity concerning the benefits of significant weight loss. Numerous reports have described amelioration and even resolution of many risk factors, including diabetes, hypertension, and pulmonary disease.[11–15]

A multitude of conservative therapies have been popularized in both the medical and nonmedical communities.[16,17] These include numerous diets, meal substitutes, pills, exercise programs, behavioral modification, hypnosis, support groups, and combinations of the above. Despite the ability of most patients to achieve significant short-term weight loss, the long-term success rate is only about 10–15%, and this only if success is viewed very narrowly.[6,16–18]

Surgical therapy for the treatment of significant obesity has been controversial since its inception in the late 1950s. Many early procedures were technically difficult and had significant operative risks. In addition, some were prone to failure or had the potential for serious late complications. To many, the overall risks of such surgery did not seem to justify the benefits.

The recent refinements in these operations to decrease perioperative complications and reduce failure rates, and the greater recognition of the medical consequences of obesity, have made surgical therapy more acceptable. This chapter will address the role of surgery in the treatment of obesity, including indications, complications, the treatment of failures, and a discussion of the various operative procedures performed.

SURGICAL OPTIONS

The interest in developing surgical procedures for the treatment of medically significant obesity came from the growing recognition of its health consequences and from frustration with the poor long-term results seen with medical therapy. A wide variety of operations were designed to either reduce food intake or limit its absorption.

Intestinal Bypasses

The early surgical approaches to obesity were directed toward limiting nutrient absorption. In the mid-1950s Kremen et al. demonstrated, in a group of dogs and one patient, that bypass of a significant length of intestine can promote weight loss.[19] This initial report led to a number of procedures aimed at detouring the nutrient stream away from a predetermined length of absorptive surface area. These operations are often referred to as *jejunoileal bypass* (*JIB*). Weight loss was directly related to the length of small intestine bypassed. The two most popular variations were the end-to-side shunt of Payne and DeWind[20] and the end-to-end shunt of Scott et al.[21] Both of these procedures excluded approximately 90% of the small intestine from the nutrient stream (Figure 15–1). Tens of thousands of patients had these operations in the 1960s and 1970s. This broad experience confirmed that surgeons could perform these procedures with acceptable risk. Operative mortality was reported to be less than 3%. While perioperative complications were frequent (about 30%), most were minor, including wound infections and phlebothrombosis.[18]

Interestingly, weight loss was discovered to be due primarily to reduction in food intake and, to a lesser extent, to nutrient malabsorption. Appetite normalization was hypothesized to be related to the avoidance of gastrointestinal symptoms

Figure 15–1. The JIB (A) Payne and DeWind technique. (B) Scott et al. technique.

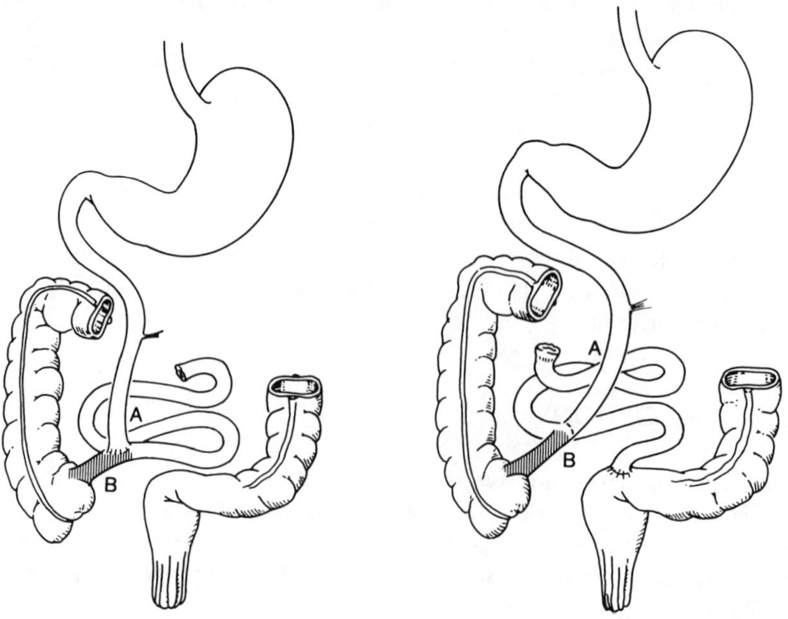

TABLE 15–1 Late Complications of JIB

Liver disease	Nephrolithiasis
Cholelithiasis	Arthropathies
Vitamin deficiencies	Chronic diarrhea
Protein malnutrition	Dermatitis
Bone demineralization	Electrolyte deficiencies
Mineral deficiencies	Intussusception

such as diarrhea, which was induced by eating. Other explanations included loss of taste for sweets and changes in hormonal or metabolic balance.[16,18]

Despite the seemingly good results, these operations fell from favor due to the development of serious late complications (Table 15–1) discovered during long-term follow-up.[22,23] Approximately 25% of patients required hospitalization sometime within the first 2 years for control of severe diarrhea, abdominal pain, and vomiting. More serious complications included liver dysfunction, protein malnutrition, renal disease, and stone formation. Most of these problems were related to either nutrient malabsorption or bacterial overgrowth in the bypassed segment. Hepatic disease, the most potentially life-threatening problem, was reported in about 29% of patients and progressed to cirrhosis in about 7%.[22,24] The fatty deposition and fibrosis were described to be quite similar to alcoholic liver changes.[18]

Despite the benefits of weight loss, many patients required reoperation for bypass reversal due to these complications. It has been reported that as many as 26–41% of patients developed symptoms significant enough to require takedown within 3–5 years after bypass.[24] Simple takedown of the bypass led to significant weight gain in nearly all patients.[24–26] Many surgeons recommend that a gastric partitioning procedure be performed at the time of takedown to prevent weight gain.[25,27–31] The severity of these complications and the high rate of subsequent reversal led to the abandonment of these procedures.[32]

Other modifications of JIB have also been reported. These procedures were designed to match the ability to reduce weight but produce fewer chronic complications. Two of the more popular ones are the biliary-intestinal bypass of Eriksson[33] and the biliopancreatic bypass of Scopinaro and associates.[34] The former involved the anastomosis of the bypassed small bowel with the gallbladder, the later a gastrectomy with Roux-en-Y gastroenterostomy. Both of these operations are described as superior to JIB because they maintain the normal enterohepatic circulation. Unfortunately, there is little evaluation of the long-term results.

Gastric Partitioning Procedures

The significant problems encountered with the malabsorptive procedures prompted the search for alternatives. Gastric partitioning procedures were developed to limit food intake without affecting absorption. The first such procedure was the *gastric bypass* (*GBP*), described by Mason and Ito in 1967.[35] After observing weight loss in patients after extensive gastrectomy, they developed a procedure that partitioned the stomach into a small proximal pouch and a larger distal pouch. The proximal, or functional, pouch was drained by a loop of jejunum. Weight loss was due to the extremely small pouch, which caused symptoms of early satiety after consuming small quantities of food. Unfortunately, the procedure was difficult to perform and had both a significant perioperative complication rate and a high percentage of failures. Several technical modifications, including the introduction of stapling equipment, improved its operative safety and long-term results. Presently, the procedure (Figure 15–2) involves the stapled partition of the stomach without division and Roux-en-Y gastrojejunos-

Figure 15–2. Roux-en-Y GBP.

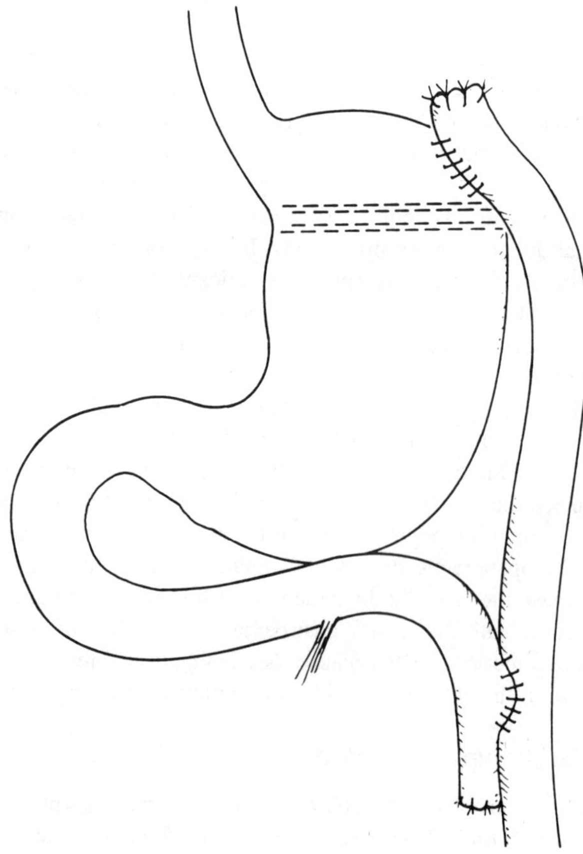

tomy drainage through a 1-cm stoma.[15] Today GBP is the gold standard, the procedure for the treatment of obesity against which all others are judged.[12,15] Weight loss is reported to be about 60% of excess weight within the first 2 years. The patients of Halverson and Koehler lost about 30–35% of excess weight 1 year after bypass and about 60% after 2 years.[36] In another report, Glysteen et al. described a 61% weight loss after the first postoperative year.[11] At our institution, Benotti et al. reported a 50–64% excess weight loss, with a failure rate of about 5%.[14] To date, few studies have published long-term follow-up data. Therefore, gastric partitioning for morbid obesity is still considered advanced therapy.

Recently, significant improvements in technique and decreased perioperative complications have been reported. Operative mortality has been reported to range from less than 1% to 5% but to be as high as 19% in older patients.[13,32] Perioperative complications include splenic injuries, pulmonary and cardiac events, wound infections, thromboembolic disease, anastomotic leaks, intra-abdominal sepsis, and even death.[13,14,37,38] Serious complications are rare, but wound problems are more common.[13,14,36] At our institution, the mortality was reported to be 0.008%. Wound problems were seen in 23% of patients. One patient had a nonfatal pulmonary embolus, 14 patients developed atelectasis, and another 4 had pneumonia. There were no myocardial infarctions, but four patients had superventricular arrhythmias. Only 16 patients (6%) required reoperation.[14] The most threatening early complication is an anastomotic leak. This occurred in 4% of our patients.[14] Patients may manifest few physical signs.[39] Elevated pulse and abdominal, back, or left shoulder pain are the most common findings. Chest x-ray may display a left pleural effusion. There may even be a leukocytosis. Water-soluble contrast studies often can document a leak. Unfortunately, the leak may not always be demonstrated, and a high index of suspicion is required. In many of these cases, prompt, immediate operative exploration is necessary.

Long-term complications are also quite common but are easily managed. These include anemia, vitamin and mineral deficiencies, dehydration, persistent vomiting, and dumping syndrome.[13,14,37,40] Weight loss failures are usually due to dietary indiscretion, which may manifest as pouch dilatation or staple line disruption. Some patients present with intractable vomiting. The workup often revealed stomal stenosis. These anatomic problems often require revision.

The significant morbidity seen with the earlier gastric bypass procedures led to an effort to simplify the technique but maintain the basic design of diminishing the gastric reservoir. A new class of such operations, called *gastroplasties*, first became popular in the 1970s. These procedures were designed to partition the stomach without the gastrojejunostomy, thereby eliminating the potential for an anastomotic leak. Some of the earlier varieties, including the horizontal gastroplasty of Gomez and the gastrogastrostomy, were prone to failure secondary to pouch dilatation and/or staple line disruption and were abandoned.[41]

The vertical banded gastroplasty (VBG), described by Mason in 1982, has become widely popular.[42] It has been shown to be safe and effective. Simply put, it involves the creation of a 30-ml pouch by the application of two double-rowed staple lines. The pouch outlet has a external circumference of 5 cm and is reinforced by a Marlex band. This small channel delays emptying, thereby causing the sensation of early satiety (Figure 15–3).

The vertical banded gastroplasty has been used with variation in the size of the pouch, the size of the outlet, and the type of stapling techniques used to create the pouch. The results are varied but there has been the concern about the high failure rate over time. This has predominately been related to the breakdown of the staple line.[58,64] In addition these studies found that the VBG

Figure 15–3. VBG as described by Mason and Ito.[35]

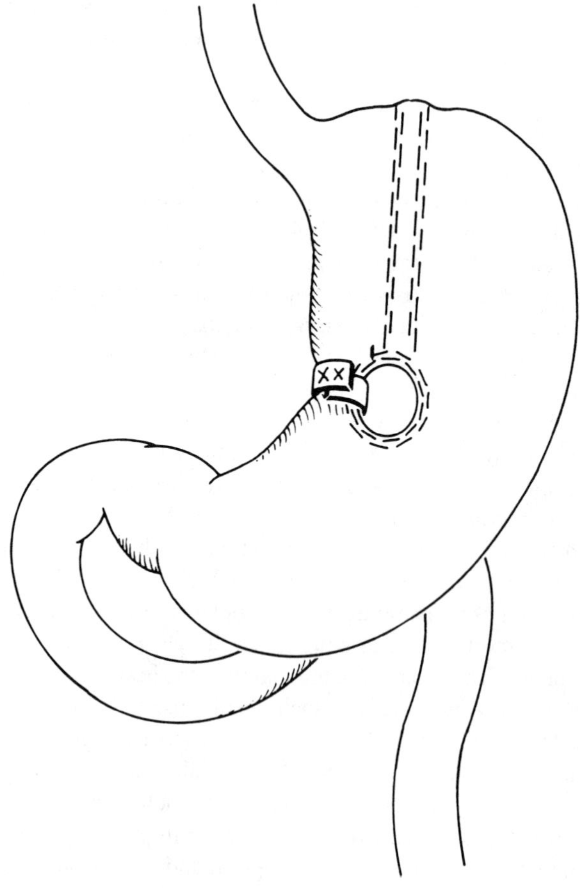

was not effective with the superobese patients. Finally the quality of eating has some problems with the VBG, as the success of the operation usually means that the patient will be consuming predominantly soft or liquid diets.

There are now several studies comparing the gastroplasty to the gastric bypass.[12,15,65] The evidence indicates that the gastric bypass results in a significantly greater weight loss, with fewer patients requiring subsequent revisions for structural failure. Major complications were similar in the two groups. Despite these findings the gastroplasty is still an effective operation with relatively low morbidity. Selection of the operation is predominately done by the surgeon in discussions with the patient, but may be based on the patients nutritional behavior with those consuming more sweets generally doing better with a gastric bypass.[14,15]

Miscellaneous Procedures

A few other techniques were popular in the past but deserve only brief mention. Fat excision, jaw wiring, waist banding, and intragastric balloons have all been reported to induce weight loss. These procedures have been shown to be successful only in the short run or have had major complications.[43] Few bariatric surgeons offer them to their patients.

INDICATIONS FOR SURGERY

The goals of any procedure for weight loss must include the reduction of sufficient excess weight such that associated risk factors are ameliorated or eliminated. The procedure must be able to be performed with acceptable morbidity and mortality rates, and there must be measurable improvement in the quality of the patient's life. The degree to which these goals are achieved often depends on the establishment of rational indications for surgery.

Careful patient selection is the cornerstone of long-term success. Although many postoperative failures can be traced to technical errors, there is still a significant number of patients whose poor results can be attributed to noncompliance. Dietary indiscretion can lead to staple line disruption or pouch dilatation. In addition, some patients display maladaptive eating behavior and have been seen to abuse high-calorie drinks that empty rapidly and induce weight gain without causing structural abnormalities.

The selection process is quite comprehensive. Most centers restrict the procedures to patients who have 100% excess body weight or who, at a minimum, have medically significant obesity.[16,44] Clearly, these technically challenging procedures should not be performed merely for cosmetic reasons. In addition, all potential candidates should have demonstrated repeated failure to control their weight by medical means, including supervised dietary programs.

Careful medical and neuropsychiatric evaluations are performed. Patients with significant medical or psychiatric disease may not be appropriate operative candidates. A strong history of substance abuse may preclude consideration. Some patients who respond favorably to psychiatric or psychological therapy can be reëvaluated for surgery. Extremes of age, on the other hand, are only a relative contraindication in otherwise healthy individuals.

A detailed dietary history is obtained. Patients considered for surgery must not display evidence of eating behavioral patterns (e.g., bulimia) that will preclude compliance with the postoperative dietary restrictions. In addition, they must show evidence of stress and environmental dietary control.

After the initial screening process is completed, many centers rely on a multidisciplinary group including internists, nurses, psychiatrists, dietitians, and surgeons to evaluate potential candidates. A consensus opinion is required to accept a patient for surgery. This process is designed to prevent poor candidates from undergoing surgery. In one report, as many as 50% of all candidates were denied surgery.[45]

PREOPERATIVE ASSESSMENT

Preoperative evaluation to identify significant comorbidity includes the standard surgical laboratory and radiographic studies, as well as pulmonary function tests, gallbladder ultrasonography, cardiac evaluation, and upper gastrointestinal fluoroscopy when indicated. During this period, extensive teaching, counseling, and supervised dietary instructions are provided. A videotape of the procedure and the postoperative course is viewed, which helps to answer many of the most commonly asked questions. Patients are also encouraged to lose weight prior to the operative date. By demonstrating the ability to lose about 10% of their excess weight preoperatively, patients benefit not only psychologically but also physiologically. This weight loss leads to decreased insulinemia, fluid retention, and sympathetic stimulation.

All operative candidates are admitted to the hospital the day prior to surgery. Minidose heparin prophylaxis is administered, and any further workup is completed. On route to the operating room, 2 g of cefalozin antibiotic is given intravenously. This regimen has been shown to be associated with the lowest wound infection rate.[46] At our institution, the standard Roux-en-Y GBP and VBG are performed for all primary procedures. A gastrostomy tube is often placed in the distal excluded stomach, which can be used to supply nutrition should the patient be slow to tolerate adequate oral nutrients or fluids. Cholecystectomy is performed only if there is gallbladder disease—not routinely, as recommended by Schmidt et al.[47]

POSTOPERATIVE MANAGEMENT

Typically, most patients are extubated in the operating room at the conclusion of the procedure or in the recovery room by postoperative day 1. Epidural and patient-controlled analgesia have improved early postoperative pain management and pulmonary toilet. A balanced-electrolyte, dextrose-free solution is given intravenously. The creation of a calorie-deficient state initiates the breakdown of fat and subsequent ketosis. The recovery of ketones in the urine usually occurs within the first 24–48 hr after surgery. Sepsis, on the other hand, will inhibit ketosis in favor of gluconeogenesis. Glucosuria can be used as a sensitive indicator of infection.[48] On the first postoperative day, this solution is fortified with amino acids, vitamins, and minerals. The amino acids have protein-sparing qualities.

The nasogastric tube is usually removed on the fourth day, and a barium swallow is obtained to detect any anastomotic leaks. If none is detected, a supervised dietary protocol is begun. Patients start with small volumes of water and progress to pureed food by the time of discharge. The diet is then advanced to regular food within 6 to 8 weeks. The median length of stay at our institution is 10 days.[14] Patients unable to consume sufficient quantities of food and fluids by mouth can still be discharged in a timely fashion with gastrostomy tube supplementation.

REVISIONAL SURGERY

Bariatric procedures are considered to have failed when patients do not achieve sufficient weight loss, regain weight after initial loss, or have debilitating symptoms.

Since its inception, surgery for morbid obesity has evolved considerably. The learning curve was quite deep. The procedures have become safer and more efficacious. As previously discussed, the original bariatric operations, consisting of intestinal bypasses, were successful in achieving weight loss but often caused significant metabolic derangements. Although most were not life-threatening, some, such as liver dysfunction, had that potential. These procedures were essentially abandoned by most surgeons because the risks outweighed the benefits. Many of the patients treated by these procedures eventually came to revision.

The original gastric partitioning procedures were also plagued by a disturbingly high failure rate. The early gastroplasties and gastrogastrostomies were found to be flawed operations. While they were relatively safe to construct and had minimal metabolic abnormalities, none proved successful for reaching weight loss goals.[41] These procedures were subsequently discarded in favor of the VBG and the GBP, which have been shown to be more effective operations. The GBP is still a technically formidable operation for most surgeons but is now performed with only minimal problems.

Presently, despite careful patient selection and the use of operations that have been shown to be safe and effective, failures still occur. Some authors report a failure rate as high as 25%.[49–51] While technical mistakes do occur (e.g., constructing stomas or pouches of incorrect size), many investigators attribute most failures to patient noncompliance.[39,49,51–53] After surgery, patients are advised to adhere to strict dietary guidelines. Some patients have been found to ignore these restrictions, leading to pouch dilatation, stomal enlargement, or even staple line disruption. A few creative patients will short-circuit their procedure by abusing high-calorie drinks that empty readily. This causes inadequate weight loss without altering the surgical anatomy. Although many groups describe careful preoperative patient selection to avoid operating on those patients likely to not comply, there is no well-established selection process.[50]

Although revisional surgery is often successful in promoting weight loss, it is challenging. Dense adhesions to the spleen, diaphragm, and liver distort the anatomy and obscure the original staple line. A tenuous blood supply to a reconstructed gastrojejunostomy is prone to ischemia and leakage.[50] Many groups report a major complication rate as high as 50%.[49,50,53] While some problems such as stomal stenosis can be dealt with endoscopically, avoiding major surgery, most require operative correction.[54–56] Since failure is often due to patient noncompliance, and since revisional surgery is fraught with potential complications, some surgeons question whether it should be performed routinely.[46–50] Unfortunately, the consequences of ongoing obesity remain. In our experience and in that of others, patients with demonstrated anatomic abnormalities who are deemed capable of following dietary guidelines will be offered revision. Patients with no demonstrable abnormalities, or those who have proven anatomic derangements but who are thought to be incapable of adhering to postoperative dietary restrictions, may be denied surgery.[51]

Presently, many surgeons, including those at this institution, revise all gastric partitioning procedures to gastric bypasses.[39,41,52,57] Failed gastric bypasses usually require reconstruction of the gastrojejunostomy, restapling of the stomach pouch, or both. Maclean et al.[58] favor reconstruction of a failed VBG without conversion to GBP unless there is outlet obstruction or erosion of the mesh into the gastric lumen. In those cases, they recommend conversion of the VBG to the GBP by removal of the Marlex band, stapled closure of the pouch, and side-to-side anastomosis of the lesser curvature to a Roux-en-Y loop of jejunum brought up in a retrocolic and retrogastric position. (Figure 15–4A). Another variation of this technique involves the anastomosis of the gastric pouch end-to-side to the Roux-en-Y loop of jejunum, with suture closure of the distal channel (Figure 15–4B).

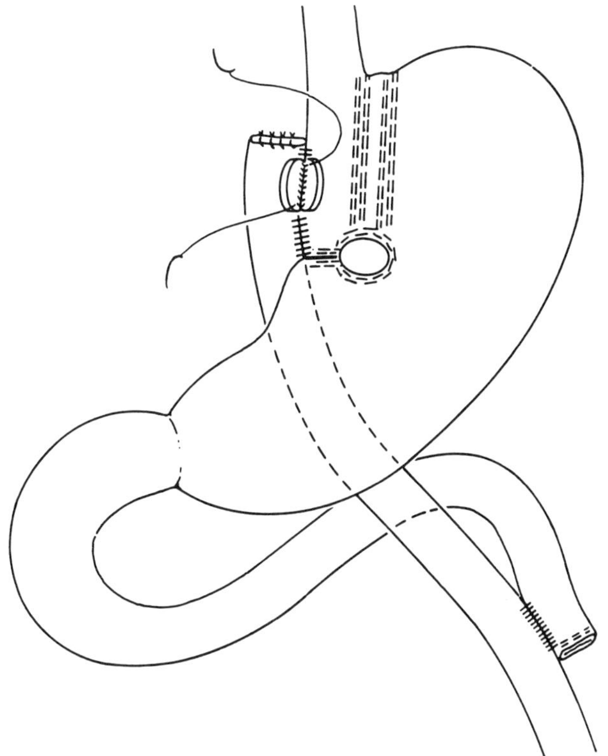

Figure 15–4. Conversion of the VBG to a Roux-en-Y GBP, as described by Maclean et al.[58] The end of the vertical pouch maybe closed (A) or used for the anastomosis (B).

LONG-TERM CONSIDERATIONS

A good surgical result does not ensure a successful outcome. Surgery is only one aspect of the comprehensive management needed to maximize weight loss. Bothe et al. described the process as involving three priorities: cue control and food avoidance behavior change, establishment of increased activity patterns, and weight-reducing surgery.[48] Despite anatomically limiting the gastric storage capacity, patients are still required to modify their eating behavior. Strict guidelines are often necessary to prevent the tendency to resume inappropriate eating habits and the potential for staple line disruption or pouch/stomal dilatation. One such set of eating guidelines dictates that patients consume three small solid meals daily. These are eaten very slowly, with approximately 5 min between

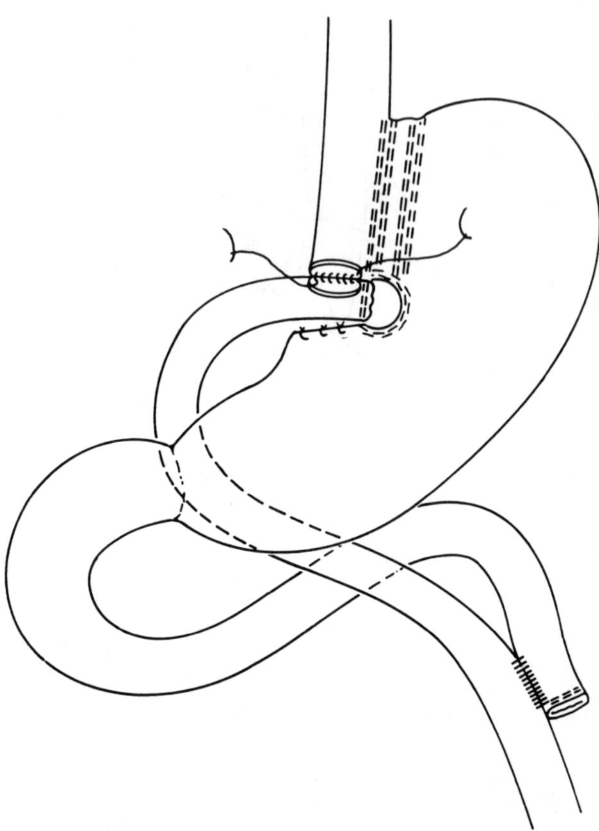

Figure 15–4. *Continued*

each bite. No liquids are allowed with meals, and the meal should cease when the sensation of hunger passes.[36]

As expected, patient compliance and outcome are directly related to the number of postoperative follow-up office visits.[36] Follow-up should address psychological issues and outgoing nutritional concerns and should screen for signs of potential failure. Patients given access to weekly seminars, tutorial sessions, and group meetings develop a sense of partnership in their weight loss program and are more eager to participate. Again, the vast resources of a multidisciplinary team are quite useful.

Although postoperative malnutrition was common following intestinal bypasses, it seems to be a much less serious issue following gastric restrictive procedures. After JIB, there is a significant loss of lean body tissue. These patients resemble those suffering from kwashiorkor malnutrition. In contrast, the gastric procedures produce marked loss of fat with only minimal changes in lean body tissue.[48] Therefore, fewer long-term nutritional sequelae are encountered. On the other hand, vitamin deficiencies are prevalent after gastric bypass.[59] Serum iron, folate, and vitamin B_{12} levels must be closely and chronically monitored. Most patients will require lifelong supplementation. Since the VBG does not produce these vitamin deficiencies, it may be the procedure of choice for menstruating women.

OUTCOME

The primary goal of surgery for morbid obesity is to induce weight loss sufficient to ameliorate associated medical problems such as diabetes, heart disease, and respiratory abnormalities. There is no consensus among bariatric surgeons as to the magnitude of weight loss necessary to achieve this goal.[60] Some authors feel that the loss of as much as 50–70% of excess weight is necessary.[14] There are a number of reports describing improvement and even resolution of morbid obesity–associated diseases with surgically induced weight loss of even a lesser magnitude.

Herbst and coworkers[61] reported improvement in blood sugar control in 23 morbidly obese patients with adult-onset diabetes mellitus 6 weeks after surgery. Fourteen of these patients no longer required insulin, and another seven were able to reduce their insulin requirements by 72%. Weight loss in this group averaged only 30 kg. In addition, the authors noted that the improvement in glucose control persisted over a follow-up period that averaged about 20 months. Similar results were described by others.[11,12,15]

The beneficial effects of weight loss on cardiovascular disease has also been described. Gleysteen et al.[11] reported decreased serum triglyceride levels and improved lipid profiles in 42 morbidly obese patients 1 year after surgery. The group had a mean weight loss of 61% of excess weight. They also noted persistent improvement as long as 5 to 7 years postoperatively despite a 12% weight regain. Alpert and coworkers[62] studied ventricular function using echocardiography in morbidly obese patients both preoperatively and after weight loss. They reported significant improvement in left ventricular ejection fraction and lesser improvements in chamber size and ventricular wall thickness. In addition, they reported improvement in blood pressure. This has also been described by others.[11,12,15]

Pulmonary manifestations of morbid obesity include the obesity-hypoventilation syndrome and the sleep apnea syndrome. Both problems are life-threatening and can occur together (Pickwickian syndrome). Sugarman and coworkers[63] reported an incidence of at least one of these disorders in 14% in their patients. They described improvement or cure in most of their patients after weight loss. Their group had a mean loss of 45% of excess weight. They found improvements in arterial blood oxygenation, decreased carbon dioxide retention, decreased episodes of sleep apnea, increased lung volumes, and resolution of polycythemia vera.

A number of other associated medical problems, such as infertility, arthritis, and venous stasis disease, have also been shown to improve with weight loss.[60]

In a recent study morbidly obese patients were studied with echocardiography, nuclear scans, and right heart catheterizations.[66] The patients were challenged with both fluid and physical exercise. After 100 pounds of weight loss, the patients returned and had the studies including the right heart catheterization repeated. The initial studies demonstrated the presence of the obese cardiomyopathy with both structural and functional changes. These cardiac alterations improved with the magnitude and the maintenance of the weight loss. The improvement included decreases in the thickness of the heart, and an improvement in the exercise response, with increased ventricular work.

CONCLUSION

Presently, morbid obesity is an incurable disease. Since the biologic basis for this illness remains unknown, specific therapy is still not available. The consequences of the comorbidities are significant. The cost in terms of shortened life expectancy, need for chronic health care, and poor overall quality of life mandates ongoing efforts to treat the disease. The limited success achieved by the various nonsurgical approaches has fueled interest in promoting the surgical option. The state-of-the-art procedures to date, GBP and VBG, have been shown to be safe and efficacious. The proceedings of the National Institutes of Health Consensus Development Conference on *Gastrointestinal Surgery for Severe Obesity*[67,68] states that GBP or VBG, as part of a comprehensive weight management program, offers the best long-term therapy for severe obesity. Until science finds a cure to the underlying biologic derangements that cause obesity, surgery to assist weight loss will continue to be necessary.

REFERENCES

1. Van Itallie TB. Health implications of overweight and obesity in the United States. *Ann Intern Med* 103(6 pt 2):983, 1985.
2. National Institutes of Health Consensus Development Conference statement. Health implications of obesity. *Ann Intern Med.* 103:147, 1985.
3. Bray GA. Complications of obesity. *Ann Intern Med.* 103(6 pt 2):1052, 1085.

4. Drenick EJ. Sudden cardiac arrest in morbidly obese surgical patients unexplained after autopsy. *Am J Surg* 155:720, 1988.
5. Van Itallie TB. Obesity: Adverse effects on health and longevity. *Am J Clin Nutr* 32:2723, 1979.
6. Fitzgerald FT. The problem of obesity. *Annu Rev Med* 32:221, 1981.
7. Kral JG. Morbid obesity and related health risks. *Ann Intern Med* 103(6 pt 2):1043, 1985.
8. Hubert HB, Feinleib M, McNamara PM, et al. Obesity as an independent risk factor for cardiovascular disease: A 26-year follow-up of participants in the Framingham Heart Study. *Circulation* 67:968, 1983.
9. Drenick EJ, Bale GS, Seltzer F, et al. Excessive mortality and causes of death in morbidly obese men. *JAMA* 243:443, 1980.
10. Van Itallie TB, Kral JG. The dilemma of morbid obesity. *JAMA* 246:999, 1981.
11. Gleysteen JJ, Barboriak JJ, Sasse EA. Sustained coronary-risk-factor reduction after gastric bypass for morbid obesity. *Am J Clin Nutr* 51:774, 1990.
12. Hall JC, Watts JM, O'Brien PE, et al. Gastric surgery for morbid obesity. The Adelaide study. *Ann Surg* 211:419, 1990.
13. Halverson JD. Gastric restriction procedures for morbid obesity. *Surgical Rounds* 49, 1988.
14. Benotti PN, Hollingshead J, Mascioli EA, et al. Gastric restrictive operations for morbid obesity. *Am J Surg* 157:150, 1989.
15. Sugarman HJ, Londrey GL, Kellum JM, et al. Weight loss with vertical banded gastroplasty and Roux-Y gastric bypass for morbid obesity with selective versus random assignment. *Am J Surg* 157:93, 1989.
16. Lerman RH, Cave DR. Medical and surgical management of obesity. *Adv Intern Med* 34:127, 1989.
17. Forse A, Benotti PN, Blackburn GL. Morbid obesity: Weighing the treatment options-surgical intervention. *Nutrition Today* 10, 1989.
18. Adibi SA, Stanko RT. Perspectives on gastrointestinal surgery for treatment of morbid obesity: The lesson learned. *Gastroenterology* 87:1381, 1984.
19. Kremen AJ, Linner JH, Nelson CH. An experimental evaluation of the nutritional importance of proximal and distal small intestine. *Ann Surg* 140:439, 1954.
20. Payne JH, DeWind LT. Surgical treatment of obesity. *Am J Surg* 118:141, 1969.
21. Scott HW, Dean RH, Shull HJ, et al. New considerations in use of jejunoileal bypass in patients with morbid obesity. *Ann Surg* 177:723, 1973.
22. Hocking MP, Duerson MC, O'Leary P, et al. Jejunoileal bypass for morbid obesity. Late follow-up in 100 cases. *N Engl J Med* 308:995, 1983.
23. Jewell WR, Hermreck AS, Hardin CA. Complications of jejunoileal bypass for morbid obesity. *Arch Surg* 110:1039, 1975.
24. Pessa ME, Hocking MP, Woodward ER. Management of the patient with a jejunoileal bypass. *Infect Surg* 110, 1988.

25. Hitchcock CT, Jewell WR, Hardin CA, et al. Management of the morbidly obese patient after small bowel bypass failure. *Surgery* 82:356, 1977.
26. Halverson, JD, Gentry K, Wise L, et al. Reanastomosis after jejunoileal bypass. *Surgery* 84:241, 1978.
27. Ackerman NB. Metabolic consequences from conversion of jejunoileal bypass to gastric bypass. *Ann Surg* 196:553, 1982.
28. Junker K, Jensen JB, Jensen HE. Simultaneous small-intestinal reconstruction and gastric partitioning as treatment for complications after jejunoileal bypass for morbid obesity. *Scand J Gastroenterol* 16:433, 1981.
29. Tapper D, Hunt TK, Allen RC, et al. Conversion of jejunoileal bypass to gastric bypass to maintain weight loss. *Surg Gynecol Obstet* 147:353, 1978.
30. Pessa M, Robertson J, Woodward ER, et al. Surgical management of the failed jejunoileal bypass. *Am J Surg* 151:364, 1986.
31. Griffen WO, Hostetter JM, Bell RM, et al. Experiences with conversion of jejunoileal bypass to gastric bypass. Its use for maintenance of weight reduction. *Arch Surg* 116:320, 1981.
32. Halverson JD, Scheff RJ, Gentry K, et al. Jejunileal bypass. Late metabolic sequelae and weight gain. *Am J Surg* 140:347, 1980.
33. Eriksson F. Biliointestinal bypass. *Int J Obes* 5:437, 1981.
34. Scopinaro N, Gianetta E, Civalleri D, et al. Bilio-pancreatic bypass for obesity. II. Initial experience in man. *Br J Surg* 66:618, 1979.
35. Mason EE, Ito C. Gastric bypass in obesity. *Surg Clin North Am* 47:1345, 1967.
36. Halverson JD, Koehler RE. Gastric bypass: Analysis of weight loss and factors determining success. *Surgery* 90:446, 1981.
37. Buckwalter JA, Herbst CA. Complications of gastric bypass for morbid obesity. *Am J Surg* 139:55, 1980.
38. Peltier G, Hermreck AS, Moffat RE, et al. Complications following gastric bypass procedures for morbid obesity. *Surgery* 86:648, 1979.
39. Eckhauser FE, Knol JA, Strode WE. Remedial surgery following failed gastroplasty for morbid obesity. *Ann Surg* 198:585, 1983.
40. Marcuard SP, Sinar DR, Swanson MS, et al. Absence of luminal intrinsic factor after gastric bypass surgery for morbid obesity. *Dig Dis Sci* 34:1238, 1989.
41. Sugarman HJ, Wolper JL. Failed gastroplasty for morbid obesity. Revised gastroplasty versus Roux-Y gastric bypass. *Am J Surg* 148:331, 1984.
42. Mason EE. Vertical banded gastroplasty for obesity. *Arch Surg* 117:701, 1982.
43. Munro JF, Stewart IC, Seidelin PH, et al. Mechanical treatment for obesity, in Wurtman RJ, Wurtman JJ (eds), *Human Obesity. Annals of the New York Academy of Sciences*, Vol. 499. New York, 1987, p. 305.
44. Buckwalter JA. Nonsurgical factors important to the success of surgery for morbid obesity. *Surgery* 91:113, 1982.
45. Halverson JD, Zuckerman GR, Koehler RE, et al. Gastric bypass for morbid obesity. A medical-surgical assessment. *Ann Surg* 194:152, 1981.

46. Forse RA, Karam B, MacLean LD, et al. Antibiotic prophylaxis for surgery in morbidly obese patients. *Surgery* 106:750, 1989.
47. Schmidt JH, Hocking MP, Rout WR, et al. The case for prophylactic cholecystectomy concomitant with gastric restriction for morbid obesity. *Am Surg* 54:269, 1988.
48. Bothe A, Bistrian BR, Greenberg I. Energy regulation in morbid obesity by multidisciplinary therapy. *Surg Clin North Am* 59:1017, 1979.
49. MacArthur RI, Smith DE, Hermreck AS, et al. Revision of gastric bypass. *Am J Surg* 140:751, 1980.
50. Schwartz RW, Strodel WE, Simpson WS, et al. Gastric bypass revision: Lessons learned from 920 cases. *Surgery* 104:806, 1988.
51. Halverson JD, Koehler RE. Assessment of patients with failed gastric operations for morbid obesity. *Am J Surg* 145:357, 1983.
52. Buckwalter JA, Herbst CA, Khouri RK. Morbid obesity. Second gastric operations for poor weight loss. *Am Surg* 51:208, 1985.
53. Cates JA, Drenick EJ, Abedin MZ, et al. Reoperative surgery for the morbidly obese. A university experience. *Arch Surg* 125:1400, 1990.
54. Sataloff DM, Lieber CP, Seinige UL. Strictures following gastric stapling for morbid obesity. Results of endoscopic dilatation. *Am Surg* 56:167, 1990.
55. Kretzschmar CS, Hamilton JW, Wissler DW, et al. Balloon dilation for the treatment of stomal stenosis complicating gastric surgery for morbid obesity. *Surgery* 102:443, 1987.
56. Rajdeo H, Bhuta K, Ackerman NB. Endoscopic management of gastric outlet obstruction following surgery for morbid obesity. *Am Surg* 55:724, 1989.
57. Torres JC, Oca CF, Honer HM. Gastroplasty conversion to roux-en-Y gastric bypass at the lesser curvature due to weight loss failure. *Am Surg* 51:559, 1985.
58. MacLean LD, Rhode BM, Forse RA. Late results of vertical banded gastroplasty for morbid and super obesity. *Surgery* 107:20, 1990.
59. Printen KJ, Halverson JD. Hemic micronutrients following vertical banded gastroplasty. *Am Surg* 54:267, 1988.
60. Brolin RE. Results of obesity surgery. *Gastroenterol Clin North Am* 16:317, 1987.
61. Herbst CA, Hughes TA, Gwynne JT, et al. Gastric bariatric operation in insulin-treated adults. *Surgery* 95:209, 1984.
62. Alpert MA, Singh A, Terry BE, Kelly DL, el-Deane MS, Mukerji V, Villarreal D, Artis AK. *Am J Card* 64:1361, 1989.
63. Sugarman HJ, Fairman RP, Baron PL, et al. Gastric surgery for respiratory insufficiency of obesity. *Chest* 90:81, 1986.
64. MacLean LD, Rhode BM, Forse RA. A gastroplasty that avoids stapling in continuity. *Surgery* 113:780, 1993.
65. MacLean LD, Rhode BM, Forse RA, et al. Results of the surgical treatment of obesity. *Am J Surg* 165:155, 1993.

66. Alaud-din A, Meterissian S, Lisbana P, MacLean LD, Forse RA. Assessment of cardiac function in patients who were morbidly obese. *Surgery* 108:809, 1990.
67. Consensus Development Conference Panel, Gastrointestinal Surgery for Severe Obesity. *Ann of Int Med* 115:956, 1991.
68. Gastrointestinal Surgery for Severe Obesity: National Institutes of Health Consensus Development Conference Statement. *Am J Clin Nutr* 55:6155, 1992.

Pharmacologic Therapy for Obesity

CHAPTER

16

Myrlene A. Staten, M.D.

BACKGROUND AND BARRIERS

Obesity remains one of the greatest public health hazards for which there are no effective prevention strategies or treatments. Conventional approaches to weight reduction include voluntary restriction of energy intake or voluntary increases in energy output through physical activity. Reduction of caloric intake can be done moderately, as with slimming groups or traditional nutritional counseling, or it can be drastically, as with very low-calorie-diet regimens. Although data on long-term success rates (greater than 5 years) are reported infrequently,[1] the best weight loss maintenance results have been achieved with food restriction combined with various behavior modification techniques. However only 10–30% of patients maintained at least 50% of the weight reduction 4 years after treatment.[2] This lack of success has led many patients to resort to more drastic measures such as surgical intervention. However, despite the severity of the problem and the lack of success with available therapies, pharmacologic approaches for treating obesity remain poorly accepted by most medical professionals.[3,4] The negative attitude toward pharmacologic therapy of obesity results from a number of factors, the most obvious of which is the abuse potential of the earlier amphetamine-related compounds.[5] Other factors working against the acceptance of drugs for obesity are the unrealistic expectations of both the patient and the health care provider.[6] Most obese patients want the "magic pill," one that will allow, without any negative effects, unrestricted eating while the fat melts away. Most obese patients have a desire for large amounts of weight loss to achieve thinness, with little knowledge of the evidence that 5 to 10 kg of weight loss can provide a significant medical benefit.[7,8] Additionally, both the patient and the physician want a pill that can be taken for short periods (weeks or months) and that will take care of the problem for the duration of the patient's life. Generally, a pharmacologic therapy for a chronic medical condition such as hypertension is considered effective if the drug controls the condition when an adequate amount of the drug is present. The ameliorating effect of the drug is expected to disappear when it is no longer present. Why the expectation is different for antiobesity drugs when obesity is a well-recognized chronic condition is not clear.

Another factor that impedes the acceptance of antiobesity drugs is the lack of physician familiarity with available agents. Most medical students in the United States do not receive formal training in the treatment of obesity, and when it is included in the curriculum, the methods traditionally taught as acceptable are diet, exercise, and behavioral modification regimens.

Ideal characteristics of an antiobesity drug are as follows:

1. No potential for abuse or dependence.
2. Produces loss of body fat without significant loss of lean body mass.
3. Maintains or continues weight loss during chronic administration.
4. Can be taken safely with chronic administration.

An optimal agent does not yet exist. All of the pharmacologic agents currently available are recommended only for short-term administration.

A pharmacologic agent effective for treating obesity can either decrease energy availability or increase energy output. Decreased energy availability can be accomplished by decreasing appetite or increasing satiety (with decreased food intake) or by decreasing nutrient absorption from the gastrointestinal tract. Increased energy output can be accomplished by increasing the basal metabolic rate or thermogenesis in response to stimulants or by increasing physical activity. Increased energy outflow through thermogenesis could be achieved by decreasing the efficiency of intermediary metabolism as a result of increasing energy wasting or futile cycling, resulting in increased heat production.

AVAILABLE AGENTS

Currently, most of the agents approved by the Food and Drug Administration (FDA) for the treatment of obesity are available only by prescription. They decrease appetite and consequently help the patient control food intake.[9] These agents act centrally and affect either the catecholamine system or the serotonergic system (Table 16.1). Initially introduced in the late 1930 and early 1940s, the first of these agents, dextroamphetamine and methamphetamine, were derivatives of phenylethylamine. (See Table 16.2 for the structure of phenylethylamine and other anorectic compounds.) Although these agents are not recommended because of the potential for drug dependency and abuse,[10] chemical modifications of the basic phenylethylamine structure have led to drugs with decreased central nervous system stimulation without alteration of the anorexigenic effects. The anorexigenic effect of phenylethylamine depends on the presence of two carbons between the amino and phenyl groups and on the absence of a hydroxyl group in the phenyl ring.[3,10] The most common modifications of phenylethylamine are listed in Table 16.3 and include the following:

1. A methyl group on the alpha carbon (position 5).
2. An ethyl, methyl, or phenyl group on the amino nitrogen (position 6).
3. A chloride or fluoride on the phenyl ring (positions 1, 2, or 3).

Diethylpropion and phentermine are chemically related to amphetamine and still have some central stimulation but have less potential for abuse. Phentermine is widely used in Europe. Mazindol and ciclazindol (an investigational drug) are structural analogues of each other and are central stimulants that decrease appetite, but they are not chemically related to amphetamine.[3,11–13] There is evidence that the hypothalamic sites mediating anorexia may be $beta_2$ receptors, and albuterol (World Health Organization's recommended name, salbutamol), an asthma drug, is a beta-2-adrenergic agonist that has been shown to decrease food intake in rats.[14] No studies have been reported on its effect on food intake in humans.

Phenylpropanolamine is a amphetamine derivative that is available over the counter for the treatment of obesity. The anorectic effect of phenylpropanolamine was first described in 1939.[15] However, it was not until 1972 that phenylpropanolamine was widely marketed over the counter as an aid to weight reduction. Clinical trials demonstrated the efficacy of phenylpropanolamine,[6,16–18] and in 1982 a FDA panel found that it was safe and effective as an aid for weight reduction.[19] Its potential for abuse is very low. Phenylpropanolamine has been known to increase blood pressure in some patients, especially when administered with other agents with cardiovascular stimulation properties,[20,21] and recently the

TABLE 16–1 Pharmacologic Agents for the Treatment of Obesity

Generic or Proprietary Name	Common Trade Names	DEA* Schedule	Usual Administration Regimen	Half-Life in Blood (hr)
		DRUGS ACTING ON CATECHOLAMINE NEUROTRANSMITTERS		
Amphetamine	Dexedrine	II	5–10 mg before meals	5–10
Methamphetamine	Desoxyn	II	2.5–5.0 mg before meals or 10–15 mg in the morning (sustained release formulation)	4–5
Phenmetrazine	Preludin	II	75 mg qd (prolonged action formulation)	
Phendimetrazine	Bontril	III	105 mg before breakfast (slow release)	2–4
	Plegine		35 mg before meals	
Benzphetamine	Didrex	III	25–50 mg before meals	2
Diethylpropion	Adipex-P	IV	35 mg qd	8–13
	Tenuate		25 mg before meals or 75 mg in the morning (controlled release)	4–6
	Tepanil			
Mazindol	Mazanor	IV	1 mg before meals or 2 mg in the morning	13
	Sanorex			
Phentermine	Ionamin	IV	15 or 30 mg in the morning	7–8
	Fastin			
Phenylpropanolamine	Dexatrim	OTC	75 mg qd (sustained release)	
	Acutrim			
		DRUGS ACTING ON SEROTONERGIC TRANSMITTERS		
Fenfluramine	Pondimin	IV	20–40 mg before meals	20
Dexfenfluramine (not available in the United States)	Isomeride	—	15 mg bid	17

TABLE 16–2 Structure of Catecholamines and Anoretic Agents

Phenylethylamine

(ring with R at sites 1, 2, 3) —CH(R)—CH(R)—NH-R

Sites: 1 2 3 4 5 6

Compound	Site 1	Site 2	Site 3	Site 4	Site 5	Site 6
Schedule II						
Amphetamine	H	H	H	H	CH_3	H
Methamphetamine	H	H	H	H	CH_3	CH_3
Schedule III						
Benzphetamine	H	H	H	H	CH_3	$CH_2\phi$
Schedule IV						
Diethylpropion	H	H	H	=0*	CH_3	$(C_2H_5)_2$*
Phentermine	H	H	H	H	$(CH_3)_2$*	H
Fenfluramine	H	CH_3	H	H	CH_3	C_2H_5
Over-the-counter						
Phenylpropanolamine	H	H	H	OH	CH_3	H
Catecholamines						
Dopamine	OH	OH	H	H	H	H
Epinephrine	OH	OH	H	OH	H	CH_3
Norepinephrine	OH	OH	H	OH	H	H

* = H shown in the figure is not present with this substitution.

TABLE 16–3 Functional Properties of Structural Modifications of Phenylethylamine

Structure	Site	Function	Examples
$-OH$ or OCH_3	1,2,3 (phenyl ring)	↓ anorexigenic potential of the drug	Dopamine, epinephrine
Cl or CF_3	1,2,3	↓ CNS stimulation with moderate ↓ in appetite suppression activity	Mazindol
$=O$	4	↓ CNS stimulation with moderate ↓ in appetite suppression activity	Diethylpropion
cyclization	4,5	↓ cardiovascular and CNS stimulation without ↓ anorexigenic potential	Phenmetrazine, phendimetrazine
$-CH_3$	5	Protects against monoamine oxidase ↑ affinity for CNS membranes ↓ CNS stimulation with only slight ↓ anorectic effect	Amphetamine
$-CH_2\phi$, CH_3, or benzyl group	6	↓ CNS stimulation without ↓ appetite suppression activity	Benzphetamine

CNS, central nervous system.

wisdom of its availability over the counter has been questioned in open public hearings. The FDA has reopened its investigation of phenylpropanolamine, but at this time the drug is still available and its safety record has been excellent.[18]

OTHER APPROACHES TO PHARMACOLOGIC THERAPY FOR OBESITY

Agents Affecting Serotonin

Serotonin is a neurotransmitter thought to play a role in appetite regulation, specifically for carbohydrate craving. Of the agents that affect the serotonergic system, fenfluramine was the first approved for use in humans. Fenfluramine promotes the release of serotonin and is reputed to increase satiety rather than reduce hunger.[12,22] Unlike the amphetamine-related appetite suppressants, fenfluramine is associated with sedation, depression, and dry mouth rather than central nervous system stimulation. More recently, the dextro-isomer of fenfluramine, dexfenfluramine, has been approved for use in 32 countries, including France, the United Kingdom, and Italy. The dextro-isomer is thought to contain the active agent for satiety, with minimal side effects of sedation and depression. In one 2-weeks study, subjects who reported carbohydrate craving selected fewer high-carbohydrate snacks when treated with dexfenfluramine, suggesting that there was a nutrient specificity to the decreased food intake associated with dexfenfluramine therapy.[23] In another recent study, 822 patients were placed on a diet combined with either dexfenfluramine (15 mg bid) or placebo.[24] Approximately 40% of patients dropped out of the study. Of those patients who completed the 1-year study, the 256 patients taking dexfenfluramine ($N = 256$) lost approximately 2 kg more weight than the 227 patients on placebo and diet alone.[24] All of the weight loss was achieved by 6 months and most of the weight loss was then maintained for the next 6 months. More patients ($N = 89$) in the placebo group withdrew due to dissatisfaction with weight loss than in the group treated with dexfenfluramine ($N = 49$). The only complaints reported more often by the patients receiving drug therapy than by those receiving placebo were fatigue, diarrhea, polyuria, dry mouth, and drowsiness. Of concern are reports of pulmonary hypertension in patients treated with dexfenfluramine, and recently Servier agreed to add a warning of the possibility of pulmonary hypertension with chronic therapy to its prescribing information.[25] Additionally, a recent study showed that dexfenfluramine caused degeneration of axons and decreased the number of serotonin-immunoreactive axons in the brains of squirrel monkeys. However, the dose that decreased the number of axons was approximately 20 times the usual dosage for humans.[26]

Fluoxetine is another drug that affects serotonin and acts by preventing its reuptake, thus increasing the concentration of serotonin in the synaptic region.[27] Although fluoxetine is approved in the United States only for the treatment of depression, some depressed patients treated with it lose weight. Clinical trials are currently in progress to examine the role of fluoxetine in the treatment of obesity. In one report, nondepressed, obese patients given minimal dietary advice lost approximately 3 kg more with fluoxetine (40 to 80 mg/day) than with placebo after 8 weeks of treatment.[27] The only complaint reported more frequently in the group receiving active treatment was asthenia. In a subsequent 8-week study of fluoxetine at dosages of 10, 20, 40, or 60 mg/day, weight loss was greater in the group treated with 60 mg/day (3.9 ± 3.9 kg) compared with the placebo group (0.5 ± 2.3 kg).[28] Intermediate weight losses were noted with the lower doses. Dose-dependent increases in the reports of asthenia, somnolence, and sweating were reported. Interestingly, a critical review of the methodology of the study follows the article. Femoxitine is another serotonin-uptake inhibitor that has been suggested as a agent for obesity. However, one clinical trial showed a trend toward weight loss that was not significant (7.9 ± 4.4 vs. 6.2 ± 5.5 kg).[29]

Agents Affecting Other Regulators of Food Intake

In addition to the compounds related to the catecholamine and serotonergic pathways in the central nervous system (CNS), there are many other factors that act either primarily in the CNS or in the periphery (the gastrointestinal tract) to regulate meal frequency, composition, and size.[30] Other compounds also affect CNS regulation of food intake and appetite, such as neuropeptide Y, bombesin, opioids, corticotropin-releasing factor, and possibly cholecystokinin. Some are being investigated as possible agents for new pharmacologic approaches to control energy input.[31] The opioid system is thought to play a role in appetite regulation, with selectivity for regulation of fat intake; however, the results of clinical trials with naltrexone, an opioid antagonist, are not promising.[6,32] Cholecystokinin receptors are found in both the CNS and the gastrointestinal tract, and cholecystokinin has been shown to enhance satiety in animals and to reduce meal size and frequency.[33,34] Single-dose administration in humans has resulted in smaller food intake at subsequent meals, but to date, clinical trials with more than single-dose administration in humans have not been reported.

Peripheral inputs such as taste and neuronal input from the gastrointestinal tract to the CNS can affect food intake. Benzocaine, a topical anesthetic that presumably acts by numbing the mouth and taste buds, has been added to over-the-counter products such as hard candy and chewing gum. Very little data are available on the weight loss effects of benzocaine. However, based on the results of two unpublished double-blind studies, the Advisory Committee to the FDA reported in 1982 that benzocaine was probably safe and effective as an aid to weight reduction.[19,21] Additionally, on August 7, 1991, when the FDA announced a ban on 111 ingredients found in diet pills that were not generally recognized as safe and effective for weight loss, benzocaine was not banned.[35] However, similarly to the reevaluation of phenylpropanolamine, the agency is currently investigating its prior position regarding the efficacy of benzocaine for weight loss.

Fiber or bulking agents have been proposed as weight reduction aids, presumably because of their ability to delay gastric emptying and alter neuronal and hormonal gastrointestinal responses. Since the therapeutic response to fiber depends on its type, source, amount, and method of administration, the published data on the weight loss effect of fiber are difficult to interpret,[36,37] and the clinical usefulness of the currently available over-the-counter fiber agents remains unclear. Chlorocitrate is a therapeutic agent that was thought to work by delaying gastric emptying, thus increasing satiety.[38] However, in human subjects, despite the effect of decreased food intake, there was no delay in gastric emptying.[39] No recent studies of this compound have been reported.

In summary, the central and peripheral pathways of appetite regulation are complex, with many redundant and compensating mechanisms.[30,40] The likelihood of any single agent adequately controlling appetite without significant side effects seems unlikely. As continued studies on the regulation of food intake provide insights into pathways that integrate the overall response, specific targets for intervention will likely be revealed.

Agents That Decrease Nutrient Availability

In addition to decreasing appetite and food intake, another way to decrease nutrient availability significantly is to decrease the usable calories from ingested food. Two general approaches have been tried. One method involves food substitutes that provide either the sweetness (saccharin or aspartame), or the consistency of fat (Simplesse or sucrose polyester) without providing significant usable energy. The other method is to inhibit absorption from the intestine of utilizable nutrients.[41] Both methods assume that the patient will not compensate for the lack of usable nutrients by consuming more food than usual.

Artificial sugar substitutes have been on the market for many years. They are widely used in soft drinks and convenience foods, with net sales in the United States of approximately $10 billion per year.[42] One study that examined the efficacy of aspartame in improving weight loss on a low-calorie diet showed that consumption of aspartame may have helped women to achieve weight loss, but not men.[43]

Artificial, low- or nonnutritive fat substitutes have been developed, such as Simplesse and Olestra. Simplesse, a hydrolyzed protein with the consistency of fat, was approved by the FDA for use in frozen desserts in 1990. Olestra, a sucrose polyester, is still not approved. No clinical trails of the efficacy of Simplesse in enhancing weight loss have been reported. Additionally, since the food additive Simplesse is available only in frozen desserts, it is unlikely that decreasing the calories consumed in frozen desserts will have a significant impact on body weight for the majority of obese patients. Olestra, sucrose polyester, is a lipid with physical properties of triglycerides, is synthesized from fatty acid methyl esters and sucrose.[44] Because most of it is not hydrolyzed in the intestine, it is not absorbed and has little, if any nutritive value. However, unlike Simplesse, which is a protein, sucrose polyester can be exposed to heat and therefore used in cooking and in prepared snack foods. Clinical trials of treatment with sucrose polyester suggest that it can decrease the plasma cholesterol level and utilizable caloric and fat intake.[45] However, it is unclear if the treated patients try to compensate for the caloric dilution by increasing their intake.[46] Sucrose polyester is still being evaluated by Proctor and Gamble and by the food additive section of the FDA and is not yet available. In 1990, Proctor and Gamble limited its application for the proposed use of Olestra to snacks foods. At this time, a decision has not been made by the FDA.[47]

Presently, no pharmacologic agents that inhibit absorption of normal nutrients are available. In July 1991 the results of clinical trials of acarbose, a glycoside hydrolase inhibitor, were presented to the FDA at a public Advisory Committee hearing for approval for the treatment of diabetes. These studies showed that acarbose slowed but did not block absorption of carbohydrate. Consequently, acarbose would not be expected to cause weight loss through caloric deficit. In one small clinical trial in which the weight loss effect of acarbose was studied,[48] five obese patients were given 1500 mg of acarbose as outpatients. Two patients lost no weight and were lost to follow-up at 5 and 8 months. The three other patients lost between 9 and 11 kg with treatment for 10 to 30 months. Since all patients were prescribed a low-calorie (4600 kJ/day) diet, no conclusion could be drawn concerning acarbose as a weight reducing agent, but the results did not indicate faster weight loss than would be achieved by diet alone. Except for complaints of meteorism, borborygmi, and flatulence, acarbose was considered safe. In a more recent trial, 47 patients with diet-resistant type II diabetes treated for 24 weeks with 100 mg tid acarbose had slightly improved glycemic control but had no difference in body weight compared to a comparable group treated with placebo.[49]

Because of the increased caloric density of fat, decreased absorption of fat would be a more efficient method of inducing a caloric deficit. One approach currently being studied is the inhibition of dietary fat absorption by blocking intestinal lipase. The first reported fat absorption inhibitors were discontinued early in their development due to safety concerns, including the finding of an accumulation of chylomicrons in the wall of the small intestine, or due to lack of efficacy in initial clinical trials.[41] Ro 18–0647 is a intestinal lipase inhibitor currently in development[50] that showed an increased weight loss in its initial evaluation.[51] Ro 18–0647 works by blocking the action of intestinal lipase to cleave intact triglycerides into monoglycerides and free fatty acids, an essential step in the absorption of dietary fats. Consequently, a portion of dietary fat is not absorbed and is excreted in the feces as intact triglyceride. Clinical trials are currently underway to determine the potential of Ro 18–0647 for the treatment of obesity.

Agents That Increase Energy Output

Apart from decreasing energy input, the other major mechanism for increasing weight loss and facilitating weight maintenance is increased energy outflow. Increasing the energy burned by the organism, or thermogenesis, is a logical approach. The thermogenesis of an individual consists of three components: basal metabolic rate; stimulated thermogenesis in response to food, stress, cold, and so on; and energy expenditure from physical activity. Increased physical activity through exercise is a proven way to increase total energy expenditure and improve weight loss maintenance. Unfortunately, the amount of energy expended by most people in exercise can easily be compensated for by one extra serving of food. Additionally, many people encounter difficulty in maintaining a long-term exercise program.

Since the largest component of an individual's daily energy expenditure is the energy required to keep the cells and organs of the body functioning, an obvious intervention would be an increase in the basal metabolic rate. Consequently, many pharmacologic agents have been developed to increase energy expenditure by increasing the resting metabolic rate—for instance, the catecholamines and thyroid hormone. Thyroid hormone, one of the first antiobesity drugs, increased the resting metabolic rate. However, administration of excess thyroid hormone wasted nitrogen and calcium and caused tremor and tachycardia.[52] Its use is not recommended.

Several companies have studied agents that increase thermogenesis through stimulation of beta-adrenergic receptors. Beta-1 receptors are common in the heart and adipose tissue (both white and brown), and beta-2 receptors are common in skeletal muscle, vascular beds, and bronchi.[53] More recently, beta–3 receptors, also known as *atypical beta* receptors, have been identified that are present in brown fat.[54] Drugs that nonselectively stimulate all beta receptors, such as epinephrine and ephedrine, are thermogenic but are associated with significant tremor, tachycardia, and palpitations.[55,56] Indeed, most agents of this type developed to stimulate thermogenesis produce excess cardiovascular stimulation. Drugs that are relatively specific for the beta-3 receptors have been studied more recently. These drugs are very effective in increasing thermogenesis and subsequent weight loss without significant cardiac effects in animals.[54] Clinical trials have been completed in humans, with mixed results.[57–60] The obvious question is whether these drugs, which primarily stimulate brown fat thermogenesis in small animals, will be effective in adult humans who have very little brown fat. Is it possible that chronic exposure to these beta–3 agonists might produce hypertrophy of brown fat in humans, allowing the atypical beta agonist to have significant thermogenic effect? Or is muscle stimulation (i.e., tremor) necessary for stimulation of thermogenesis in humans?

Another method to increase total energy expenditure is to increase facultative (sympathetic nervous system–induced) thermogenesis. One study, using ephedrine, found no increase in basal thermogenesis but did find increased thermogenesis in response to ephedrine.[61] The authors suggested that if the thermogenic response was increased not only to ephedrine but also to biologic catecholamines, facultative thermogenesis would be increased and weight loss might result.[61] However, no clinical trials have been reported on the effect of long-term ephedrine administration on weight loss.

Another approach to increasing energy outflow is to decrease metabolic efficiency by increased futile cycling in the intermediary pathways of metabolism. One example of futile cycling is the interconversion of fructose–6-phosphate to fructose-diphosphate, in which energy in the high-energy bonds of adenosine triphosphate is consumed without apparent change in the system.[62] By increasing the activity of these less fuel-efficient processes, energy would be wasted and therefore not available for fuel storage as fat. Agents that work to shift the handling of ingested nutrients from more energy-efficient pathways to less efficient ones, thereby wasting heat, have been and are being developed. For example, administration of yohimbine, an alpha–2 antagonist, causes fatty acids to be released from adipocytes.[63,64] The fatty acids not needed for energy will be returned to storage, thus forming a futile cycle that will waste energy.[62] Two clinical trials have reported the effect of yohimbine on weight loss, with conflicting results that were attributed to the timing of its administration.[65,66] More studies are in progress.

Agents are also being developed that inhibit uptake of fatty acids into adipocytes.[67] Elevation of free fatty acids in the plasma is associated with their increased oxidation as an energy source. With increased fat oxidation, less carbohydrate would be oxidized, and thus more carbohydrate would be stored as glycogen or synthesized into fat, both very energy-costly procedures.[62] Thus, by either increasing the cycling of fatty acids out of and back into adipocytes or by diverting the normal oxidation of carbohydrate to carbohydrate storage, more energy would be wasted.

Another approach has been to decrease fatty acid synthesis. Associated with decreased fatty acid synthesis, lipolysis was increased, and consequently fatty acid oxidation increased. This approach was shown to have antiobesity effects in animals, potentially through the mechanism described for yohimbine.[38]

Another way in which a drug could lower energy efficiency would be to uncouple the oxidation of nutrients from phosphorylation, resulting in heat generation rather than adenosine-triphosphate production. As heat is generated, the organism becomes more inefficient. Dinitrophenol is such as compound, but unfortunately it is too toxic. To date, no drug has been developed that is capable of uncoupling oxidative phosphorylation without significant toxicity.

SUMMARY

For the present, the mainstays of obesity treatment remain dietary caloric reduction and lifestyle change through behavior modification and exercise. Given the complexity of obesity, the ideal situation for adjunctive pharmacologic therapy would be to have agents available that affect energy input as well as energy output. At present, the only pharmacologic agents available primarily affect energy input. However, physicians should not shy away from judicious use of the anorectic agents on Schedule IV or even presently available over-the-counter agents for use in selected patients. With consideration of the cardiovascular stimulatory effects of some of the anorectic agents, one of the catecholamine-related agents might be appropriate for the slightly depressed, overweight patient. For the overweight, anxious patient with no signs or history of depression, fenfluramine might be the appropriate agent. The presently approved recommended use of these agents is only for short periods (weeks). However, the likelihood of weight regain is high when the drug is stopped. Consequently, some patients might be followed carefully over extended periods of weight loss, and if weight regain occurs, consideration given to readministering the therapy.

In summary, considerable interest persists in the development of drugs for the treatment of obesity. As greater knowledge of the complex pathways of appetite control and body weight regulation emerge, more specific agents will be developed. Obesity remains one of the last major unresolved health problems and a fertile field for future developments.

REFERENCES

1. Wing RR, Jeffery RW. Outpatient treatments of obesity: A comparison of methodology and clinical results. *Int J Obes* 3:261, 1979.

2. Kramer FM, Jeffery RW, Forster JL, et al. Long-term follow-up of behavioral treatment for obesity: Patterns of weight regain among men and women. *Int J Obes* 13:123, 1989.
3. Samuel PD, Burland WL. Drug treatment of obesity, in Bray GA (ed), *Obesity in Perspective*. Bethesda, MD, National Institutes of Health, 1973, pp. 419–428.
4. Munro JF. Drug treatment of obesity: An overview. *Int J Obes* 11:13, 1987.
5. Silverstone T. Appetite-suppressant drugs in the management of obesity: The current view. *Int J Obes* 11:135, 1987.
6. Weintraub M, Bray GA. Drug treatment of obesity, in Bray GA (ed), *The Medical Clinics of North America*. Philadelphia, WB Saunders, 1989, pp. 237–249.
7. Reisin E, Abel R, Modan M, et al. Effect of weight loss without salt restriction on the reduction of blood pressure in overweight hypertensive patients. *N Engl J Med* 298:1, 1978.
8. Blackburn GL, Kanders BS. Medical evaluation and treatment of the obese patient with cardiovascular disease. *Am J Cardiol* 60:55G, 1987.
9. Scoville BA. Review of amphetamine-like drugs by the food and drug administration: Clinical data and value judgments, in Bray GA (ed), *Obesity in Perspective*. Bethesda, MD, National Institutes of Health, 1973, pp. 441–443.
10. Bray GA. Drug therapy for the obese patient, in Smith LH (ed) *The Obese Patient*. Philadelphia, WB Saunders, 1976, pp. 353–410.
11. Dallosso HM, Davies HL, Lean MEJ, et al. An assessment of ciclazindol in stimulating thermogenesis in human volunteers: A detailed metabolic study. *Int J Obes* 8:413, 1984.
12. Burland WL. A review of experience with fenfluramine, in Bray GA (ed), *Obesity in Perspective*. Bethesda, MD, National Institutes of Health, 1973, pp. 429–440.
13. Wyllie MG, Fletcher A, Rothwell NJ, et al. Thermogenic properties of ciclazindol and mazindol in rodents, in Sullivan AC, Garattini S (eds), *Novel Approaches and Drugs for Obesity*. London, John Libbey, 1985, pp. 85–92.
14. Garattini S, Samanin R: D-Fenfluramine and salbutamol: Two drugs causing anorexia through different neurochemical mechanisms, in Sullivan AC, Garattini S (eds), *Novel Approaches and Drugs for Obesity*. London, John Libbey, 1985, pp. 151–157.
15. Hirsch LS. Controlling appetite in obesity. *J Med (Cincinnati)* 20:84, 1939.
16. Weintraub M, Ginsberg G, Stein EC, et al. Phenylpropanolamine OROS (Acutrim) vs placebo in combination with caloric restriction and physician-managed behavior modification. *Clin Pharmacol Ther* 39:501, 1986.
17. A nasal decongestant and a local anesthetic for weight control? *Med Lett* 21:65, 1979.
18. Morgan JP. *Phenylpropanolamine*. Fort Lee, NJ, Jack K Burgess, 1986, pp. 1–80.
19. Establishment of a monograph for weight control products for over-the-counter human use. *Fed Register* (Doc No 81N-0022) 47:8466, 1982.

20. Brown NJ, Ryder D, Branch RA. Pharmacodynamics and drug action: A pharmacodynamic interaction between caffeine and phenylpropanolamine. *Clin Pharmacol Ther* 50:363, 1991.
21. Appelt GD. Weight control products, in Edward Feldmann (ed), *Handbook of Nonprescription Drugs*. Washington, DC, American Pharmaceutical Association, 1990. pp. 563–580.
22. Jung RT. Appetite Suppressants, in *Color Atlas of Obesity*. St Louis, Mosby Year Book, 1990, pp 157–158.
23. Wurtman JJ, Wurtman RJ. D-Fenfluramine selectively decreases carbohydrate but not protein intake in obese subjects, in Sullivan AC, Garattini S (eds), *Novel Approaches and Drugs for Obesity*. London, John Libbey, 1985, pp. 79–84.
24. Guy-Grand B, Crepaldi G, Lefebvre P, et al. International trial of long-term dexfenfluramine in obesity. *Lancet* 2:1142, 1989.
25. Servier's dexfenfluramine ADRs. *SCRIP* 1646:22, 1991.
26. Ricaurte GA, Martello MB, Wilson MA, et al. Dexfenfluramine neurotoxicity in brains of non-human primates. *Lancet* 338:1487, 1991.
27. Levine LR, Rosenblatt S, Bosomworth J. Use of a serotonin re-uptake inhibitor, fluoxetine, in the treatment of obesity. *Int J Obes* 11:185, 1987.
28. Levine LR, Enas GG, Thompson WL, et al. Use of fluoxetine, a selective serotonin-uptake inhibitor, in the treatment of obesity: A dose–response study (with a commentary by Michael Weintraub). *Int J Obes* 13:635, 1989.
29. Bitsch M, Skrumsager K. Femoxetine in the treatment of obese patients in general practice. *Int J Obes* 11:183, 1987.
30. Bray G. Nutrient balance and obesity: An approach to control of food intake in humans. *Med Clin North Am* 73:29, 1989.
31. Leibowitz SF. Hypothalamic neurotransmitters in relation to normal and disturbed eating patterns. *Ann NY Acad Sci* 499:137, 1987.
32. Atkinson RL, Berke LK, Drake CR, et al. Effects of long-term therapy with naltrexone on body weight in obesity. *Clin Pharmacol Ther* 38:419, 1985.
33. Stacher G, Steinringer H, Schmierer G, et al. Cholecystokinin octapeptide decreases intake of solid food in man. *Peptides* 3:133, 1982.
34. Dourish CT, Rycroft W, Iversen SD. Postponement of satiety by blockage of brain cholecystokinin (CCK-B) receptors. *Science* 245:1509, 1989.
35. Nonprescription diet drug products banned. *Fed Register* 56:37792, 1991.
36. Evans E, Miller DS. Bulking agents in the treatment of obesity. *Nutr Metab* 18:199, 1975.
37. Solum TT, Ryttig KR, Solum E, et al. The influence of a high-fibre diet on body weight, serum lipids, and blood pressure in slightly overweight persons: A randomized, double-blind, placebo-controlled investigation with diet and fibre tablets (Dumo Vital). *Int J Obes* 11:67, 1987.
38. Sullivan AC, Hogan S, Triscari J. New developments in pharmacological treatments for obesity. *Ann NY Acad Sci* 499:269, 1987.

39. Heshka S, Nauss-Karol C, Nyman A, et al. Effects of chlorocitrate on body weight in obese men on a metabolic ward. *Nutr Behav* 2:233, 1985.
40. Wilber JF. Neuropeptides, appetite regulation, and human obesity. *JAMA* 266:257, 1991.
41. Puls W, Krause HP, Muller L, et al. Inhibitors of the rate of carbohydrate and lipid absorption by the intestine, in Sullivan AC, Garattini S (eds), *Novel Approaches and Drugs for Obesity*. London, John Libbey, 1985, pp. 181–190.
42. The American diet market. *New York Times*, Nov 26, 1989, p. F17.
43. Kanders BS, Lavin PT, Kowalchuk MB, et al. An evaluation of the effect of aspartame on weight loss. *Appetite* 11:73, 1988.
44. Jandacek RJ. Studies with sucrose polyester. *Int J Obes* 4:13, 1984.
45. Glueck CJ, Jandacek R, Hogg E, et al. Sucrose polyester: Substitution for dietary fats in hypocaloric diets in the treatment of familial hypercholesterolemia. *Am J Clin Nutr* 37:347, 1983.
46. Mellies MJ, Vitale C, Jandacek RJ, et al. The substitution of sucrose polyester for dietary fat in obese, hypercholesterolemic outpatients. *Am J Clin Nutr* 41:1, 1985.
47. Shapiro E. The long, hard quest for foods that fool the palate. *New York Times*, Sept 29, 1991, pp. F5–F6.
48. William-Olsson T, Sjostrom L. Acarbose—a safe drug? *Curr Ther Res* 31:786, 1982.
49. Hanefeld M, Fischer S, Schulze J, et al. Therapeutic potentials of acarbose as first-line drug in NIDDM insufficiently treated with diet alone. *Diabetes Care* 14:732, 1991.
50. Hauptman JB, Jeunet FS, Hartmann D. Initial studies in humans with the novel gastrointestinal lipase inhibitor Ro 18–0647 (tetrahydrolipstatin). *Am J Clin Nutr* 55:309S, 1992.
51. Drent ML, van der Veen EA. Tetrahydrolipstatin treatment in obese patients. *Int J Obes* 15:24, 1991.
52. Bray GA. Thyroid hormones in the treatment of obesity, in Bray GA (ed), *Obesity in Perspective*. Bethesda, MD, DHEW Publ No. 75–708, 1973, pp. 449.
53. Garcia-Sainz JA, Fain JN. Regulation of adipose tissue metabolism by catecholamines: Roles of alpha–1, alpha–2, and beta-adrenoceptors. *TIPS* 201, 1982.
54. Arch JR, Ainsworth AT, Cawthorne MA, et al. Atypical β-adrenoceptor on brown adipocytes as target for anti-obesity drugs. *Nature* 309:163, 1984.
55. Pasquali R, Baraldi G, Cesari MP, et al. A controlled trial using ephedrine in the treatment of obesity. *Int J Obes* 9:93, 1985.
56. Sjostrom L, Schutz Y, Gudinchet F, et al. Epinephrine sensitivity with respect to metabolic rate and other variables in women. *Am J Physiol* 245:E431, 1983.
57. Connacher AA, Jung RT, Mitchell PEG. Weight loss in obese subjects on a restricted diet given BRL 26830A, a new atypical β adrenoceptor agonist. *Br Med J* 296:1217, 1988.
58. Beecham's BRL 26830A in obesity. *SCRIP* 1307:24, 1988.

59. MacLachlan M, Connacher AA, Jung RT. Psychological aspects of dietary weight loss and medication with the atypical beta agonist BRL 26830A in obese subjects. *Int J Obes* 15:27, 1991.
60. Connacher AA, Bennet WM, Jung RT. Clinical studies with the β-adrenoceptor agonist BRL 26830A. *Am J Clin Nutr* 55:258S, 1992.
61. Astrup A, Lundsgaard C, Madsen J, et al. Enhanced thermogenic responsiveness during chronic ephedrine treatment in man. *Am J Clin Nutr* 42:83, 1985.
62. Flatt JP. The biochemistry of energy expenditure, in Bray GA (ed), *Recent Advances in Obesity Research*, Vol. II. London, Newman, 1978, pp. 211–228.
63. Curtis-Prior PB, Tan S. Application of agents active at the α2-adrenoceptor of fat cells to the treatment of obesity—a critical appraisal. *Int J Obes* 8:201, 1984.
64. Berlan M, Galitzky J, Riviere D, et al. Plasma catecholamine levels and lipid mobilization induced by yohimbine in obese and non-obese women. *Int J Obes* 15:305, 1991.
65. Zahorska-Markiewica B, Kucio C, Piskorska D. Adrenergic control of lipolysis and metabolic responses in obesity. *Horm Metab Res* 18:693, 1986.
66. Berlin I, Stalla-Bourdillon A, Thuillier F, et al. Absence d'efficacite de la yohimbine dans le traitement de l'obesite. *J Pharmacol* 17:343, 1986.
67. Triscari J, Sullivan AC. Anti-obesity activity of a novel lipid synthesis inhibitor, in Sullivan AC, Garattini S (eds), *Novel Approaches and Drugs for Obesity*. London, John Libbey, 1985, pp. 227–239.

CHAPTER

17

Promoting Long-Term Weight Maintenance

John P. Foreyt, Ph.D.
and G. Ken Goodrick, Ph.D.

For relatively short periods of time, obese patients can be motivated to alter their eating and exercise patterns to achieve significant weight loss. However, very few maintain these losses. Using behavior modification treatment, only about 5% keep their weight off beyond a few years posttreatment.[1] The long-term success rate for very-low-calorie diets (VLCDs) programs is about 10%.[2] Unless losses can be maintained, treatment seems to provide only temporary relief. However, the subsequent regain often leads to weight cycling, which may be deleterious to physical[3] and psychological[4,5] health.

Health professionals who offer treatments that do not have good long-term outcomes may be contributing to weight cycling and doing more harm than good. The ethical dilemma of what to offer obese patients is highlighted when it is recognized that a majority of obese patients present with symptoms of food dependence[6] such as nonpurging bulimia.[7] This aspect of obesity suggests that

Preparation of this chapter was supported in part by Grant No. 1 RO1-DK 43109 from the National Institute of Diabetes and Digestive and Kidney Diseases, National Institutes of Health.

many patients may have a dysfunctional relationship with food and that behavioral self-management instruction may be inadequate to overcome eating urges.[8]

This discussion of maintenance will focus on the implications that stem from the assumption that many obese patients suffer from food dependence. The applications of the proposed methods should also have value for those patients who have control over eating urges but who may slowly slip back into old habits. The recommended treatment components emphasize the need for a lifetime commitment with continued social support, in the same way that chemically dependent patients are viewed as being in "recovery" rather than "cured." It is no longer ethically feasible for therapists to allow obese patients to attend a clinic for a fixed period of instruction, only to be released on their own after achieving weight loss.

Our recommendations will focus on strategies to motivate the obese patient to take a lifetime perspective, to break free of weight-cycling habits, to make lifestyle changes designed to minimize inappropriate eating and nonexercising urges, and to accept the need for social support. These recommendations are largely speculative, since there is scant research on which to base a treatment approach. Treatments today are multicomponent; research to evaluate which individual components are efficacious is difficult. Much of what we have to say in this chapter is based on clinical experience, although we give evidence that suggests the appropriateness of new directions in treatment.

LIFETIME COMMITMENT

For patients who have a history of weight cycling, treatment dependency may have developed, that is, the patient depends on treatments to get a temporary "fix" of weight loss. Rather than maintain an ongoing treatment perspective, the patient may leave against medical advice once the goal weight is achieved. Since the obese may attribute weight loss to treatment but blame themselves for regain,[9] they may be hesitant to return to treatment until a considerable amount of weight is regained. Patients may switch clinics to avoid the stigma of failure.

This tendency on the part of patients to abuse therapy might be thwarted if therapists could convince patients of the need for a lifetime perspective, the acceptance of a treatment and maintenance plan that includes preventive measures for all exigencies, and the need for social support through peer groups on an indefinite basis. The fact that many patients seem so fixated on the idea of quickly losing excess weight, without regard for long-term consequences, is a reflection of the irrational behavior of many of the obese[10] and parallels the behavior of the chemically dependent. Such patients will flee to clinics offering the quick and easy path, until such time as regulation imposes strictures on what kinds of treatment can be offered.

At a minimum, we believe that patients should be required to enter into a contract at the beginning of treatment that specifies the following:

1. Treatment/maintenance must be a lifetime effort; short-term approaches almost always lead to relapse and cycling, and cycling is harmful.
2. Without regular exercise, relapse is almost unavoidable.
3. Without a structured social support system, relapse is likely.

Family, friends, and coworkers of the patient should be similarly advised and included in maintenance plans.

Assessing for symptoms of nonpurging bulimia[7,11] and reviewing the typical history of repeated failures are often useful. These methods help patients admit that they are unable to control their eating or exercise behaviors, and that short-term approaches are not only futile but iatrogenic.

Another approach that is sometimes useful in eliminating weight cycling is to focus on the social pressure to be thin and to learn how to accept one's body as it is, without letting body image affect self-esteem.[12] This may help reduce the impulse to try to lose weight too quickly by using overly restrictive and self-punishing techniques, which are associated with the highest likelihood of regain. A careful pretreatment screening to assess weight-loss motivations can be helpful.[13,14] For patients who appear to be motivated by urgent cosmetic needs, counseling to reduce the sense of urgency is usually needed before behavioral treatment begins.

LIFETIME EXERCISE COMMITMENT

The evidence for the relationship between regular aerobic exercise and successful maintenance of weight loss is so convincing[15–18] that exercise should be ranked as equally important with dietary changes in the treatment of obesity. There has been little controlled research on adherence to exercise among the obese; what little there is shows that the obese do less well than thinner persons.[19] Obese persons rate themselves as less able to self-motivate for exercise than thinner individuals.[20] Our clinical experience shows that with a regimen of walking with self-regulated intensity,[21] many obese persons seem to enjoy exercise and report that they feel better and have more energy. However, cessation of regular exercise seems to occur during periods of increased life stress. Injury, work, family demands, and lack of time are often cited as reasons for quitting.[22,23]

Cessation of exercise can be construed as part of a vicious cycle, since the resultant reduction in physical capacity may decrease perceived energy, making exercise less likely.[24] Exercise can become a positive "addiction,"[25] but this is less likely among the obese. Maintenance of the exercise habit may require structured exercise programs or regular exercise support groups with peers.

In order to instill a lifetime commitment to exercise, we emphasize that exercise is a positive, enjoyable activity that also helps to control excess body fat by minimizing metabolic showdown due to dieting[26,27] and by burning calories. We stress that exercise increases the feeling of energy and can be beneficial for mild depression[28]; low perceived energy level and depression have been related to early dropout from weight-loss programs.[29] We continuously tell our patients that if they choose to stop exercising, they are choosing to fail in their weight-loss efforts. Even those whose obesity has damaged their lower extremities are helped to exercise with equipment that uses only the upper body.

A treatment program requires participation in a structured exercise program with behavior therapy methods for several months. Thereafter, patients can exercise at other facilities or at home, so long as fitness tests show evidence of exercise adherence. A system for matching up patients geographically can be used to assign exercise buddies. Support groups should be designed to maximize constructive social pressure and peer help with problem solving.

We try to get patients involved in fitness by recommending that they subscribe to fitness magazines, such as *Walking*, join fitness organizations, and participate with their fellow patients in identifying exercise facilities in the community. The idea is to help them develop a new, positive identity as fitness enthusiasts, to replace their old, negative obese identity.

Therapists should also work with patients to lobby governmental bodies to increase access to safe recreational facilities and parks. Many of our female patients enjoy walking but feel unsafe. Walking in shopping malls is one alternative; walking paths monitored by the police is another.

LIFETIME COMMITMENT TO LOW-FAT EATING

We assume that most obese patients need to reduce their dietary fat to less than 30% of total calories. A very gradual reduction in fat in the diet may lead to reduction in body fat through metabolic[30] and appetitive[31] mechanisms. A focus on fat reduction rather than calorie restriction may be indicated since an emphasis on caloric restriction may lead to psychological and physiological deprivation, making control of eating very difficult and perhaps even exacerbating symptoms of an eating disorder.[32]

Thorough longitudinal studies of the processes of regain have yet to be reported. It is unclear how many patients have regains characterized by distinct episodes of loss of eating control leading to nonadherence or how many regain through a gradual relaxation of dietary strictures over time. The relapse research literature focuses on specific episodes and shows that self-control is lost under tempting situations involving negative emotions when alone, positive emotions in social situations, or when very hungry.[33]

If urges to eat inappropriately could be reduced, long-term maintenance would be easier. The behavioral management of the variables associated with relapse is discussed elsewhere in this volume. Treatment strategies need to be developed that minimize inappropriate eating urges. Gradual reduction of fat in the diet may reduce the frequency and intensity of such urges.[34] A gradual rate of weight loss during treatment may also be indicated for the development of better eating control. Studies of those who have succeeded in long-term maintenance show a rate of weight loss of less than 0.5 kg/week.[35]

Another approach to reducing inappropriate eating urges is to help the patient develop a positive attitude toward low-fat food alternatives. If the patient can experience a low-fat diet as satisfactory without a feeling of deprivation, then the battle against high-fat foods is won. A program of food preference training has achieved short-term maintenance in a majority of patients using very-low-fat foods.[36] Reduction in the resting metabolic rate was much less than expected; the metabolic rate may be less influenced during caloric restriction if the diet has a very low fat:carbohydrate ratio. Insull et al.[37] reported success in helping women at high risk of developing breast cancer reduce the fat content of their diet from the typical 39% to 20%, with good maintenance after 2 years. This was achieved using behavior self-management training and social support.

A related issue is the negative attitude many patients have toward food. Food is seen as the enemy, which is unfortunate given the need to eat. This approach–avoidance conflict over food builds up anxiety, which triggers loss of eating control. A low-fat food preference training program may foster long-term compliance by making eating a pleasurable activity rather than a cause for alarm.[38]

Another factor most likely responsible for relapse and regain is the attempt to maintain an unrealistic goal weight. Many therapists give patients goal weights based on weights from insurance company tables, which are based on nonobese population samples. Some goal weights are based on ideal weight (IW), which is sometimes calculated as 100 lb plus 5 lb for every inch in height over 5 ft for women and 105 lb plus 6 lb for every inch over 5 ft for men. However, for individuals who have had a weight problem with a history of dieting cycles, the body fat percentage that corresponds to a tolerable and maintainable eating and exercise lifestyle may have been altered upward relative to the normal population. A more realistic goal weight formula has been developed that is based on the experience of patients who comply with treatment recommendations and keep a constant weight for more than 6 months.[39]

This possible weight (PW) is calculated as follows:

$$PW = IW + (0.22)(\text{age} + \text{no. of years overweight}) + (0.1)(\text{max. weight}) - 4.4$$

Using this formula, a patient's weight may be 150 lb rather than 120 lb. Careful counseling may be needed to help the patient accept the heavier figure as a goal. Ciliska[12] has outlined a treatment program that focuses on helping patients grieve over the loss of their thin self and develop a positive body image and higher self-esteem. Such self-acceptance is needed to replace the irrational and self-destructive desire to be thinner. In treating obese patients, the goal of the health professional should be to help them optimize their psychological and physical health. Physical health is maximized when the patient adheres to a regimen of low-fat eating and regular exercise. The weight at which a patient stabilizes under such a regimen is what he or she should weigh, regardless of any calculations of goal weight. Psychological health is maximized when therapy leads to the acceptance of this weight.

About 10 years ago, some case studies appeared to have had success in reducing eating urges using techniques to break the chain of behaviors leading to inappropriate eating,[40,41] but this line of research did not continue. Recently, cue exposure[42] and cognitive-behavioral approaches[7] have been suggested as strategies to enhance eating self-control. These strategies, combined with more realistic goal weights and peer social support, show the most promise for future research to improve eating control.

To provide continuing cues to proper eating behavior, we recommend to our patients that they join nutrition/consumer advocacy groups such as the Center for Science in the Public Interest (Washington, D.C.). This organization works to promote more healthful practices in the food industry, such as fat and sodium reduction, and publishes a monthly newsletter. We also recommend magazines such as *Cooking Light* so that patients are reminded on a monthly basis of their new identity as prudent eaters.

To help restructure the eating environment in which patients must live, health professionals should attempt to work toward better government regulation of the food industry. This may involve mandatory nutrition labeling to show the percentage of calories from fat or taxation of foods that are adulterated with added fat. It would be helpful if there were grocery stores that sold only foods recommended on a prudent diet. Clearly, if foods were lower in fat, adherence would be easier.

A NETWORK MODEL

As discussed above, the time has passed when health professionals could allow patients to attend a clinic for a short time, only to be released to follow their own devices after having achieved some weight loss. The high long-term relapse rate and the evidence of eating disorder symptoms among the obese dictate a more comprehensive approach to weight management. A stepped-care strategy using a network of treatment systems has been used for over 25 years in Argentina.[39] This network is based on an addictive model of obesity and includes three intervention modalities. The medical clinic offers VLCD and other structured diet/exercise protocols. A "diet club" provides weekly group meetings with education and advice; a self-help organization provides weekly group meetings for the support of individuals trying to control compulsive eating.

To complement these three modalities, the network includes (1) a self-help organization for the families of compulsive overeaters, based on the principles of AL-ANON; (2) self-help groups for persons with bulimia and anorexia nervosa; (3) a Walkers Club; (4) a delivery service providing prepared meals; (5) a weekend crisis hotline; and (5) a health cruise and diet resort. The network is also active in providing advice through the mass media and educational programs for school children.

This network claims to help over 90% of patients achieve a body mass index within normal limits for those who remain active; however, the dropout rate at 1 year is 75% for the self-help groups and 40% for the diet club. Nonetheless, the network model does provide for continuing support of patients, who can enter the network at any point and change to different modalities as appropriate. This network model parallels current treatment for chemical dependency and appears to be a more ethical approach than the old treat/release model.

The use of peer social support groups may be one of the more important methods of improving maintenance. There is very little meaningful outcome research on any of the 12-step self-help programs for addictive disorders. According to a survey conducted by Overeaters Anonymous (OA),[43] the average member who had attended for more than 6 months had lost about 24 lb, and about 25% of respondents said they had achieved a "satisfactory normal" weight. This survey was based on a 26% return rate, so the results may be unrepresentative of the average OA member. Our patients tell us that some of the OA groups are dominated by members who push rather strict and sometimes bizarre diet recommendations. Others state that OA is depressing, as the content of the group discussion focuses on members' failures rather than their successes.

Eating relapse episodes are associated with cognitive distortions and irrational behavior.[44] If patients can be convinced of the use of peer support to help get through temptation crises, they might fare better than by trying to rely on their own devices. The mental wherewithal needed to perform self-management techniques, which seems to be lacking under conditions of temptation,[45,46] may be augmented through the help of a peer who is not undergoing a crisis. Peer support groups set up by therapists have shown promise of good weight loss maintenance.[47] Peer self-help groups that are organized and controlled by a clinic might be a fruitful approach.

RELAPSE PREVENTION PROGRAMMING

In the chemical dependency treatment field, *relapse prevention planning* refers to a system of patient support that is negotiated at the onset of treatment and activated when there is a risk of dropout from treatment or relapse to old behaviors.[48] In the case of obesity treatment, we believe that such programming involves the following steps:

1. Helping patients to admit that they cannot achieve lasting adherence to prudent eating and exercise habits on their own without a support system.
2. Negotiating contracts with patients, family, friends, and coworkers that specify constructive intervention if any of the following occur: (a) a predetermined weight gain; (b) failure to attend treatment or support groups; (c) obvious uncontrolled eating; or (d) failure to exercise for a predetermined period.
3. Involving patients in constructive intervention with directed social pressure to return to adherence or treatment. It may also involve the use of financial contingencies such as forfeiting deposits to a charity.

The patient's progress is monitored on the clinic's computer tracking system. This database includes all treatment information, as well as attendance records at diet club meetings and peer self-help meetings. The parties involved in the relapse prevention contract would be contacted when the computer flags a member as nonadherent. This can be based on weight regain or failure to report behavioral or weight data. This approach may seem draconian; however, most patients will agree that a system of monitoring and policing of their behavior is a good idea if it will help motivate them to stay in control or help them return to control after they have strayed. In fact, it has been our clinical experience that patients like the idea of being watched; it reduces their anxiety about relapsing, since there is a perceived "safety net." This reduction of anxiety alone may enhance self-control. Furthermore, it makes sense to us that social pressure should be used to maintain healthful eating and exercise habits, since it is perceived social pressure that has driven many patients into desperate yet self-damaging attempts to be thinner.[49]

MAINTENANCE AND MENTAL HEALTH

Controlled studies have concluded that the obese are no more psychologically disturbed than the nonobese.[50,51] However, many obese patients may show psychopathology secondary to the intense social pressure to be thin. Repeated failure at maintenance may be viewed by the patient as an indication of an underlying disturbance.[52] Many obese patients suffer from binge eating and depression, which may be due to the application of overly restrictive diets and unrealistic goal weights. Patients who suffer from more severe binge eating and chaotic eating patterns are more likely to have significant personality disturbance.[53]

Patients who have such problems cannot be expected to show the self-control required to maintain prudent eating and exercise habits. Binging, depression, and failure in weight loss programs go hand in hand.[54,55] Screening for such symptoms may allow the matching of obese patients to programs with more emphasis on cognitive therapy for depression and body image problems.[7]

Many patients may be seeking weight loss as a means of solving relationship or other personal problems. When weight loss fails to be the answer, the posttreatment disillusionment might affect the patient's willingness to continue maintenance behaviors. The hidden agenda of patients should be probed before treatment to ensure that expectations about the effects of weight loss on personal functioning, as well as the amount of weight loss that can be maintained, are realistic.

Weight loss is better maintained if patients are helped to adjust to their new, thinner identity.[56] In addition to helping make expectations realistic, this entails assisting patients in dealing with the new coping skills they may need as their social environment changes. Persons who have adapted over many years of discrimination because of their size may have difficulty interacting without some residue of distrust. Unprepared patients may find the new reactions of others to their thinner appearance uncomfortable or even anxiety-provoking. The combination of such negative emotions together with the perhaps unconscious knowledge that eating will return them to their previous adapted state may lead patients to relapse.

SUMMARY

Since maintenance of lost weight is the most important issue in the treatment of the obese, major changes in the traditional delivery of treatment are needed to improve the current situation. We suggest the following approaches, which need empirical verification:

1. Establishing a lifetime commitment to exercise and low-fat eating.
2. Addressing symptoms of food dependence.
3. Providing a stepped-care approach with clinics, educational follow-up meetings, and self-help groups, along with community involvement.
4. Setting more realistic weight loss goals and slower rates of weight loss.
5. Planning for social intervention on the risk of relapse.
6. Assessing and addressing depression or personality disturbances that might interfere with the ability to adhere to eating and exercise recommendations.

REFERENCES

1. Kramer FM, Jeffery RW, Forster JL, et al. Long-term follow-up of behavioral treatment for obesity: Patterns of weight regain among men and women. *Int J Obes* 13:123, 1989.
2. Wadden TA, Stunkard AJ, Liebschutz J. Three-year follow-up of the treatment of obesity by very-low-calorie diet, behavior therapy, and their combination. *J Consult Clin Psychol* 56:925, 1988.
3. Rodin J, Radke-Sharpe N, Rebuffe-Scrive M, et al. Weight cycling and fat distribution. *Int J Obes* 14:303, 1990.
4. Garrow JS. Very low calorie diets should not be used. *Int J. Obes* 13:145, 1889.
5. Wooley SC, Wooley OW, Dyrenforth SR. Theoretical, practical and social issues in behavioral treatment of obesity. *J Appl Behav Anal* 12:3, 1979.
6. Loro AD, Orleans CS. Binge eating in obesity: Preliminary findings and guidelines for behavioral analysis and treatment. *Addict Behav* 6:155, 1981.
7. Telch, CF, Agras WS, Rossiter EM, et al. Group cognitive-behavioral treatment for the nonpurging bulimic: An initial evaluation. *J Consult Clin Psychol* 58:629, 1990.
8. Foreyt JP, Goodrick GK. Factors common to successful therapy for the obese. *Med Sci Sports Exerc* 23:292, 1991.
9. Jeffery RW, French SA, Schmid TL. Attributions for dietary failures: problems reported by participants in the hypertension prevention trial. *Health Psychol* 9:315, 1990.
10. Sash SE. Why is the treatment of obesity a failure in modern society? *Int J Obes* 1:247, 1977.
11. Gormally J, Black S, Daston S, et al. The assessment of binge eating severity among obese persons. *Addict Behav* 7:47, 1982.
12. Ciliska D. *Beyond Dieting*. New York, Brunner/Mazel, 1990, p. 1.
13. Laporte DJ, Stunkard AJ. Predicting attrition and adherence to a very-low-calorie diet: A prospective investigation of the eating inventory. *Int J Obes* 14:197, 1989.
14. Brownell KD. Dieting readiness. *Weight Cont Dig* 1:1, 1990.
15. Colvin RH, Olson SB. Winners revisited: An 18-month follow-up of our successful weight losers. *Addict Behav* 9:305, 1984.
16. Hoiberg A, Bernard S, Watten RH, et al. Correlates of weight loss in treatment and at follow-up. *Int J Obes* 8:457, 1984.
17. Marston AR, Criss J. Maintenance of successful weight loss: Incidence and prediction. *Int J Obes* 8:435, 1984.
18. Pavlou KN, Krey S, Steffee WP. Exercise as an adjunct to weight loss and maintenance in moderately obese subjects. *Am J Clin Nutr* 49:1115, 1989.
19. Dishman RK (ed). *Exercise Adherence*. Champaign, Ill, Human Kinetics, 1988.
20. Schlundt DG, Zimering RT. The Dieter's Inventory of Eating Temptations: A measure of weight control competence. *Addict Behav* 13:151, 1988.

21. Foreyt JP, Goodrick GK. Health maintenance through exercise and nutrition, in Blechman EA (ed), *Behavior Modification with Women*. New York, Guilford Press, 1984, pp. 221–244.
22. Sallis JF, Hovell MF, Hofstetter CR, et al. Lifetime history of relapse from exercise. *Addict Behav* 15:573, 1990.
23. Goodrick GK, Hartung GH, Warren DR, et al. Helping adults stay physically fit: preventing relapse following aerobic exercise training. *JOPERD* 55:48, 1984.
24. Sims EAH. Exercise and energy balance in the control of obesity and hypertension, in Horton ES, Terjung RL (eds), *Exercise, Nutrition, and Energy Metabolism*. New York, Macmillan, 1988, pp. 242–257.
25. Glaser W. *Positive Addiction*. New York, Harper & Row, 1976.
26. Van Dale D, Saris WHM, ten Hoor F. Weight maintenance and resting metabolic rate 18–40 months after a diet/exercise treatment. *Int J Obes* 14:347, 1990.
27. Frey-Hewitt B, Vranizan KM, Dreon DM, et al. The effect of weight loss by dieting or exercise on resting metabolic rate in overweight men. *Int J Obes* 14:327, 1989.
28. Greist JH, Eischens RR, Klein MH, et al. Antidepressant running. *Psychiatr Ann* 9:134, 1979.
29. Pekarik G, Blodgett C, Evans RG, et al. Variables related to continuance in a behavioral weight loss program. *Addict Behav* 9:413, 1984.
30. Dreon DM, Frey-Hewitt B, Ellsworth N, et al. Dietary fat: Carbohydrate ratio and obesity in middle-aged men. *Am J Clin Nutr* 47:995, 1988.
31. Ramirez I, Tordoff MG, Friedman MI. Dietary hyperphagia and obesity: What causes them? *Physiol Behav* 45:163, 1989.
32. Polivy J, Herman CP. Dieting and bringing: A causal analysis. *Am Psychol* 40:193, 1985.
33. Schlundt DG, Sbrocco T, Bell C. Identification of high-risk situations in a behavioral weight loss program. Application of the relapse prevention model. *Int J Obes* 13:223, 1989.
34. Lissner L, Levitsky DA, Strupp BJ, et al. Dietary fat and the regulation of energy intake in human subjects. *Am J Clin Nutr* 46:886, 1987.
35. Wing RR, Jeffery RW. Successful losers: A descriptive analysis of the process of weight reduction. *Obes Bar Med* 7:190, 1978.
36. Kreitzman SL, Kreitzman SN. Weight control with a very low fat diet: Novel food preference training programme. *Int J Obes* 14:106, 1990.
37. Insull W, Henderson MM, Prentice RL, et al. Results of a randomized feasibility study of a low-fat diet. *Arch Intern Med* 150:421, 1990.
38. Jordan HA. Behavioral approaches to obesity treatment, in Storlie J, Jordan HA (eds), *Behavioral Management of Obesity*, New York, Spectrum, 1982, pp. 1–18.
39. Cormillot A, Fuchs A, Zuckerfield R. A network for multifaceted treatment of obesity based on the addictive behavior model, in Berry EM, Blondheim SH, Eliahou HE, et al (eds), *Recent Advances in Obesity Research*, Vol. V. London, John Libbey, 1987, pp. 375–382.

40. Youdin R, Hemmes NS. The urge to eat—the initial link. *J Behav Ther Exp Psychiatry* 9:227, 1978.
41. Rosen LW. Self control program in the treatment of obesity. *J Behav Ther Exp Psychiatry* 12:163, 1981.
42. Wardle J. Conditioning processes and cue exposure in the modification of excessive eating. *Addict Behav* 15:387, 1990.
43. Overeaters Anonymous. A survey of Overeaters Anonymous groups and membership in North America. Torrance, Calif, Author, 1988.
44. Sjoberg L, Persson L. A study of attempts by obese persons to regulate eating. *Goteb Psychol Rep* 7:12, 1977.
45. Foreyt JP, Goodrick GK, Gotto AM. Limitations of behavioral treatment of obesity: review and analysis. *J Behav Med* 4:159, 1981.
46. Grilo CM, Shiffman S, Wing RR. Relapse crises and coping among dieters. *J Consult Clin Psychol* 57:488, 1989.
47. Perri MG, McAdoo WG, Spevak PA, et al. Effect of a multicomponent maintenance program on long-term weight loss. *J Consult Clin Psychol* 52:480, 1984.
48. Gorski TT. The CENAPS model of relapse prevention: Basic principles and procedures. *J Psychoactive Drugs* 22:125, 1990.
49. Bennett W. Dietary treatments of obesity. *Ann NY Acad Sci* 499:250, 1987.
50. Crisp AH, McGuiness B. Jully fat: Relation between obesity and psychoneurosis in a general population. *Br Med J* 1:7, 1976.
51. McReynolds WT. Toward a psychology of obesity: Review of research on the role of personality and level of adjustment. *Int J Eat Disorders* 2:37, 1982.
52. Garner DM, Rockert W, Olmsted MP, et al. Psychoeducational principles in the treatment of bulimia and anorexia nervosa, in Garner DM, Garfinkel RE (eds), *Handbook of Psychotherapy for Anorexia Nervosa and Bulimia*. New York, Guilford Press, 1985, pp. 513–572.
53. Fitzgibbon ML, Kirschenbaum DS. Heterogeneity of clinical presentation among obese individuals needing treatment. *Addict Behav* 15:291, 1990.
54. Kolotkin RL, Revis ES, Kirley BG, et al. Binge eating in obesity: Associated MMPI characteristics. *J Consult Clin Psychol* 55:872, 1987.
55. Gormally J, Rardin D, Black S. Correlates of successful response to a behavioral weight control clinic. *J Counsel Psychol* 27:179, 1980.
56. Morton CJ. Weight loss maintenance and relapse prevention, in Frankle RT, Yang M-U (eds), *Obesity and Weight Control*. Rockville, Md, Aspen, 1988, pp. 315–332.

CHAPTER

18

Relapse Prevention in the Treatment of Obesity

Robert I. Berkowitz, M.D.

INTRODUCTION

Although important advances have been made in the behavioral treatment of obesity in the last 20 years, the maintenance of new health habits that promoted weight loss remains problematic.[1] Long-term follow-up studies have typically shown relapse difficulties following short-term treatment.[2] Brownell and Wadden[3] estimated in their review that just in the first year following weight reduction, there is a 36% average regain of weight that had been lost in treatment.

Any medical or psychological benefits obtained from the treatment of obesity generally require weight loss maintenance. Attempts to develop appropriate therapies for comorbid conditions, such as hypercholesterolemia, type II diabetes mellitus, hypertension, orthopedic difficulties, obstructive sleep apnea, and so forth[4] depend on long-term maintenance of weight loss. A major challenge will be to develop therapies aimed at long-term weight loss stabilization. This chapter will examine some factors related to relapse and the use of relapse prevention techniques.

RELAPSE IN CLINICAL POPULATIONS

Follow-up studies have shown considerable difficulty in maintaining weight losses following short-term behavioral treatment. After treatment, participants in clinical weight loss programs tend to stop practicing their new health habits and gain back their lost weight.[5–7]

One recent study chronicled the problem graphically. In a 5-year follow-up of participants initially treated for 1 year by very-low-calorie-diet (VLCD), behavior therapy, and their combination, Wadden and his colleagues[8] found that most of the participants in all three conditions returned to their pretreatment weight. There were no longer significant differences among participants in the three groups by 5-year follow-up. Of note, these participants did not receive any maintenance therapy following the initial 1 year of treatment. However, this study points out that in a clinical population with serious obesity (mean body mass index = 39), short-term treatment (even 1 year) by itself does not promote long-term maintenance.

Relapse may be conceptualized from several viewpoints, ranging from the biologic to the environmental. Set point theory suggests that weight is regulated very carefully and that attempts to change it inevitably result in a return to the baseline weight level.[9] Other biologic influences may be related to fat cell physiology and metabolic rate. The genetic hypothesis strongly suggests a physiologic drive toward obesity that may only briefly be contended with.

Though the presence of obesity may relate to inheritance, the degree of obesity may be dependent on environmental factors.[10] Environmental factors such as the prevalence of tasty food with a high fat content and a sedentary lifestyle set the stage for a greater level of obesity in the population.[11] In addition, it may be more difficult than was originally anticipated to continue healthy eating and exercise habits under the influence of an environment that reinforces behaviors contributing to both the development and maintenance of the obese state.

The patient attempting longer-term weight loss maintenance therapy may thus be enduring a form of double jeopardy. On the one hand, there is a sizable biologic component (set point, metabolic rate, genetic vulnerability, and so forth) to be contended with. On the other hand, environmental factors related to the Western lifestyle strongly reinforce behaviors contributing to and maintaining the obese state in vulnerable persons. In such an environment, sedentary activities (such as TV watching) are reinforcing, minimal physical activity is required in tasks of daily living (riding vs. walking or cycling to school or work), and high fat, tasty food is relatively inexpensive and all too prevalent. Both the physiologic-genetic and environmental forces may place overwhelming burdens on many patients attempting to maintain a lower body weight using behavioral techniques, leading to regain of lost weight.

In the Wadden et al. study[8] noted earlier, at the first year following treatment, 50% of the members of the combined VLCD and behavioral modification group had kept off 10 kg compared to 23% for the behavioral group and only 14% for the VLCD-alone group. Thus, behavioral treatment improved the 1-year follow-up outcome. Unfortunately, by the 3-year follow-up (without maintenance treatment), participants in both behavioral treatment groups had gained back 75% of their weight loss.

Twenty-three of the 76 participants were assessed regarding the frequency with which various weight control behaviors were practiced. Behaviors probably instrumental in the early phases of treatment for weight loss appeared to be infrequently reported at the 3-year follow up: Exercise (other than daily activity) was reported to occur on average once or twice a month (when a minimal recommendation for weight loss maintenance is most likely to be three or four times per week); keeping high-calorie foods out of sight (a common stimulus control procedure) was reported to occur one or two times a month; eating more slowly was practiced about twice a month; and substituting low-calorie for high-calorie foods was practiced perhaps only once a week on average. Occurring less than once a month on average were planning eating in advance, employing social support to promote weight management, and keeping a diary of food intake.

The lack of weight loss maintenance may then be related, in part, to the lack of continued practice of the new weight management techniques and behaviors learned in the early phase of behavioral treatment. Again, it is important to note that these patients were not receiving maintenance treatment during this follow-up period. As noted earlier, this study and others,[6,7] suggest that participants in clinical weight loss programs stop practicing behaviors aimed at weight loss and maintenance without continued treatment and thus regain their lost weight. Of further note, in the Wadden et al. study[8] in which seriously overweight women were treated, 18% of all participants maintained a loss greater than 5 kg and 5% maintained all their weight loss at 5 years. One important feature of this study is the very instructive longitudinal nature of the follow-up, certainly an example for future studies.

SUCCESSFUL MAINTAINERS

Another view of the relapse issue comes from the literature describing successful maintainers following weight loss. Schacter[12] (1982) reported that obese individuals make repeated efforts to lose weight before they are successful (true also, he suggested, of cigarette smokers). An episode of weight loss and regain may be a learning experience for an individual developing self-management strategies useful for longer-term weight control.

Most reports of obesity treatment come from studies of patients seeking treatment, and relatively little is known about those who attempt to manage their weight outside formal programs.[13] Perhaps those who have a more serious or more complicated disorder are seen in professionally led programs. Kayman et al.[14] and others[13–17] have found some trends in those who tend to maintain and relapse.

Kayman et al.[14] studied a population of women selected from a general medical clinic in a health maintenance organization who were defined as (1) *relapsers,* who had lost at least 20% of their weight at least once and had regained it and were at least 20% overweight (based on the 1959 Metropolitan Life Insurance Tables); (2) *maintainers,* who were of average weight, had previously been at least 20% overweight but who had lost and maintained their weight for at least 2 years; and (3) *control* participants, who were of average weight. Information was elicited by self-report regarding weight lost, including whether participants had enrolled in formal programs or had managed their own weight loss.

Maintainers had a greater rate of finishing college than did relapsers (30% vs. 20%), and more had salaried jobs (77% vs. 46%). There were no differences between maintainers and controls regarding education or employment.

Kayman et al. further found that maintainers and control participants exercised regularly (90% and 82%), while few relapsers did (34%). Most maintainers and controls were conscious of their behavior, while the relapsers tended to "eat unconsciously in response to emotions." The maintainers tended to use coping strategies that they designed for themselves, while the relapsers tended to attend organized weight management programs or to see their physicians or other professionals. Most maintainers and controls sought social support at problematic or stressful times (70%, 80%), while relapsers used social support less often (38%).

In addition, Kayman et al. reported differential responses to stressful problems. Although all the women reported some difficulties, the maintainers and controls used problem-solving or confrontational techniques (95% and 60%). Relapsers, however, used less problem solving (10%) and tended to use escape-avoidance ways of coping with stress, such as by eating, smoking, or taking tranquilizers. These investigators report that weight regain was often reported as related to negative emotional states and stressful life events. They suggest that these findings may further support the relapse theory of Marlatt and Gordon,[18] which states that once someone makes a behavioral change, relapse (return to the previous behavior) occurs when a high-risk situation, problem, or emotional state occurs in the face of insufficient coping skills.

THE RELAPSE PROCESS

In an earlier study, Rosenthal and Marx[19] interviewed 28 women 2 months following their participation in a behavioral weight reduction program. The investigators were evaluating dieters in terms of the relapse hypothesis proposed by Marlatt and Gordon noted above. A "slip" was defined when a dieter did not use a method typically relied on for at least 24 hr. A "relapse" was considered if a 5-lb gain occurred in the 2-month period following treatment.

Rosenthal and Marx found that 48% of the slips were intrapersonal: negative emotional states (32%), negative physical states (5%), and positive emotional states (11%). Interpersonal determinants (52%) related to initial slips were categorized as well: positive emotional states (32%), interpersonal conflict (10%), and social pressure (10%). Thus, their findings suggest two main types of high-risk situations for those trying to maintain weight loss: *negative emotional states while alone* (anxiety, depression, boredom) and *positive emotional states involving others* in celebrations, parties, and socializing. These two main types of situations accounted for 64% of the initial slips and perhaps were instrumental in further slips. Sternberg[20] observed similarities reported by Marlatt and Gordon[21] regarding initial slips by those addicted to alcohol, cigarettes, and heroin to those by patients attempting to maintain weight loss.

In summary, there are at least two features of relapse around which further cognitive and behavioral interventions have developed:

1. Shorter-term treatment (including 1 year of treatment) in clinical populations alone is prone to high relapse rates. Thus, investigators are beginning to examine longer-term treatment and to view obesity as a chronic difficulty requiring continued therapist contact and programmatic support.
2. Patients who tend to relapse may have certain characteristics and/or skills deficits, such as eating when experiencing negative affective states while alone or when experiencing positive emotional states in social situations. Further, they may have problems adhering to an ongoing behavioral protocol, including changing their eating habits, continuing to exercise, and continuing to monitor their weight. The behavioral protocol may be particularly demanding considering the environmental pressure related to sedentary lifestyle and the prevalence of high-fat, tasty foods.

These findings suggest that a cognitive-behavioral approach aimed at developing coping skills may be useful for relapse prevention.

RELAPSE PREVENTION TREATMENT APPROACHES

Duration of Treatment

As the findings regarding "booster sessions" following short term treatment were found to have mixed results,[22] investigators began to evaluate the benefit of more frequent treatment sessions during the maintenance period. Bennett[23] reviewed over 100 treatment studies, revealing a relationship with the duration of treatment and the amount of weight loss.

To investigate duration of treatment in the maintenance period, Perri and his colleagues[24] first used behavioral treatment (20 weeks) for weight loss, followed by three different conditions: a peer-support maintenance program (15 biweekly sessions), a therapist-contact maintenance program (15 biweekly sessions), or no treatment following the initial behavioral treatment. The therapist-led maintenance program, incorporating a problem-solving approach, revealed greater maintenance of weight loss than either the peer-led group or the no-contact condition at 7 months of follow-up. Questionnaire responses suggested that the therapist-led groups may have adhered more to self-control strategies.

Thus, it may be that longer-term treatment led by a professional therapist is helpful. But by the 18-month follow-up of this same study,[24] following a period without treatment, even the clients from the therapist-led group gained weight, with relapse rates now the same across all three conditions.

Perri and colleagues[25] again assessed the effect of length of treatment on weight loss by administering the same behavioral program in either 20 or 40 weekly sessions. Thus, the same program content was reviewed, but more gradually, in the 40-week treatment group. The longer-treatment group again had greater weight losses at 40 and 72 weeks. Further, adherence measures suggested that the group receiving only 20 weeks of treatment was not adhering as well to the program by 40 weeks as was the 40-week treatment group.

Longer-term therapist led treatment appears to encourage greater adherence to behavioral procedures with improved weight loss stabilization. Thus, continuing therapist contact appears necessary for behavioral interventions to be useful in weight loss maintenance.

Relapse Prevention Training

As described earlier, Marlatt and Gordon[18] have written extensively about long-term relapse prevention strategies for addictive behaviors, including weight loss management. They suggest that relapse (return to a previous behavior) occurs when a person is confronted with a high-risk situation, problem, or emotional state in the face of insufficient coping skills. A relapse prevention program thus would include the development of awareness for high-risk triggers for overeating and practicing alternate ways to cope.

Marlatt[26] has also described the *abstinence violation effect,* defined as a feeling of terrible guilt or discouragement following a behavior (such as overeating or binge eating) that is felt to be off limits to the behavioral program. After such a "lapse," Marlatt proposes, a reduction in self-efficacy about weight management follows, which may then trigger further overeating. Perhaps even small lapses may trigger such an abstinence violation effect, with resultant disbelief in one's own ability to follow through with self-control procedures. The result may lead to relapse and weight regain.

A cognitive-behavioral approach was developed[20,27] to focus on relapse prevention and was added to a standard weight control program. A randomized design assessed a 9-week standard behavioral program compared with a standard program to which a cognitive relapse-prevention (RP) program had been added. The RP program focused on changing cognitions and self-talk related to high-risk eating situations (as described earlier, negative affective states while alone and positive affective states in social situations). A problem-solving approach was taken to develop new strategies (instead of eating) to cope with these high-risk situations. Further, participants were encouraged to include rewarding activities in their schedules.

Although health professionals were aware of the problem of relapse, it was uncommon for behavioral programs to bring up this issue. In their study, Rosenthal and Marx[19] actively discussed relapse issues, including slips, lapses, and past relapses. Participants were encouraged to become aware of their cognitions and feelings at these times and to change their ways of thinking about them. A very negative reaction (the abstinence violation effect) to a lapse may have been worse than the lapse itself, triggering discouragement and, thus, further overeating. Participants were encouraged to analyze the situation and to see new ways to cope. Members of the standard and RP groups lost the same amount of weight initially. Two months following treatment, the RP group had lost further weight, while the standard treatment group had begun to regain. This suggested that the RP approach may have been useful in helping weight loss patients maintain their losses. Longer-term results, though, were unavailable from this study, making it impossible to judge whether these differences persisted.

Studies by Perri and his colleagues have investigated the continued use of therapist contact and a variety of strategies, including a problem-solving approach similar to the RP approach used above. One major finding from their most comprehensive study[28] is that continued contact with a therapist resulted in maintenance of weight loss in a 1-year, biweekly program following a 20-week weight loss program. The control group, which received no therapy that year, had a significant regain (about half their weight lost).

In addition, Perri et al.[28] studied a variety of techniques to examine whether any one or a combination might improve weight loss maintenance. They included a problem-solving approach (similar to the relapse prevention approach), social support, and exercise during the sessions and their combination. These different treatment groups all maintained their weight loss (the control group regained), but none was significantly different from the others. This study too suggests that both continued therapist contact and a behavioral program incorporating a problem-solving approach will lead to maintenance of weight lost at least for the 1 year of the maintenance program.

Perri et al.[28] suggest that the group that tended to do the best was the one that received the entire multicomponent package: cognitive-behavioral treatment, therapist contact, social support (from other group members), and aerobic exercise. This was the only group that continued to lose weight in the maintenance period and maintained 99% of their initial weight loss by the 18-month follow-up. Still, it is important to note that all groups in this study regained weight in the 6-month period when no therapist contact or group sessions continued. Again, we are left to wonder just how long and how much therapist support and programming will be required to see long-term weight loss maintenance using these cognitive-behavioral strategies.

USE OF NUTRITIONAL PRODUCTS

An interesting feature of the very-low-calorie-diet is the use of nutritional supplements as total meal and food replacements, while eliminating all regular foods during the acute weight loss phase. Participants in these programs in the short term generally are able to adhere, with successful weight reduction of 20 kg or more. My colleagues (W.S. Agras and B. Arnow) and I have speculated that this approach removes participants from the stimuli regulating eating behavior—the sight, smell, and taste of palatable foods. This may be yet another form of stimulus control,[29] reducing the number of situations triggering eating behavior by focusing on "narrowing the stimuli" of food itself.

The quality of food itself in our Western culture may be a major problem, related to the great variety of choices and the palatability of the food. As previously noted, a high-fat, tasty, and relatively available diet may lead to weight gain and obesity.[11] Great variety in the diet can induce overeating and the consequent development of obesity both in animal studies[30,31] and in human studies.[32]

During the VLCD using nutritional supplements alone, food choices are limited, with a major reduction in food variety; thus the stimuli triggering eating are narrowed. Participants are able to adhere to the protocol and lose considerable weight. It may be that this and other similar approaches induce sensory-specific satiety[33]; that is, a more uniform, less varied, lower-fat diet may reduce hunger and food intake.

Following the VLCD or other weight reduction programs, return to the typical Western diet, with its increased variety and fat content, may again induce increased eating. Another possibility may be to continue the use of prepackaged food products, both supplements ("shakes") and prepackaged meals, to some degree in long-term treatment. At this time, despite the booming commercial market for such products, there exist almost no data to support their use during the maintenance period.

My colleagues (W.S. Agras and B. Arnow) and I have piloted the use of prepackaged supplements and meals (rather than regular foods) following a 12-week VLCD for a 6-week period in a group of 12 patients. A matched group who followed the standard return to regular foods had lost the same amount of weight at the end of the VLCD. The group continuing to use prepackaged food products in the next 6 weeks lost significantly more weight during this time than did the standard treatment group. Longer-term follow-up was not possible. Though short term and uncontrolled, this study suggested that the use of prepackaged food products may be useful in longer-term treatment.

Studies are ongoing regarding the use of nutritional products in the maintenance period. A balanced, low-fat diet with only moderate variety, using some prepackaged products, requires further testing to evaluate its usefulness for long-term treatment of obesity. A potential difficulty may be adherence to a diet viewed as less palatable or tasty in order to maintain lower fat or caloric consumption. On the other hand, these products may provide a important aid in complying with such a dietary prescription.

SUMMARY

The maintenance of weight loss following behavioral programs remains a major challenge. Factors related to relapse include biologic, psychological, environmental, and programmatic issues. The typical Western lifestyle may be instrumental in the development and maintenance of the obese state in vulnerable individuals.

Successful weight loss maintenance in clinical populations is promoted by ongoing therapist-led behavioral treatment programs. A variety of programs including cognitive-behavioral techniques to cope with relapse, problem solving, social support, and exercise programs all seem to improve compliance with the maintenance program and thus with weight loss maintenance. A model of relapse prevention strategies drawn from the literature is presented in Table 18–1.

Future research in the long-term treatment area, though challenging, is extremely important. A number of years ago, it appeared as difficult to help patients lose weight as it may now appear to help them maintain their weight losses. Such long-term treatment research is essential to investigate techniques to promote weight loss maintenance.

Areas for further investigation include: ongoing long-term cognitive-behavioral approaches combined with "crisis intervention" directed at acute weight gain, therapy for binge eating, individualization of treatment, adherence strategies, social support, exercise programs developed in the clinical setting, use of specialized nutritional products, and combined treatment with pharmacotherapy.

TABLE 18–1 Model of Relapse Prevention and Long-Term Weight Loss Maintenance Treatment Using Cognitive, Behavioral, and Nutritional Techniques

1. *Continued therapist contact*. Studies suggest that ongoing, long-term treatment (*maintenance treatment*), with a minimal frequency of contact every 2 weeks, is required for weight loss maintenance. Further research is needed to evaluate the optimal length of treatment, including individualization for specific needs.
2. *Continued review and reinforcement of the basic behavioral program,* perhaps with greater individualization, to include:
   A. *Self-monitoring*. This includes continued or periodic monitoring of dietary intake, exercise, weight, and problem areas.
   B. *Stimulus control procedures*. These include keeping foods out of sight, eating in specifically designated dining areas, keeping foods away from the workplace, avoiding eating while involved in another activity such as reading or TV watching, and so forth.
   C. *Nutrition education*. This needs to be ongoing, with a focus on adherence to a low-fat, balanced diet. Use of nutritional products such as supplements and prepackaged meals requires more investigation during the maintenance period.
   D. *Changing eating habits*. Changes include eating more slowly, choosing moderate to small portions, eating only when hungry, eating regular meals, planning eating in advance, and avoiding excessive snacking.
   E. *A regular, moderate exercise program is essential*. Individualization may be crucial, with a focus on both lifestyle and structured approaches. A long-term exercise adherence program will require more research.
3. *A relapse prevention program with a cognitive-behavioral orientation* has proven useful in studies of up to 1 year during maintenance treatment. Longer studies are needed. Such programs would include:
   A. *Identifying high-risk situations triggering lapses,* especially overeating episodes and stopping exercise. These include:
      i. *Negative feeling states while alone,* such as anxiety, boredom, and depression.
      ii. *Positive feeling states in social gatherings,* such as holiday gatherings, parties, and celebrations focused around meals or food.
      iii. *Environmental stimuli,* such as seeing very attractive foods as at a restaurant or at home.
   B. *Learning alternative ways to cope with the triggers to slip or relapse, ways to stay on one's program, and ways to return to the program as soon as possible following a lapse*. Such strategies may be role-played in a group format. Alternative strategies include exercise, relaxation training, problem solving, communication, and development of greater social support.
   C. *Individuals with comorbid states* (anxiety, depression, binge-eating disorder, or social isolation) will need more specific treatment for these other difficulties.
4. *Combined treatments need to be explored,* including pharmacotherapy, and surgical approaches with the extremely obese.
5. *Obesity needs to be viewed from a long-term, chronic disease point of view*. Adherence and compliance research is needed to aid long-term treatment.

Note: This model has been drawn from the work of many investigators, many of whom are referenced in this chapter.

REFERENCES

1. Council on scientific Affairs, American Medical Association. Treatment of obesity in adults. *JAMA* 260:2547, 1988.
2. Stunkard AJ, Penick SB. Behavior modification in the treatment of obesity: The problem of maintaining weight loss. *Arch Gen Psychiatry* 36:801, 1979.
3. Brownell KD, Wadden TA. Behavior therapy for obesity: Modern approaches and better results, in Brownell KD, Foreyt JP (eds), *Handbook of Eating Disorders: Physiology, Psychology and Treatment of Obesity, Anorexia and Bulimia*. New York, Basic Books, 1986, pp. 180–197.
4. Pi-Sunyer FX. Health implications of obesity. *Am J Clin Nutr* 53:1595S, 1991.
5. Kramer M, Jeffery RW, Forester JL, et al. Long-term follow-up of behavioral treatment for obesity: Patterns of weight regain among men and women. *Int J Obes* 13:123, 1989.
6. Foreyt JP. Issues in the assessment and treatment of obesity. *J Consult Clin Psychol* 55:677, 1987.
7. Perri MG. Maintenance strategies for the management of obesity, in Johnson WG (ed.), *Advances in Eating Disorders: Treating and Preventing Obesity*. Greenwich Press, 1987, pp. 177–194.
8. Wadden TA, Sternberg JA, Letizia KA, et al. Treatment of obesity by very-low-calorie-diet, behavior therapy, and their combination: A five year perspective. *Int J Obes* 13 (Suppl. 2):39, 1989.
9. Stallone DD, Stunkard AJ. The regulation of body weight: Evidence and clinical implications. *Ann Behav Med* 13:220, 1991.
10. Price RA, Ness R, Sorensen TIA. Changes in commingled body mass index distributions associated with secular trends in overweight among Danish young men. *Am J Epidemiol* 133:501, 1991.
11. Jeffrey RW. Population perspectives on the prevention and treatment of obesity in minority populations. *Am J Clin Nutr* 53:16215, 1991.
12. Schachter S. Recidivism and self-cure of smoking and obesity. *Am Psychol* 37:436, 1982.
13. Brownell KD, Marlatt GA, Lichtenstein E, et al. Understanding and preventing relapse. *Am Psychol* 41:765, 1986.
14. Kayman S, Bruvold W, Stern JS. Maintenance and relapse after weight loss in women: behavioral aspects. *Am J Clin Nutr* 52:800, 1990.
15. Wilson GT. Psychological prognostic factors in the treatment of obesity. In Hirsch J, Van Itallie TB. (eds.), *Recent advances in obesity research: IV*. London, John Libbey and Co Ltd, 1985, pp. 301–311.
16. Wing RR, Jeffery RW. Successful losers: A descriptive analysis of the process of weight reduction. *Obes Bar Med* 7:190, 1978.
17. Gormally J, Rardin D, Black S. Correlates of successful response to a behavioral weight control clinic. *J Counsel Psychol* 27:179, 1980.

18. Marlatt GA, Gordon JR (eds). *Relapse Prevention: Maintenance Strategies in Addictive Behavior Change*. New York, Guilford Press, 1985.
19. Rosenthal BS, Marx RD. Determinants of initial relapse episodes among dieters. *Obes Bar Med* 10:94, 1981.
20. Sternberg B. Relapse in Weight control: Definitions, processes and prevention strategies, in Marlatt GA, Gordon JR (eds.), *Relapse Prevention: Maintenance Strategies in the Treatment of Addictive Behaviors*. New York, Guilford Press, 1985, pp. 521–541.
21. Marlatt GA, Gordon JR. Determinants of relapse: Implications for the maintenance of behavior change. In Davidson PO, Davidson SM (eds.), *Behavioral Medicine: Changing Health Life-styles*. New York, Brunner/Mazel, 1980.
22. Wilson GT, Brownell KD. Behavior therapy for obesity: An evaluation of treatment outcome. *Adv Behav Res Ther* 3:49, 1980.
23. Bennett GA. Behavior therapy for obesity: A quantitative review of the effects of selected treatment characteristics on outcome. *Behav Ther* 17:554, 1986.
24. Perri MG, McAdoo WG, McAllister DA, et al. Effects of peer support and therapist contact on long-term weight loss. *J Consult Clin Psychol* 55:615, 1987.
25. Perri MG, Nezu AM, Patti ET, et al. Effect of length of treatment on weight loss. *J Consult Clin Psychol* 57:450, 1989.
26. Marlatt GA, Gordon JR (eds). *Relapse Prevention: Maintenance Strategies in Addictive Behavior Change*. New York, Guilford Press, 1985.
27. Rosenthal BS, Marx RD. A comparison of standard behavioral and relapse prevention weight reduction program. Paper presented at the meeting of the Association for Advancement of Behavior Therapy, Chicago, December 1979.
28. Perri MG, McAllister DA, Gange JJ, et al. Effects of four maintenance programs on the long-term management of obesity. *J Consult Clin Psychol* 56:529, 1988.
29. Bandura A. *Principles of Behavior Modification*. New York, Holt, Rinehart and Winston, 1969, p. 255.
30. Sclafani A, Springer D. Dietary obesity in normal adult rats: Similarities to hypothalamic and human obesity syndromes. *Physiol Behav* 17:461, 1976.
31. Kanarak RB, Hirsch E. Dietary-induced overeating in experimental animals. *Fed Proc* 36:154, 1977.
32. Rolls BJ, Rowe EA, Kinston B, et al. Variety in a meal enhances food intake in man. *Physiol Behav* 26:215, 1981.
33. Rolls BJ. Sensory specific satiety. *Nutr Rev* 44:93, 1986.

CHAPTER

19

Models for Multidisciplinary Treatment Programs

The Physician's Office

Jaimy F. Honig, M.D.

The acknowledgment that obesity is a disease that contributes to the severity of many other chronic diseases has led to the blossoming of a new medical specialty: nutritional medicine. Indeed, the complex interrelationships between obesity and its co-morbidities emphasize the importance of treatment being executed by specially trained physicians and dietitians if there is to be favorable long-term patient outcome. Currently, 50 million Americans are spending nearly $10 billion annually[1] to lose excess weight by using commercial diet products or programs with little or no medical support or scientific basis. Implementation of dietary modification and instructions for beginning an elementary exercise program can be facilitated by many of the lay and commercial programs, but medical evaluation, assessment, and weight-loss management must be provided by physicians involved in primary care medicine and health promotion.

The physician with training in nutritional medicine can develop a successful and sound practice in the office setting either full-or part-time. The professional staff should include a registered nurse, a registered dietitian, a consulting exercise physiologist, and a counselor skilled in behavioral and psychological counseling. It is an extremely rewarding specialty, since implementing nutritional medicine principles can reverse the pathogenesis and altered metabolism involved in the chronic diseases associated with obesity. This is quite different, for example, from the pharmacologic treatment of obese hypertension, because many antihypertensive medications, while reducing blood pressure, have little effect on the pathogenesis of essential hypertension.[2] Further, the recently described *syndrome x* is uniquely reversed by weight reduction.[3] Similarly, weight reduction can be expected to have profound effects on many other such illnesses,[4,5] and it has the potential to save $100 million that otherwise would have been spent on treatment.[6]

Practicing nutritional medicine is a challenge given the poor preparation of physicians in the use of nutrition therapy, prescription of foods for special dietary and medical purposes, and evaluation and treatment of obesity and its health sequelae. However, maintaining an individual in a postobese state requires comprehensive, multidisciplinary ongoing treatment. Physicians can begin to gain expertise in nutritional medicine by means of fellowships and continuing medical education (CME) courses and by treating 25–50 patients longitudinally. Nutritional medicine uses the science and technology available today from the fields of metabolism, endocrinology, nutritional biochemistry, preventive medicine, genetics, behavioral medicine, and epidemiology to facilitate change in the energy/body weight set point and to train patients in the development of new skills that are consistent with maintaining a lower set point and improving their quality of life. Much of the practice involves the transfer of knowledge to the patient. This requires a partnership among the patient, physician, and dietitian, with each member contracting to fulfill his or her obligations. Patients thus become empowered to take an essential proactive role in their lifelong health care, constantly attending to lifestyle changes and self-reinforcement through self-monitoring and behavioral techniques. Recruiting a patient to participate in this partnership is indeed a worthy challenge to the primary care physician.

Organization and planning are crucial to the success of a nutritional medicine practice. Although the physician may have expertise in the field of nutrition, weight control, behavioral medicine, internal medicine, or general surgery, this unique practice must be effected through a multidisciplinary team approach for time, cost, and outcome effectiveness. The clinic/office manager, registered nurse, and registered dietitian each has a distinct role that helps ensure patient success. Group orientation sessions by the entire staff eliminate the need to repeat basic principles to each patient. The physician is the team leader and is responsible for establishing a patient–physician relationship. This begins with an informative introduction to the science of nutritional medicine and the effect of obesity on health and well-being at the onset of the group orientation. Patients should be encouraged to ask general questions at this time. Interactive discussion with the physician fosters the principles of partnership and mutual responsibility crucial to success in developing a postobese plan for living.

After the introductory session, each patient is seen individually for a comprehensive health and obesity history and medical evaluation.[7] Later this information will be used to develop a specific nutritional medicine prescription tailored to his or her specific needs and goals. At each step the patient learns that the major difference between a nutritional medicine practice and a weight-loss clinic is that nutritional medicine considers the total person, nutrition, fitness, stress management, and disease prevention under its auspices. Weight loss is just one piece of the whole, not an end in itself.

INITIAL MEDICAL EVALUATION

As part of the comprehensive medical evaluation, the patient's motives and goals for treatment should be explored. Often the patient is unaware that emotional and psychological factors contribute to disordered eating. Focusing solely on food intake and lack of physical activity diverts attention from the investigation of potentially greater barriers the patient may face in making changes in his or her lifestyle. Occasionally patients' psychological problems are so overwhelming that they must begin psychological counseling prior to starting or concurrently with a nutritional and exercise regimen; antidepressant medication may be required as an adjunct. These patients are so stressed that to remove their only coping mechanism, food, would be too great a challenge without professional support. Consulting psychologists should be available as necessary. Psychological screening questionnaires, such as the Profile of Mood Status (POMS),[8] Beck's Depression Inventory (BDI),[9] and the Eating Attitudes Test (EAT),[10] are efficient and reliable tools to assist in identifying patients for psychological consultation.

The health and obesity history focuses on conditions and diseases related to being overweight. It should be reinforced that weight losses of 10–15% make significant improvements in many of these comorbidities, and that aspiring to reduce to an "ideal" weight may be unrealistic for many obese people and unnecessary from a medical viewpoint.[11] Stressing realistic goals from the onset of treatment prepares patients for making permanent changes in eating, activity, and stress management. To identify periods of significant weight cycling and weight stability, the patient's weight history can be charted on a graph that covers 20 years. Observing longitudinal trends in weight helps identify energy/weight set points for formulating short-and long-term weight goals. This type of graph also identifies periods when low weights achieved through dieting were followed by rapid and excessive regain and therefore may have been unrealistic for a particular patient. Thus, this low weight should not serve as a goal weight.

Included in the physical exam are anthropometrics, waist:hip ratio, and body composition analysis. Careful measurement of supine and upright blood pressure and attention to physical signs consistent with genetic or endocrine forms of obesity and pathology resulting from obesity, such as sleep apnea, degenerative joint disease, diabetes, and other conditions, are basic components of the medical evaluation. If indicated, arrangements can be made for basal energy expenditure measurement and genetic or endocrine testing. Laboratory investigation should include a complete chemistry panel, thyroid function tests, total cholesterol, urinalysis, and an electrocardiogram. The physician or an exercise physiologist should conduct fitness testing, and nutritional assessment should be performed by a registered dietitian. Table 19–1 provides a sample nutritional medicine history and physical form. Table 19–2 shows the essential components of a physical activity form.

Assessment of a patient's motivation to undertake a long-term weight reduction and fitness program is best conducted during a 2- to 4-week introductory period before beginning a formal dietary regimen. Patients begin to identify their problematic eating, activities, and emotional habits through the use of highly structured recordkeeping procedures so that they can target what needs to be changed in their lives in order to develop a postobese lifestyle. Coping mechanisms are also recorded and examined. Rather than implementing a formal dietary regimen in this introductory phase, the patient is given general guidelines to begin to eliminate high-fat foods from the diet by means of a three-column sheet that divides foods into categories by fat level. If patients are unable, after up to 3 weeks of orientation, to make efforts at significant change in food selection, physical activity, and high-risk eating situations, their level of motivation should be reevaluated and alternative plans used until the patient has developed the determination to continue with an active weight loss plan. This investment of time on the part of the physician and patient will help to distinguish between those who are truly ready to make a commitment to health improvement and those who are in search of the elusive "magic bullet." The latter will continue to seek therapies more in line with those offered by commercial weight loss enterprises. Additional information on the medical evaluation and classification of the obese patient can be found in chapter 2.

OVERVIEW OF NUTRITIONAL AND EXERCISE INTERVENTIONS

The registered dietitian and/or behaviorist can most efficiently conduct nutrition, exercise, and behavioral education in a group format, with each group having between 8 and 12 patients. The physician must continue to be involved with patients throughout the active weight loss phase so that medical progress can be monitored, intercurrent health events identified and treated, and adjunctive treatments prescribed if necessary, such as medication or surgical consultation. It is also imperative that a strong maintenance program be created, since it is after patients undergo an initial period of weight reduction and lifestyle change

TABLE 19–1 Sample Medical History and Physical Examination Form

Name: ______________________ Date: ___/___/___

1. MEDICAL HISTORY BY SYSTEM (Check if symptom present and explain if presence or history of the condition exists.)

RESPIRATORY	YES	NO	COMMENTS
Shortness of breath (at rest)	___	___	______
DOE	___	___	______
Night sweats	___	___	______
Productive cough	___	___	______
Hemoptysis	___	___	______
h/o Tuberculosis	___	___	______
Pneumonia	___	___	______
Asthma	___	___	______
Pulmonary emboli	___	___	______
COPD	___	___	______
CARDIOVASCULAR			
Chest pain (undiagnosed)	___	___	______
h/o HTN	___	___	______
ASHD (MI)	___	___	______
Angina	___	___	______
CHF	___	___	______
Heart murmur	___	___	______
Hypotension	___	___	______
Edema	___	___	______
Peripheral vascular disease	___	___	______
GASTROINTESTINAL			
Nausea	___	___	______
Vomitting	___	___	______
Abdominal pain (undiagnosed)	___	___	______
Black stools	___	___	______
Rectal bleeding	___	___	______
"Heartburn"	___	___	______
Belching	___	___	______
h/o Constipation	___	___	______
Diarrhea	___	___	______
Hemorrhoids	___	___	______
Ulcer disease	___	___	______
Cholelithiasis	___	___	______
Hyperlipidemia	___	___	______

Continued

TABLE 19–1 *Continued*

GENITOURINARY			
Nocturia	___	___	___
Urgency	___	___	___
Difficult starting stream	___	___	___
Burning on urination	___	___	___
h/o Enlarged prostate	___	___	___
Hematuria	___	___	___
Recurrent urinary tract infection	___	___	___
Infertility	___	___	___
MUSCULOSKELETAL	YES	NO	COMMENTS
Aching muscles or joints	___	___	___
Low back pain	___	___	___
Limitations on mobility	___	___	___
h/o Arthritis	___	___	___
Muscle cramps	___	___	___
NEUROLOGICAL			
Numbness	___	___	___
Dizziness	___	___	___
Headaches	___	___	___
h/o Epilepsy	___	___	___
Seizure disorder	___	___	___
Syncope	___	___	___
Visual limitations	___	___	___
Auditory limitations	___	___	___
SKIN			
Chronic rashes	___	___	___
Broken areas	___	___	___
Bruises easily	___	___	___
OTHER			
h/o Diabetes	___	___	___
Gout	___	___	___
Thyroid	___	___	___
Psychiatric Illness	___	___	___

2. Allergies: ______________________________
3. Number of children: ______________________________
4. ETOH: ______________________________
5. Smoking: __________ Packs/day ________ Number of years ________
6. Surgical history (please list dates and surgeries):

____

____

____

Continued

TABLE 19–1 *Continued*

7. Current medications—include prescription and over-the-counter drugs:

Drug name	Dose	Frequency	Reason

8. (Women) Last menses: _____/_____/_____
9. Postmenopausal (Y/N): _____
10. Last Pap smear: _____/_____/_____ Results: __________
11. Last breast exam: _____/_____/_____ Results: __________
12. Birth control: __________ 13. Gravida/pari: __________
14. Do you currently have a primary-care physician? Yes _____ No _____ If yes, give name, address, and phone number below:

____

____

Abbreviations: DOE, dyspnea or exertion; COPD, chronic obstructive pulmonary disease; HTN, hypertension; ASTD (MI), ASHD (Atherosclerotic heart disease); CHF, congestive heart failure; ETOH, (Ethanol intake)

PHYSICAL EXAMINATION FORM DATE __________
(assumed normal unless otherwise noted) Name __________

BP right: _____/_____/_____
BP left: _____/_____/_____
Temp: _____
Pulse: _____
Resp: _____
Height: _____
Weight: _____
General
Orientation
Mood
Skin
Hair
Nodes
Head
Eyes
Fundi

Ears
Nose
Mouth
Throat
Cranial nerves
Thyroid
Neck
Carotids
Back
Chest
Lungs
Heart
Rhythm
Breast
Abdomen
Hernia

TABLE 19–1 *Continued*

Aorta-iliacs	LABORATORY
Genitalia	CBC
Vagina	Urinalysis
Cervix	Chemical screen
Pap smear	Lipid screen
Uterus	ECG
Adnexae	Thyroid screen
Anus	Other:
Rectum	OPTIONAL EXAMINATIONS
Arms	Tonometry
Branchial arteries	Laryngoscopy
Hands	Anoscopy
Legs	Proctoscopy
Femoral-popliteal	X-ray
Feet	RECOMMENDATIONS
Posterior tibial–dorsalis pedis	Immunizations
Superficial reflexes	Tuberculin test
Deep reflexes	
Toe signs	
Motor function	
Sensory function	NEXT OFFICE VISIT
Vibration sense	ANNUAL EXAMINATION
IMPRESSIONS	

Abbreviations: CBC, complete blood count; ECG, electrocardiogram.

TABLE 19–2 Sample Physical Activity Form

Patient Name: ____________________ Visit Date: __________

1. How many days in the last week did you participate in any of the following physical activities and
2. On the average, how many minutes of *continual* exercise per session did you do?

ACTIVITY	NUMBER OF SESSIONS THIS WEEK	MINUTES PER SESSION
Walking	______	______
Joging	______	______
Swimming	______	______
Bicycling	______	______
Rowing	______	______
Cross-country skiing	______	______
Aerobic dancing	______	______
Other (specify)	______	______
Other (specify)	______	______
TOTALS:	______	______

that reinforcement of these behaviors must continue. Contact with the nutritional medicine team no less frequently than monthly for at least 2 years during maintenance will help reinforce new behaviors; some of these contacts can be by telephone.

The physician pursuing a career in nutritional medicine can continue to serve as a primary-care physician for his or her own patients or as a consultant to internists, pediatricians, or surgeons. As a consultant, the nutritional medicine specialist has special facilities and equipment for evaluation and monitoring of obesity-related morbidities. Maintaining open lines of communication with the primary physician regarding health status and appropriate medication changes is essential for optimal patient care. Patients should have a clear understanding of each physician's role in their total health care management. The patient orientation brochure is an excellent way to describe how the practice functions and whom to contact in case of an emergency.

CONCLUSION

In nutritional medicine we cannot make people change in a way that they feel is out of character for them. To do so and force change will only produce guilt, conflict, and the very life stresses we seek to avoid. Rather, we must offer a menu of new knowledge, products, and services that will allow choices. If we can motivate individuals to stay with nutritional medicine, and undergo a catharsis of emotion, and mold into a group with a common cause of developing a new life image, we will succeed in overcoming the isolation and alienation that produce the illness and stress that brought them to us.

REFERENCES

1. Calloway CW. Testimony before the Subcommittee on Regulation and Business Opportunities, Committee on Small Business, U.S. House of Representatives, March 26, 1990.
2. Hebert PR, Fiebach NH, Eberlein KA, et al. The community-based randomized trials of pharmacologic treatments of mild-to-moderate hypertension. *Am J Epidemiol* 127:581, 1988.
3. Ferrannini E, Buzzigoli G, Bonnadonna R, et al. Insulin resistance in essential hypertension. *N Engl J Med* 317:350, 1987.
4. Manson JE, Colditz GA, Stampfer MJ, et al. A prospective study of obesity and risk of coronary heart disease in women. *N Engl J Med* 322:882, 1990.
5. Maclure KM, Haves KC, Colditz GA, et al. Weight, diet, and the risk of symptomatic gallstones in middle-aged women. *N Engl J Med* 321:563, 1989.

6. Cutler JA, Horan MJ, Roccella EJ, et al. guest eds. The National Heart, Lung, and Blood Institute Workshop on Antihypertensive Drug Treatment: The benefits, costs, and choices. *Hypertension* 13 (Suppl 1):1, 1989.
7. Blackburn GL, Kanders BS. Medical evaluation and treatment of the obese patient with cardiovascular disease. *Am J Cardiol* 60:55G, 1927.
8. McNail DM, Lorr M. An analysis of mood in neurotics. *J Abnorm Social Psychol* 69:620, 1964.
9. Beck AT, Beck RW. Screening depressed patients in family practice: A rapid technique. *Postgrad Med* 12:81, 1972.
10. Garner DM, Garfinkel PE. The Eating Attitudes Test: An index to the symptoms of anorexia nervosa. *Psychol Med* 9:237, 1979.
11. Kanders BS, Blackburn GL, Lavin PT, et al. Weight-loss outcome and health benefits associated with the Optifast Program in the treatment of obesity. *Int J Obes* 13 (Suppl 2):131, 1989.

The Work Site

Karen Quitzau, B.S.

BACKGROUND

Obesity, despite the volumes of research concerning its prevention and treatment, remains one of the most prevalent and serious health risks facing Americans today.[1,2] Numerous physical and psychosocial problems have been linked to obesity.[1] They include higher mortality and an increased risk of cardiovascular disease and certain cancers.[2] Fortunately, it has been shown that a significant reduction in these and other risk factors may be achieved through weight loss in the overweight individual.[2] However, treatment programs should be carefully designed to avoid a dangerous preoccupation with dieting and an overvaluation of thinness.[3] This is especially important in light of the discovery that extreme weight fluctuations have physical and psychological consequences more serious than those of maintaining a certain degree of overweight.[3] The social support structure in which many weight loss programs are provided appears to address this problem and therefore makes the work site an exciting new avenue in weight management.[1,2]

Employer-sponsored activities to promote health grew initially from an interest in reducing the number of work site injuries.[4] This idea expanded to include areas of preventative health care so that the majority of all but the smallest companies now promote some degree of health maintenance activities.[4] The work site lends itself very well to the idea of weight loss through social support and behavior modification, and has become popular among employees for its convenience as well as its personalized quality. In fact, a study conducted by Reid and Dunkley,[2] revealed that in a survey of two high-tech companies, 75% of the men and 92% of the women with a body mass index of 25 or greater were interested in participating in a company-sponsored weight loss program.[2] Not surprisingly, 68% of nonoverweight women were interested in a weight maintenance program at the work site.[2] Apparently, work site exercise facilities and low-fat, low-calorie food choices in employee cafeterias are appropriate additions to encourage.[3]

THE WORK SITE APPROACH

The success of work site weight control and physical fitness programs has been well documented in recent years.[1,4,5] A work site program involving 80 employees of the Missouri State Highway Patrol headquarters and the Missouri Department of Health resulted in an average weight loss of 5.3 lb (2.4 kg) by participants in the 10-week program, which employed weekly seminars on positive lifestyle changes.[1] Another study showed that employees will make significant changes in health practices with a minimum of professional involvement if provided with feedback on health status and information about ways to reduce certain health risks in a supportive environment.[5] It also appears that improvements in exercise habits and physical fitness are well distributed among the participating work force, regardless of age, marital status, race, or socioeconomic status.[4] Therefore, to ensure the success of a work site weight loss program, the company must make a careful assessment of the needs and interests of its employees and focus on ways to enlist the support of key administrative personnel, as well as promote continued participation.

KEY COMPONENTS

The possible components of a work site weight loss or maintenance program are varied and will obviously depend on the needs of the particular employee population. However, three key components have been recognized as useful parts of any weight loss program: (1) lifestyle or risk-reduction seminars, (2) diet therapy or nutritional guidance, and (3) aerobic exercise prescription or access to appropriate exercise facilities.[3–5]

Lifestyle seminars take many forms, ranging from all-day educational sessions on the health risks associated with high-fat diets and sedentary lifestyles to weekly lunch-hour sessions for open discussion on promoting healthful practices through nutrition, exercise, and stress management. In many cases, programs employing the informational approach alone are sufficient for realizing significant lifestyle changes among employees.[5] Ideally, however, this component should be considered as a part of a larger, more comprehensive approach to active weight reduction in which emphasis is placed on providing a well-rounded program.[6]

It is recommended that the registered dietitian play a major role in providing the resources for nutritional management of the work site population.[3] A complete weight-loss diet plan, including regular aerobic exercise, should provide at least 1,200 kcal/day for normal adults and should provide foods that are acceptable to the dieter in terms of sociocultural background, usual habits, taste, cost, and ease of acquisition and preparation.[7] In this regard, the diet therapy component of the work site weight-loss program requires a more personal approach than the lifestyle seminars provide and must be carefully conducted by a professional.

An exercise program designed for weight loss should be combined with a low-fat, reduced-calorie diet to create a negative caloric balance of approximately 500 kcal/day, resulting in a gradual weight loss without metabolic derangements.[7] The exercise component of the work site program should employ the standard practices of exercise prescription, instruction, progression, and safety. An exercise physiologist should play an integral part in obtaining adequate medical information from each participant in regard to present health status, level of physical fitness, needs and objectives, and level of exercise expertise. The coordinator should assist in setting realistic long- and short-term goals, as well as monitor progress and reevaluate each participant on an individual basis.[6] Only in this way can proper implementation, progress, and safety be assured.

EXERCISE PRESCRIPTION

A personalized exercise prescription is integral to the long-term success of any training program. Each exercise prescription should address the following three areas: intensity, duration, and frequency.[7]

1. *Intensity:* The activity chosen should allow the individual to achieve a heart rate in the range of 65–90% of maximum. The range may be calculated by multiplying the maximal heart rate (220 − age) by 0.65 and 0.90. Activities eliciting a heart rate at the lower end of the range are recommended for individuals with a low initial fitness level.
2. *Duration:* Each exercise session should consist of 15–60 min of continuous activity in the target heart rate zone. Lower to moderate duration is recommended for nonathletic adults to avoid potential injuries and compliance problems.

3. *Frequency:* Exercise sessions should occur three to five times per week. It is recommended that individuals with low initial fitness levels alternate a day of exercise with a day of rest in the initial stages of the weight loss program.

PROGRESSION

The progression of the exercise program should be carefully monitored by the exercise physiologist to ensure safe, adequate improvement in fitness level and caloric expenditure.

1. *Starter Phase:* From 2 to 6 weeks long. The routine includes flexibility exercises and light calisthenics followed by aerobic exercise of low to moderate intensity.
2. *Slow Progression Phase:* The duration and intensity of the exercise routine are increased consistently every 1 to 3 weeks, depending on the individual's tolerance.
3. *Maintenance Phase:* After approximately 6 months to 1 year, the individual may choose to sustain the current level of exercise to maintain fitness and weight loss.[6]

MODALITY SUGGESTIONS

Any activity that meets the requirements of the exercise prescription already mentioned is appropriate for achieving increased fitness and weight loss. However, several modalities lend themselves well to the work site exercise facility. These include:

1. A clearly marked walking/jogging path on company grounds that can be used during the lunch hour or after working hours.
2. Stationary bicycles, treadmills, rowing machines, or stair machines, with adequate and available instruction on their safe operation.
3. Aerobic dance classes held during the lunch hour or immediately after working hours. Classes should be designed and led by a qualified instructor so that they can be adapted for use by individuals at various fitness levels.
4. Access to an aquatic facility where continuous lap swimming or supervised aquatic exercise classes may be conducted.

It is important to apply the standard components of each exercise session to any activity chosen to ensure a well rounded approach to conditioning and weight control.[6] These four components are:

1. *Warmup:* Ten minutes of stretching, low-level calisthenics, and walking.

2. *Muscular Conditioning:* From 10 to 20 min of calisthenics, weight training, and/or floor exercises.
3. *Aerobics:* From 20 to 40 min of exercise within the target heart rate range at a level appropriate for the individual's current level of fitness.
4. *Cool-down:* From 5 to 10 min of walking and stretching to allow gradual return of the heart rate to near-resting levels.

MAINTAINING PARTICIPATION

When implementing any employer-sponsored health promotion program, the issue of participation rates must be addressed. The immediate success of any program may be gauged by initial enrollment levels, but ongoing employee participation is integral to its long-term success.[8] Participation rates have typically been found to vary from 20% to 40% for onsite programs and from 10% to 25% for programs offered outside the workplace.[8] In addition, employee fitness programs generally experience 30 to 70% dropout rates during the first 3 to 6 months.[8] In addressing this dilemma, employers must determine the likelihood that the employee population will utilize a particular program and what factors contribute to dropout. It has been suggested that program participants tend to be persons whose job stress and body mass index are high.[9] Simple employee surveys may provide direction for the employer in the development of an acceptable program. Several researchers have suggested that participation levels are enhanced by providing weekly or daily sessions held during work time, obtaining support from key administrative personnel, establishing teams to encourage group participation, and allowing employee involvement in the planning and implementing of programs.[1,8]

CONCLUSION

Studies suggest that the expected benefits to the employer of implementing a weight control program include reduced health costs, a significant reduction in reported sick days, decreased staff turnover, and enhanced productivity and morale.[2,4,5] Participants in employer-sponsored weight loss programs have repeatedly reported reduced levels of job stress compared with non-participants.[9] In recently reviewed studies on weight reduction programs, costs per participant ranged from $41.93 to $288.66 and costs per pound of weight loss ranged from $5.37 to $15.57.[3] Considering that expected savings in health benefit costs often approach 30%, weight management programs appear to be an economically sound investment.[4] It is expected that a program consisting of any combination of lifestyle education, dietary guidelines, and exercise facilities coupled with a positive perception of management's support for the plan will help maintain a level of participation and success that will prove beneficial to both employer and employee.

REFERENCES

1. Markenson DM, Schiff WJ. Adapting a community group weight reduction program to a work-site setting. *J Am Diet Assoc* 88:1436, 1988.
2. Reid DJ, Dunkley GC. Weight control in the workplace: A needs assessment for men. *Can J Public Health* 80:24, 1989.
3. Position of the American Dietetic Association: Optimal weight as a health promotion strategy. *J Am Diet Assoc* 89:1814, 1989.
4. Breslow L, Fielding J. Herrman A, et al. Worksite health promotion: Its evolution and the Johnson & Johnson experience. *Prev Med* 19:13, 1990.
5. Ostwald SK. Changing employees' dietary and exercise practices: An experimental study in a small company. *J Occup Med* 31:90, 1989.
6. Pollock ML, Wilmore JH, Fox SM. *Exercise in Health and Disease*. Philadelphia, WB Saunders, 1984, pp. 244–269.
7. American College of Sports Medicine. *Guidelines for Exercise Testing and Prescription,* ed 3. Philadelphia, Lea & Febiger, 1986, pp. 31–44.
8. Lovato CY, Green LW. Maintaining employee participation in workplace health promotion programs. *Health Educ Q* 14:73, 1987.
9. Davis KE, Jackson KL, Kronenfeld, JJ, et al. Determinants of participation in worksite health promotion activities. *Health Educ Q* 14:195, 1987.

The Clinic

Dawn E. Norton, B.S.

INTRODUCTION

The greatest asset of the medical obesity treatment clinic is the staff's education and training. The same physician–dietitian teamwork that has succeeded in hospital nutrition support services can be used in the outpatient clinic. Only the medical community is truly qualified to handle the chronic disease of obesity; thus, medical weight-loss programs should supplant commercial ones. We have seen the results of medically unsupervised programs, and our determination to educate patients in the importance of involving their doctor and an experienced nutritional team in their weight-loss efforts has led to the development of free-standing obesity treatment clinics worldwide.

A successful outpatient obesity treatment clinic requires a multidisciplinary approach incorporating the expertise of the physician, nurse, dietitian/group leader, exercise physiologist, and clinic manager. The primary element that is critical to any successful program is established credibility within the community and a reputation for understanding this complex disease. The goal of the medical community is to establish a rapport with this population such that they seek help within the medical community first rather than as a last resort.

CHOOSING THE TARGET POPULATION

The number of programs offered in the clinic will depend on financial goals as well as the target population. Marketing surveys should be conducted prior to establishing a clinic to assess the number and demographics of potential clients. Ideally, in addition to serving the morbidly obese, services should include programs for the moderately overweight. Providing these services in addition to very-low-calorie diet (VLCD) programs will increase revenues, as well as enable the clinic to be more competitive with commercial weight-loss programs.

START-UP COSTS

The operating costs of the clinic will depend on the overall long-term financial and personal goals and available resources. Clinic employees represent the largest expense, although the clinic manager may be the only employee who works full time. Other staff members can be hired on a part-time and/or per diem basis. From a financial standpoint, one of the major advantages of offering a multidisciplinary program is that nurses can deliver primary care (i.e., medical monitoring) to patients at a much lower cost than can physicians.[1] The usual cost of physician services is approximately $75/hr, whereas nurses can be hired for roughly $15/hr. Group leaders and exercise physiologists are typically hired at $25/hr for individual consultations and for $50 per group session. No benefits are included for part-time employees. Table 19–3 provides an approximation of the yearly operating costs of a free-standing clinic. Expenses listed reflect actual costs to an existing clinic in the Boston area. Variations in cost of wages, rent, insurance, and so on, determined by geographic location, should be taken into account.

PERSONNEL

Job Descriptions

The program staff may consist of only a manager, physician, and group leader, or it may incorporate other specialists such as a nurse, exercise physiologist, and behaviorist. The size of the clinic staff will vary, depending on the program requirements, the resources available, and the goals of the team.

TABLE 19–3 Yearly Operating Costs for an Established Free-Standing Clinic

Operating Expenses	
Food purchases	(expense relative to patient flow)
Capital expenses	22,045.00
Accounting and legal fees	11,225.00
Advertising/promotional (includes brochures, newsletters, invitations, etc.)	31,248.00
Books, magazines, and subscriptions	650.00
Casual labor (cleaning)	800.00
Freight and postage	325.00
Heat, light, and power	335.00
Insurance	1,395.00
Lease expenses (office machinery)	1,550.00
Maintenance and repairs	1,550.00
Medical supplies	725.00
Office expenses, program materials, and manuals (relative to patient flow)	11,200.00
Printing	725.00
Professional fees	4,872.00
Rent (relative to space, location)	11,595.00
Telephone	2,525.00
Wages—manager	26,000.00
Wages—physician (part-time)	39,880.00
Wages—nurse (part-time)	20,800.00
Wages—dietitian (part-time)	18,000.00
Taxes—payroll	11,261.00
Administrative fees at 7% of gross	(relative to revenue)
Training at 2% of gross	(relative to revenue)
Total Expenses	$377,128.00

The clinic manager oversees the organization and management of the clinic staff, the patients, and the services provided. This is a leadership position for a dynamic and outgoing individual experienced in business and office management as well as in health care and/or a service-oriented field. At a minimum, a 4-year bachelors' degree is required, with education in business, sales, and/or marketing preferred. The ability of the manager to relate well to others is what management is all about. Success as a clinic manager results from skills in dealing with clinic employees and patients. Because managers become deeply involved in operating details and bureaucratic interface, they sometimes forget their underlying function—patient service. The clinic manager must maintain a continuing sense of responsibility to ensure that the patient remains a priority.[2]

The manager must ensure that all aspects of the program are running effectively and efficiently so that the best possible care is being provided to patients. He or she must possess strong organizational and interpersonal skills, warmth, caring, and empathy for the obese population.

The role of the physician will not be discussed here, as it is thoroughly reviewed in the first section of this chapter called *The Physician's Office*.

The group leader should be a registered dietitian, ideally one with a master's degree in nutrition, education, or counseling. A minimum of 1 year of experience with obese patients or patients with eating disorders and/or addictions, as well as a minimum of 1 year of experience in providing group therapy, is required. The dietitian must possess extensive knowledge of the physical and psychological implications of obesity, and must be able to recognize the need for psychotherapy and to make appropriate referrals.

The group leader must facilitate support and foster a sense of camaraderie within the group. It is the leader's responsibility to instill commitment and compliance of patients to the program while adhering to the program's policies and protocol. In addition, the group leader develops and maintains current resource and educational materials for reference in the clinic and works with other staff members to improve the quality of care.

The clinic nurse works closely with the physician during the initial assessment and the weekly evaluations. As a qualified professional, the nurse should have experience in working with the obese population, as well as be able to identify eating disorders that may require alternative or additional therapy. Some of the nurse's primary responsibilities include obtaining and reviewing the medical history of patients (including an organ systems review, weight history, and psychological history) and performing physical assessments, including height, weight, anthropometric measurements, determination of body mass index (BMI), vital signs, phlebotomy, and performance of electrocardiograms (ECGs) and bioelectrical impedance analysis. The nurse reviews the charts and laboratory values of patients, referring clinically significant values to the supervising physician; periodically reviews charts for quality assurance; and, with the physician, routinely communicates with the patient's primary care physician. In addition to working with the entire team, the clinic nurse must be sufficiently flexible and proficient to work independently.

The exercise physiologist should possess a master's degree in exercise physiology, sports medicine, physical therapy, or physical education or certification in exercise physiology by the American College of Sports Medicine at the exercise specialist level. This individual works with the group leader to plan and conduct sessions on the importance of exercise in both weight loss and maintenance. The exercise physiologist should also be available to help patients with their own exercise programs.[3]

The behaviorist should possess a master's or doctorate degree in psychology, public health, or counseling; a master's in social work or licensed clinical social worker, or an M.D. degree in psychiatry. This individual works with the group leader to plan and conduct group sessions on behavior modification and lifestyle change. In addition, the behaviorist counsels patients who are having difficulty adhering to the program or who require individual therapy.[3]

Performance

Forms should be developed to evaluate staff performance as well as program services. Patients should complete evaluation forms approximately every 3 months, regardless of what phase of the program they are in. Team members must meet periodically to review comments and to discuss areas in need of improvement.

CLINIC SPACE

Location

In addition to the staff, the location and layout of the clinic are critical to the overall success of the program. Proximity to a medical institution is strongly recommended. This will promote physician referrals and provide easy access to support services. The clinic should be accessible from all areas of the community by car and by public transportation. Free parking should be available.[3]

Office Layout

The layout of the site will determine how smoothly and efficiently patients move through the clinic. The more efficient the layout, the smaller the space required. At the same time, however, patients must feel comfortable. A waiting room, business office/reception area, weigh-in station, exam room, group room, storage room, and two offices are recommended for the basic clinic.[3]

The waiting room may have to accommodate up to 30 patients, depending on the size of the program and how many groups are run simultaneously; thus, it should be as pleasant and comfortable as possible. A minimum of 300 ft^2 is recommended.[3]

Patients meet with the nurse and/or physician weekly in the exam room. If the patient has not experienced any serious intercurrent health events during the week, this exam normally takes 5 min or less. To expedite this process, at least two exam rooms should be available, one for the nurse and one for the physician.

The group room should be large enough to hold 17 to 20 people comfortably. To enhance communication, chairs should be set up in a U shape or in a circle around the perimeter of the room. A chalkboard or whiteboard with markers should be available, and audiovisual/VCR equipment is recommended.[3]

Offices should be available for full-time staff members, who will be engaged in various tasks during nonpatient hours. The clinic manager's office should be located at the front of the office near the reception area. A storage room should also be located near the reception area and should be large enough to hold a 6-week supply of product as well as program material. The room should be cool, dry, and locked at all times. Approximately 200 ft^2 should be adequate.[3]

Equipment and Furnishings

Office furniture differs slightly from that of a general practice in that it must be able to accommodate the obese. All chairs in the waiting area and group rooms, for example, must be larger and free of arms to seat patients comfortably. They should be 24–26 in. wide as opposed to the standard 22-in. width, have firm padding or cushions, and be very sturdy. The covering should be cloth rather than plastic or vinyl, and there should be no castors or wheels. Couches should be avoided, as obese patients have difficulty rising from them.[3]

With a few exceptions, general office and medical equipment is essentially the same as that required for any general practice. The scale, allowing for weight of up to 800 lb, should have a wide, sturdy base, with wheels for easy storage and maneuverability. For the exam rooms, additional blood pressure cuffs (two large, one thigh cuff) should be available.[3] A bioelectrical impedance machine and skinfold calipers are also required for determining body composition.

PROGRAM OVERVIEW

To promote a successful program, all patients should go through the following steps during their course of treatment: orientation, initial evaluation, fasting, refeeding and stabilization, and maintenance. Following an initial phone contact, the patient will schedule an appointment for either an initial evaluation or an orientation.[23] It is extremely important for the clinic manager to review proper telephone techniques with all office staff. Scripts are not recommended, as they sound very commercial. The office staff should feel comfortable enough with the program to speak freely.

Orientation sessions should involve participation by the entire staff. The program components should be thoroughly reviewed, and program materials should be available for review. The prospective patient should leave with a brochure and an appointment schedule for an initial evaluation if so desired. Group orientations should be scheduled during the evening hours. It is the clinic manager's responsibility to conduct individual orientations for those who are unable to attend the group session. Attendees should be limited to 15.

The initial evaluation consists of two appointments. The first is with the nurse for a medical history review, nutritional and psychological assessment, ECG, laboratory tests, and bioelectrical impedance analysis.[3] This interview normally takes 45–60 min to complete. If at this visit the registered nurse is able to rule out any contraindications to a fasting or modified fasting program, the patient is instructed to follow a balanced deficit diet (BDD) until he or she meets with the physician for a full review of the prior physical and psychological assessment and a physical exam; the nature of this exam is explained in detail in the next section of this chapter.

The fasting phase, which lasts for approximately 12 weeks, consists of a VLCD. During this phase, patients are required to attend the clinic weekly for medical monitoring and group sessions, with an emphasis on behavior modification.[3]

During refeeding, food is gradually reintroduced into the diet over a 6-week period. This phase is then followed by an 8-week stabilization period during which caloric needs are determined for maintenance of patients' new body weights. Weekly visits for medical monitoring and group sessions continue during this period, with an emphasis on nutrition education and behavioral skill development.[3]

During maintenance, medical monitoring ceases and patients become responsible for monitoring their own weight. Group sessions continue on a weekly basis, and individual consultations are scheduled with the group leader when additional support is needed. A minimum of a 12-month commitment is expected.[3]

SOME MANAGERIAL GUIDELINES

Patient Flow

Patient flow begins at the reception desk, where patients sign in and complete any necessary forms in the waiting room. Following clinical and medical assessment, weekly payments are collected and product orders are placed. Patients then attend the group session for 1 hr. Early morning and evening groups should be offered to meet the scheduling needs of patients.[4] Groups should contain no more than 15 and no fewer than 8 participants for cost effectiveness and group cohesiveness. At the end of the session, patients obtain their 1-week supply of supplement (prebagged during the group meeting) and are free to leave. It is recommended that product be distributed following the group session to ensure commitment.

Weekly Attendance

Clinic visits are weekly, and patients should expect to be at the clinic for approximately 1.5 to 2 hr. It is best to establish an attendance policy and to make patients aware of it, both orally and in writing, at screening and during the first group session. A reasonable policy would be to allow two absences during active weight loss and refeeding. If more absences occur, the patient and group leader should meet privately to address any problems and to re-evaluate the patient's commitment.[4]

Any patient who is absent on the clinic day should be contacted immediately by the group leader. It is important that the patient make arrangements to go to the clinic the following day to undergo medical monitoring and to receive the product. If, after several attempts, the group leader has been unable to reach the patient, a card or letter should be sent requesting that the patient contact the clinic and/or group leader.

Patient Education

Education is a key component of a successful program. Although most VLCD programs do provide some form of education, either in the group setting or through one-on-one counseling, it is not always mandatory. There are individual practitioners who dispense the product without providing any behavioral or nutritional counseling. Patients in such programs are at extreme risk for program failure and weight regain.[5]

Educational materials must be utilized throughout the program. The patient manual should cover a wide range of material, including behavioral issues and nutrition and exercise information. Supplementary handouts, worksheets, and videotapes should also be available, as should recommended reading lists.

PRODUCTS AND VENDORS

When selecting supplements and products for program use, it is important to interview several vendors. Request basic information about the company as well as the supplier's track record. Evaluate the quality of the product by obtaining complete nutritional information. Be sure that the entire staff samples the supplement, paying particular attention to taste and texture. Assess the vendor's commitment to providing ongoing support regarding obesity treatment and research.[6] Finally, conduct an extensive review of the program materials and manuals for content and comprehensibility.

OFFICE AUTOMATION

Choosing an office automation system can be quite a challenge. The software chosen should be designed to track inquiries, schedule patients, and manage accounts payable and all aspects of patient interaction. Reports should be generated on a daily, weekly, and monthly basis for financial accountability. As far as patient data analyses are concerned, at a minimum, the tracking system should provide data regarding average weight loss velocity and dropout rates over time.[7]

MARKETING THE CLINIC

Marketing the program demands a thoughtful, comprehensive approach. Promoting a medically supervised program seems easy at first. After all, the standard consumer ads featuring before-and-after photos of successful patients, including celebrities, are apparently effective. Why shouldn't this marketing technique be used? Simply stated, professional program ads should not focus on cosmetic weight loss.[8] Marketing should be aimed at physicians as well as potential patients; thus, the message should sound professional and stress the key components of an effective program. The seriousness of the disease should be addressed without being too alarming. Facts should be presented in such a manner as to reflect current statistics and stress what the program is doing to ameliorate the problem.

Commercial programs such as Jenny Craig, Diet Center, and Nutri/System have built multi-million-dollar operations through extensive consumer advertising. Hospital-based and free-standing medical clinics must take a different route. The obvious reason is cost.[8] For an established free-standing clinic, expect to spend approximately 9% of yearly gross income on advertising. The best place to invest most of your resources is in developing referrals within the medical community. This is particularly important during the first year of operation. It is necessary to assure doctors that you're not offering a primary-care service designed to steal their patients but rather a partnership designed to benefit the entire medical community. For example, other physicians can gain the business of a significant number of VLCD patients—as many as 40% in some programs—who do not have primary care providers.[8] Literature should be sent to physicians introducing the staff and programs offered. A thank-you letter should be sent for any referral. Update letters providing information on patient progress should be sent to active patients' physicians every 3 months.

Orientation sessions for prospective patients are an important marketing tool. Even if the person attending does not sign up for the program for any reason, you'll want to make such a positive impression that the individual discusses his or her experience with a friend, relative, or coworker. Word-of-mouth referrals are invaluable! Public relations can play a large role in marketing the program and should be utilized whenever possible. Host open houses and invite local media personnel. Keep abreast of the latest research as it is made public, and contact your local media offering to comment on the issue.[8] Distribute literature at health fairs and in waiting areas at local health centers and hospitals. Invite former patients to speak at orientations and open houses. Publish success stories in your local newspaper. One note of caution, however: If you are obtaining support from a local celebrity participating in your program, make sure that the individual does not have a history of weight cycling and that he or she will be committed to a maintenance program.[8]

FINANCIAL ISSUES

The cost of your program should be competitive with that of other hospital-based and free-standing medical clinics. Weekly fees should be established that include medical monitoring, group sessions, and product costs. If a patient misses a group meeting for any reason without approval, he or she should still be charged the full weekly fee. This will prevent patients from trying to skip groups to cut costs. For initial evaluations, it is recommended to require a deposit due 1 week prior to the scheduled appointment. This will greatly decrease your number of "no shows" and will allow the highly motivated candidates to start sooner.

Collections are always a major concern. Unfortunately, to date there are very few insurance carriers that recognize obesity as a disease; therefore, obtaining coverage of patient services may be difficult. To protect the financial integrity of the clinic, it is recommended that a fee-for-service system be established in which the patient is responsible for the charges incurred. There are a number of ways to assist the patient seeking reimbursement, and staff members should be knowledgeable and willing to help patients as needed.

Insurance coverage varies from carrier to carrier, and it is difficult to determine whether or not a given patient will receive coverage. Most carriers do not even have established guidelines for coverage; however, there are some general criteria to which most companies adhere. For example, very few carriers will even consider coverage if the patient is not at least 100% above ideal body weight. Other carriers will only pay for nutrition counseling and will not cover dietitian visits. Most insurance companies cover at least 80% of the charges for the history and physical exam, laboratory work, and ECG. Few companies will cover for the group sessions, and very few will pay for nutritional supplements.

The clinic manager must educate the staff on current policies and develop various strategies for assisting patients in the reimbursement process. The manager must first provide realistic information and hope concerning potential coverage without actually guaranteeing coverage. Patients must be reminded that the insurance coverage is very similar to that of other medical specialties and will vary, depending on the carrier and type of policy. Prospective patients should have assistance with preauthorization calls or at least be educated on how to handle the calls themselves.[9] Once patients have enrolled in the program, they should be provided with itemized receipts at each visit documenting payment and services rendered. Patients should be instructed on how to fill out insurance claim forms, and the clinic manager must be willing to provide assistance when needed. A form letter for physician updates should be designed to accompany the claim. A letter from the physician documenting the patients' baseline weight and medical condition is often requested by the carrier; thus, it is advisable to send this with the initial claim to expedite the process.

One of the major reasons patients will not enroll in medical weight-loss programs is that they feel the programs are too costly compared with commercial programs. Since insurance coverage is not usually guaranteed, patients feel that they would benefit from a lower-priced, more familiar approach. Seeking medical attention for an addictive disorder can be very frightening and intimidating. Most obese individuals will exhaust all other weight-loss programs before even considering a medically supervised program. One effective way to remedy this situation is to offer financing options. Alternative payment plans will have a major impact on the patient's perception of price. A payment plan can "reduce" a $3000 program to one that costs $50 a week or less. This type of financing will help your program be more competitive with commercial programs.[10]

In setting up any type of financing program, it is important to first evaluate your own situation and needs. The key priorities are to establish a payment plan that will reduce the weekly cost to the patient and will be as low-risk to the clinic as possible. Results must be tracked to determine the effectiveness of the financing plan.[10]

There are risks involved in offering financing options, and the advantages and disadvantages must be carefully considered before implementing any plan. The most reliable options appear to be Visa/MasterCard and bank financing programs. Patients with existing credit cards are already familiar and comfortable with them and are generally not reluctant to use them. Another advantage of using major credit cards is that the program receives the payment quickly, unlike insurance reimbursements, for which there are often delays. One disadvantage of major credit cards is that the clinic must pay a discount (surcharge) of 3–5%, although this rate tends to be lower than that for medical credit cards, and the rate is reduced for large volumes.[10]

A bank financing program that provides a competitive interest rate, no discounts to the clinic, and direct approval for the patient is ideal. More payment options may be available to the patient (i.e., secured loans), and loan rates can be negotiated that are lower than average credit card rates. The best approach when establishing bank loans is for the clinic manager to work with the bank to develop a system in which the patient can complete all the necessary forms at the clinic. A standard loan amount to cover the program expenses (e.g., $3000) should be established, and loan approval should be given within 24 hr. There should be no fees or discounts, and the clinic should not be required to accept risk of default. Setting up bank loans will initially require a great deal of effort on the part of the clinic manager. However, once the system has been instituted, the clinic will benefit greatly.[10]

EVALUATING SUCCESS

Because the weight-loss market is so fragmented, it is difficult to sustain market share and growth.[11] To thrive in this field, the program must meet all professional standards as well as patient expectations. It is important to review all program components on a current basis. Thus, if a trend or disorientation has taken place, it can be addressed in a timely fashion.[2] Patient progress and success, attrition rate, evaluations, and monthly or quarterly operating statements will enable you to make accurate assessments of the overall success of the program.

One of the greatest predictors of success, not only for patients but also for the clinic, is attendance. If you have minimized the attrition rate, you have succeeded in offering a viable program that will benefit not only the obese population but the entire medical community as well. Your multidisciplinary team can work with other specialists to address and ameliorate the variety of disorders associated with this complex disease.

REFERENCES

1. Atkinson RL, Russ CS, Ciavarella PA, et al. A comprehensive approach to outpatient obesity management. *J Am Diet Assoc* 84:439, 1984.
2. Bohlmann RC. The ABC's of clinic management. *Med Group Management* 34, 1981. Vol. 28(3).
3. *The Optifast Program Start-Up Guide*. Sandoz Nutriton Corp., Minneapolis, MN, 1987.
4. *The Optifast Program Clinical Staff Guide*. Sandoz Nutrition Corp., Minneapolis, MN, 1988.
5. Moran E. Weight loss programs still fatten profits despite competition. *Hospitals* 39, 1990. Vol. 64, No. 7.
6. Health Care Communications. Hospitals view very-low-calorie diet programs as sure-fire moneymakers. *Strategic Health Care Marketing;* 7:4, 1990.
7. Gotto AM, Foreyt JP, Goodrick GK. Evaluating commercial weight-loss clinics. *Arch Intern Med* 142:682, 1982.
8. Health Care Communications. Marketing a weight-loss program demands thoughtful, comprehensive approach. *Strategic Health Care Marketing;* 7:3, 1990.

9. Card B, Heiss D, Willette S, et al. Understanding insurance reimbursement. Paper presented at the Seventh Annual Optifast Post Graduate Seminar, San Antonio, Tex, Apr 30–May 4, 1989.
10. *The Optifast Program. Financing Options*. Sandoz Nutrition Corp, 1990.
11. Lutz S. Weight-loss market's fat profits are fading. *Modern Heathcare* 19:50, 1990.

Appendix: Multidisciplinary Model for the Assessment and Treatment of Obesity: Matching Risks and Patient Needs with Treatment Approach

A gap exists between our knowledge of obesity and its health outcome and our ability to prevent and treat this serious chronic disease. To date, trained health professionals and lay workers who treat obesity have used their own approaches to solve the problem. Obesity is a multifaceted disease whose solution demands the integration of knowledge and expertise from many different disciplines. In combining data from successful approaches, we have developed a treatment model similar to those used for other chronic diseases (e.g., hypertension, hypercholesterolemia) to provide guidance in assessing and treating the obese patient. This comprehensive treatment model emphasizes careful screening to match the patient with the most appropriate, cost-effective treatment option.

Nutrition screening and intervention cannot depend on referring all obese individuals to nutrition medicine specialists due to the shortage of such profession-

---

Sources: Academy Advisory Group; National Academy of Sciences. Institute of Medicine, Ad Hoc Advisory Group on Preventive Services, Preventive Services for a Well Population, Washington, DC, National Academy of Sciences, 1978.

Division of Consumer Affairs, New York City. 1991.

als. In addition, excellent self-help opportunities and commercial programs are available to the public. The model therefore includes four levels of care that progress from self-help to aggressive medical intervention. Treatment at any level must be multidisciplinary and must include dietary change, physical activity, and behavior or lifestyle change. Fundamental to changing behavior is teaching individuals about diet, lifestyle, and health so that they can make educated decisions.

Using the Model

Risk assessment involves the identification of characteristics known to place individuals at increased risk for obesity-related morbidity and mortality. These characteristics include excess body fat (e.g., body mass index [BMI] $\geq$ 30), upper body fat distribution (e.g., waist–hip ratio [WHR] $>$ 1), a history of weight cycling (defined as a gain or loss $>$ 10 lb in 1 year), presence of obesity-related disease (e.g., diabetes, hypertension, insulin resistance, hypercholesterolemia), early-onset obesity (defined as obesity onset prior to age 21), and/or the presence of eating disorders (e.g., bulimia, binge eating disorder, defined according to DSM-IV criteria). Results of this preliminary risk assessment will dictate whether the patient should start at Step 1 or be referred to Step 4 for more aggressive adjuvant treatment.

Once risk factors have been identified, lifestyle intervention can be undertaken to improve the patient's health, using guidelines from the U.S. Preventive Health Task Force. As always, intervention should *match* the needs and desires of the individual to promote maximum compliance with the program. Our treatment model includes a four-step treatment approach, as shown in Figure A-1.

Step One. All individuals particpate in this level during a 3- to 6-month treatment period. The minimal goal is to stop weight gain and/or effect a weight loss of 2 BMI units (2 kg/m^2 or approximately 10 lb) while at the same time incorporating healthy lifestyle changes and improving the patient's quality of life. This can be done largely through a self-help approach.

Step Two. All patients are screened first by their primary care physician and referred to a certified commercial weight loss clinic (as defined by the Division of Consumer Affairs, New York City) or a support group. Again, the goal is to stop weight gain and/or achieve a 2 kg/m^2 weight loss while incorporating healthy lifestyle changes and improving the overall quality of life.

Step Three. All patients are monitored and, if at high risk for comorbid disease, are supervised by their primary care physician. Intervention is carried out at a commercial weight loss clinic or via self-help. Treatment goals include

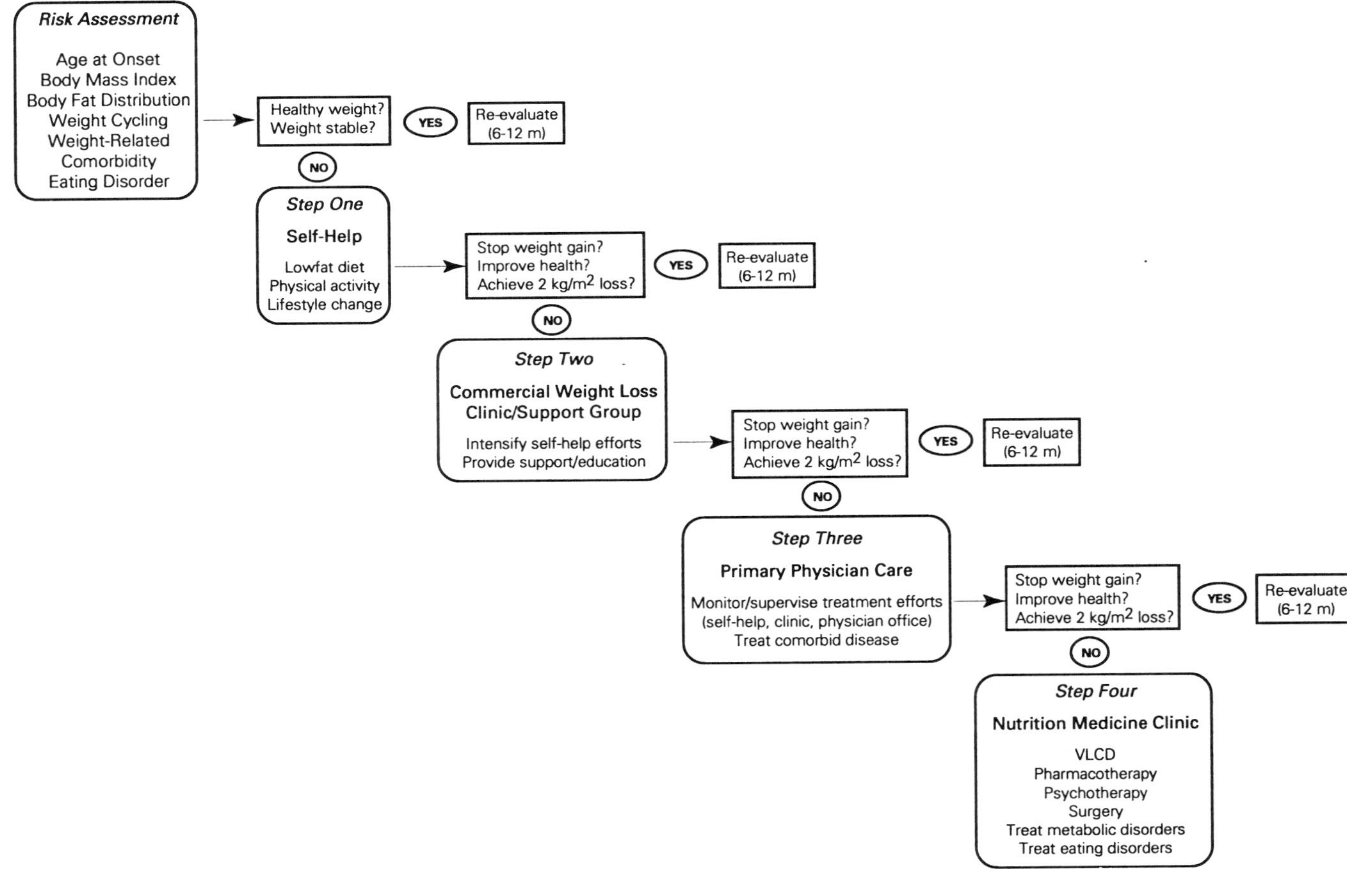

Figure A-1. Risk assessment and treatment strategies for the disease of obesity.

ameliorating obesity-related disease through improved diet and lifestyle, as well as achieving sequential 2–4 kg/m^2 weight losses. Weight loss should continue over several months or years until healthy body weight is achieved.

Step Four. All patients are referred for aggressive intervention. Specialists in obesity treatment provide intensive therapy, which can include use of a very low calorie diet, medication, surgery, and psychotherapy as necessary and appropriate. The goal of this treatment is a 30–50% reduction of excess body fat, with concomitant improvement in overall metabolic fitness (as assessed by a glucose tolerance test, respiratory function, and intra-abdominal pressure).

Index

A

T

U

V

Y